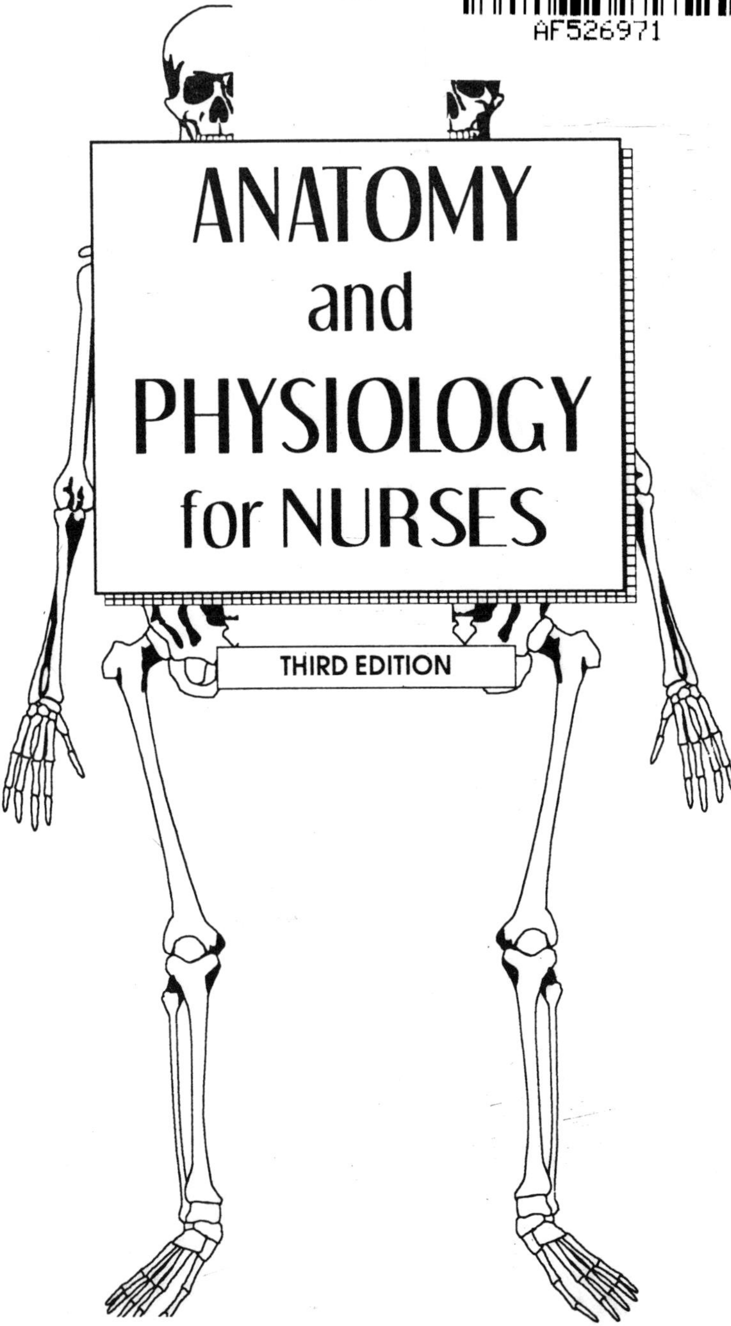
ANATOMY
and
PHYSIOLOGY
for NURSES
THIRD EDITION

ANATOMY and PHYSIOLOGY for NURSES

THIRD EDITION

N.N. YALAYYASWAMY
MSc (N), DN (Ed)
Former Professor of Nursing
Government College of Nursing
Bangalore

CBS

CBS Publishers & Distributors Pvt Ltd

New Delhi • Bengaluru • Chennai • Kochi • Kolkata • Lucknow • Mumbai
Hyderabad • Jharkhand • Nagpur • Patna • Pune • Uttarakhand

Anatomy and Physiology for Nurses

ISBN: 978-81-239-1666-8

Third Edition: 2006
Reprint: 2009, 2011, 2013, 2014, 2016, 2022

First Edition: 1996
Second Edition: 1998 Reprint: 2023 **2024**

Published by Satish Kumar Jain and produced by Varun Jain for
CBS Publishers & Distributors Pvt Ltd
4819/XI Prahlad Street, 24 Ansari Road, Daryaganj, New Delhi 110 002, India.
Ph: 23289259, 23266861, 23266867 Website: www.cbspd.com
Fax: 011-23243014 e-mail: delhi@cbspd.com; cbspubs@airtelmail.in.
Corporate Office: 204 FIE, Industrial Area, Patparganj, Delhi 110 092
Ph: 4934 4934 Fax: 4934 4935 e-mail: publishing@cbspd.com; publicity@cbspd.com

Branches

- **Bengaluru:** Seema House 2975, 17th Cross, K.R. Road, Banasankari 2nd Stage, Bengaluru 560 070, Karnataka
  Ph: +91-80-26771678/79 Fax: +91-80-26771680 e-mail: bangalore@cbspd.com
- **Chennai:** 7, Subbaraya Street, Shenoy Nagar, Chennai 600 030, Tamil Nadu
  Ph: +91-44-26680620, 26681266 Fax: +91-44-42032115 e-mail: chennai@cbspd.com
- **Kochi:** 42/1325, 1326, Power House Road, Opp KSEB, Power House, Ernakulum Kochi 682 018, Kerala, India
  Ph: +91-484-4059061-65,67 Fax: +91-484-4059065 e-mail: kochi@cbspd.com
- **Kolkata:** 147, Hind Ceramics Compound, 1st Floor, Nilgunj Road, Belghoria, Kolkata-700056, West Bengal, India
  Ph: +91-9096713055/7798394118, 9836841399 e-mail: kolkata@cbspd.com
- **Lucknow:** Basement, Khushnuma Complex, 7 Meerabai Marg (Behind Jawahar Bhawan), Lucknow-226001, UP
  Ph: +0522-4000032 e-mail: tiwari.lucknow@cbspd.com
- **Mumbai:** PWD Shed, Gala no 25/26, Ramchandra Bhatt Marg, Next to JJ Hospital Gate no. 2, Opp. Union Bank of India, Noorbaug, Mumbai-400009, Maharashtra, India
  Ph: 022-66661880/89 e-mail: mumbai@cbspd.com

Representatives

- Hyderabad 0-9885175004
- Patna 0-9334159340
- Jharkhand 0-9811541605
- Pune 0-9623451994
- Nagpur 0-9421945513
- Uttarakhand 0-9716462459

Printed at: Glorious Printers, Dilshad Garden, Delhi

Preface to the Third Edition

The warm response for the first edition of **"ANATOMY AND PHYSIOLOGY"** has encouraged me to bring out the second edition. The suggestions and comments for the improvement of the text prompted me to undertake a revision of the same, the result of which is this second edition.

The second edition contains 13 units. New facts and concepts have been added to most of the units and some parts of the text have been rewritten to update subject matter. Several illustrations have been modified and improved and several new illustrations have been included.

I hope that the systematic format and the presentation is easily palatable. It enables the students to understand the principles and mechanisms of normal body function, so that they can appreciate how these mechanisms alter in illness. Clinical applications are included in the text so that they understand why a patient has certain problem and thus the biological rationale for his medical and nursing care.

I do claim that this book is more than suffiicient for diploma nursing students. The units on skeletal systems, muscular systems, integumentary system, special senses, urinary system and nervous system have been updated to meet the requirements of B.Sc. Nursing students.

The questions at the end of each unit have been formulated to encourage students to relate and to apply the information required as their instruction progresses.

Suggestions for improving the next edition would be gratefully accepted and appreciated.

I thank M/s. Gajanana Book Publishers and Distributors for undertaking this second edition and M/s. Typograph for typesetting and illustrations.

Bangalore
14-1-1998

N. N. Yalayyaswamy

CONTENTS

UNIT 1

Introduction to the Human Body

The human body is a very complex multicellar organism in which the maintenance of life cycle depends upon a most number of physiological and biochemical activities. The total activities enable the human being to live in this world and utilise his environment, and to maintain the generation by reproducing.

ANATOMY

Anatomy is the study of the structure and architecture of the body and of the relationship of its surrounding structures.

Regional anatomy is a geographical or topographical study made on each regions. Eg. the head and neck, the chest, the arm and forearm. It consists of a number of structures to all regions such as skin, fascia, muscle, bones, nerves and vessels.

Systematic Anatomy : The body is made up of many tissues and organs, each having its own particular function to perform. The cell is the smallest unit of the body. The cells are adapted to perform the special function of the organ systems to deal with different work of the body. So these structures are studied under this heading. Eg.,

1. Osteology is the study of the bones.
2. Arthrology is the study of the joints.
3. Myology is the study of muscles.
4. Splanchnology is the study of the organs of viscera.
5. Neurology is the study of the brain and nerves.
6. Kinesiology is the study of the movements in the joints.
7. Embryology is the study of the developing embryo.
8. Cytology is the study of cells.
9. Histology is the study of cells under magnification. Eg. under microscope.

AIM OF ANATOMY

As a scientific discipline it is to study the form of body but to gain a profound understanding of the biological principles and processes of multiplication and differentiation of cells.

Macroscopic Anatomy: Certain structures are studied under naked eye examination called Macroscopic Anatomy.

Surface Anatomy is to study of organs or viscera in relation to the skin, and palpable bony points underneath the skin. Eg. to feel the radial pulse against radius bone, palpate apex beat in the left intercostal space on left side of the chest. The study of surface anatomy is very important to feel, or auscultate the viscera and diagnose the disease of human body.

Embryology is the study of the development of embryo in the uterus of mother from fertilization to delivery of the baby.

Physiology is the study of the functions of normal human body. It is closely linked with the study of all living things in the subject of biology.

Biochemistry deals with biochemical changes in haemodynamics and activities of cells and to investigating the complex chemistry of life.

Biophysics is the study of physical reaction and movements of different types of cells in the body.

ANATOMICAL NOMENCLATURE

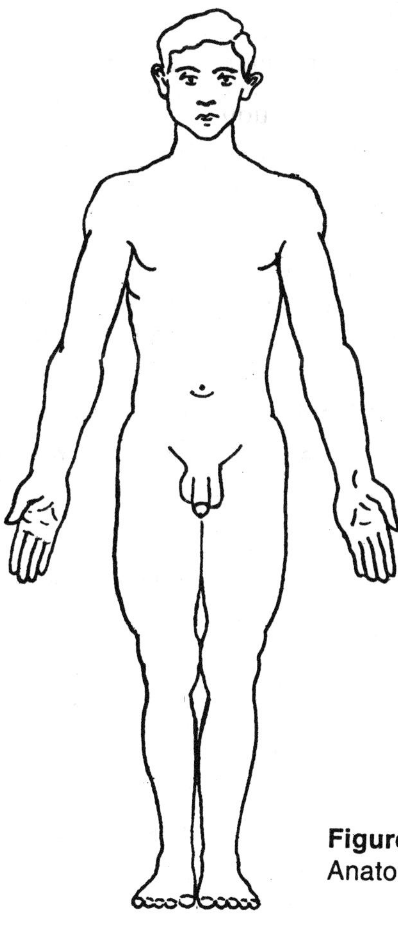

Figure 1. The Anatomical position

Words derived from Latin and Greek have also advantage of being suitable for international usage and to ensure uniform usage, made since 1895 when the Basle Nomina Anatomica was introduced.

The human body is studied from erect position with arms by the sides and the palms of the hands facing forwards, the head erect and eyes looking straight, this is described as the anatomical position.

Planes

1. Median plane is the imaginary line passes through the centre of the body.

2. Lateral plane is the imaginary line passes through the body just away or either side of median plane.

The terms superficial and deep are used to denote relative distance from the surface of the body. Superior and inferior denote positions relatively high or low.

The term anterior means front side or ventral, the term posterior or dorsal means back side; in describing the hand the terms palmar and dorsal are used instead of anterior or posterior and in describing the foot the terms plantar and dorsal are similarly employed.

UNIT 2

The Tissue Cell and Cavities of the Body

The tissue cells: A cell is a minute or microscopic mass of protoplasm. Cells are grouped together to form tissues, each of which has a specialised function. Tissues are grouped together to form organs. Eg. heart, stomach. Organs are grouped together to form systems. Systems make up the body. Cells possess the qualities of all living matter including those of self preservation and reproduction.

Cell structure: A cell consists of protoplasm composed of a centrally placed body, the nucleus and the cytoplasm, which surrounds the nucleus. Protoplasm is surrounded by cell membrane. Cytoplasm contains a number of organelles floating in watery fluid called CYTOSOL. Organelles are microscopic structures with highly specialised functions. They are the nucleus, endoplasmic reticulum, golgi apparatus, lysosomes, mitochondria, microfilaments and microtubules.

Cell membrane consists of 2 layers of phospholipids with some protein molecules embeded in them. On the outer surface of the membrane, the

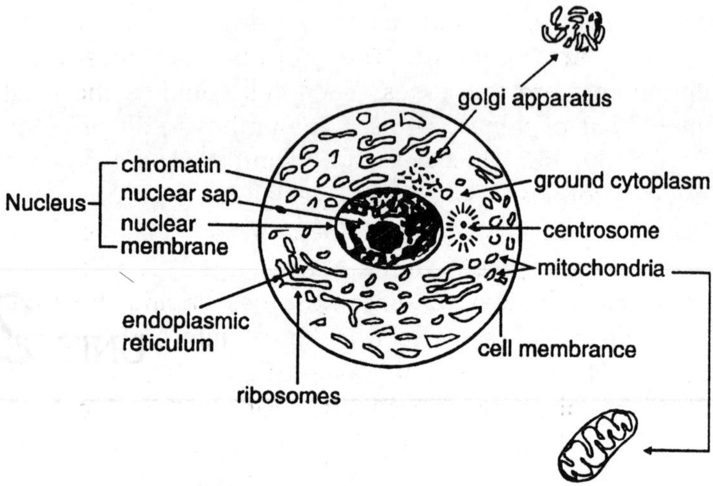

Figure 2. Structure of Cell

lipids have an electrical charge and are hydrophilic. On the inner surface they have no charge and are hydrophobic. These differences have influence on the transfer substances across the membrane, thus, it is most important in maintaining the correct chemical composition of protoplasm. Proteins give immunological identity.

Nucleus

Every cell in the body has a nucleus with the exception of mature erythrocytes. Nucleus is a more compact mass of protoplasm separated from cytoplasm by the nuclear membrane, which is selectively porous allowing substances pass in both directions. Nucleus controls the cell and its activities. The nucleus contains many protein rich threads which are collectively spoken of as chromatin. It contains genetic material in the form of large double chains of molecules (double helix) of Deoxyribonucleic acid (DNA) in a spiral arrangement. Chromosomes are cluster of dozens of DNA molecules. These chromosomes are vital to the everyday activities of the cell and are responsible for the hereditary characteristics of the human body. On the chromosomes in linear arrangement, the genetic or hereditary determinants are the genes. Each cell contains the total complement of genes required to synthesise all proteins in the body, but most cells only synthesise the defined range of proteins to their own specialised functions. This means that only part of the Genome or Genetic code is used by each cell. In human beings, there are 44 autosomes, and two sex chromosomes having the total of 46 chromosomes. The transfer of information from nuclear DNA to the site where proteins are synthesised in the cytoplasm is the function of Ribonucleic acid (RNA). The formation of RNA is controlled by genes in the DNA i.e. genetic information passes from DNA promoting protein synthesis.

Cytoplasm - It consists of

1) **Endoplasmic Reticulum** (ER)) is a series of tubules having 2 types, smooth and rough; smooth ER synthesises specialised proteins, such as, muscle proteins and steroid hormones and is associated with the detoxification of some drugs. Rough ER is studded with ribosomes, site for synthesis of proteins that are extruded from cells, i.e. enzymes and hormones.

2) **Golgi apparatus** : A series of closely folded flattened membranous sacs, larger in those that synthesise and export proteins. The proteins move from the endoplasmic reticulum to the golgi apparatus, where they form secretory granules, and move to the cell membrane.

3) **Centrosome:** A minute dense part of the cytoplasm, lying close to the nucleus. It plays an important part during cell division.

4) **Lysosomes** : These are oval bodies that produce a variety of enzymes that help in expelling waste material from the cell. Lysosomes in white blood

cells synthesise enzymes that digest foreign materials such as microbes.

5) **Mitochondria** : Small rod like structures which are involved in chemical processes by which energy is made available in the cell in the form of ATP. Adenosine triphosphate is a high energy derived from the catabolism of carbohydrates, fats and if these are in short supply, proteins are used to produce ATP.

6) **Microfilaments and Microtubules** : These are contractile structures involved in the movement of the cell and of organelles within cell that cause the movement of cilia. They also maintain the shape of the cell.

Cell Division

There are two types of cell division, mitosis and meiosis.

Mitosis : Cell division begins with fertilised egg or single cell zygote. Cells multiply and grow into all the specialities that provide the tissues or organs for the body's physiological functions. Life span of individual cells is limited, they worn out and die and are replaced by mitosis. Mitosis occurs in 2 places, replication of DNA in the form of 23 pairs of chromosomes and the division of the cytoplasm. Frequency of cell division varies with different types of cells, each daughter cells have 46 chromosomes i.e., different diploid number.

Meiosis : This is the process of cell division that occurs in the reproductive cells (gametes) i.e. ova and spermatozoa. In meiosis the chromosomes do not replicate as they do in mitosis, instead, the pairs of chromosomes separate and one from each pair moves to opposite poles of the parent cell. When it divides, each of the daughter cells has only 23 chromosomes i.e. haploid number. When it is fertilized the zygote

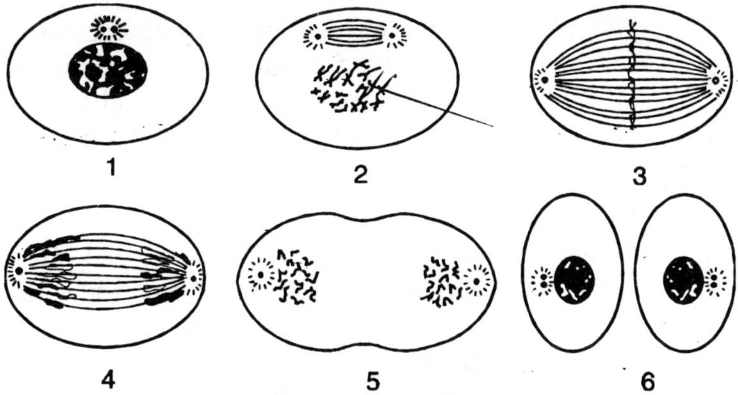

Figure 3. Cell Division

1. Cell with Nucleus and Centrosome
2. Nucleus changes. Centrosome divides
3. Spindle Fibres in position
4. Two identical sets of Chromosomes being attracted to the poles.
5. and 6. Two new Cells separating.

has the diploid i.e. 46 chromosomes, half from the father and half from the mother. Thus, the child has some characteristics inherited from the mother and some from the father. Some diseases are also inherited from the parents.

Determination of sex depends upon one pair of chromosomes, the sex chromosomes. In the female, both sex chromosomes are the same size and shape and are called X chromosomes. In the male, there is one X chromosome and a slightly smaller Y chromosome.

Sperm X + Ovum X = Child XX female.

Sperm Y + Ovum X = Child XY male.

Basic processes in the development

Two processes, growth and differentiation are involved during the conversion of single celled zygote into a multicellular complex body of the new born baby.

Growth means increase in bulk, that may take place by one of the 3 ways.

1. Multiplication (by cell division causing increase in cell number). This type of growth by a succession of mitotic division observed in most of the tissues and organs in pre-natal life. In this process, many cells may die or undergo normal contour of different systems.

2. Auxetic growth occurs by increase in cell size in some cells, particularly in oocytes and some neurons. In this, cytoplasmic volume is increased and the general nucleo-cytoplasmic ratio is disturbed eg. oocytes are surrounded by follicular cells and large neurons by neuroglia cells.

3. Accretionary growth occurs by increased accumulation of intercellular substances, eg. in connective tissues, specially, in bones and cartilages.

4. Differentiation of tissue occurs in which groups of cells assume special characteristic with specific functions to differentiate systematic anatomy. This processes of differentiation is called Histogenesis.

Tissues

The tissues of the body consist of large numbers of cells, arranged in sheets, intercellular matrix is minimum and cells are situated on basement membrane, eg: skin. They are classified into four principal types according to their function and structure.

1. Epithelial tissues
2. Connective tissues
3. Muscle tissue
4. Nervous tissue

Epithelial Tissues

They are classified into simple and compound.

Simple epithelium

Consists of single layer of cells and it is named according to the shape of the cells. They are of 4 types.

a) **Squamous or pavement epithelium:** It consists of a single layer of flattened cells arranged like the stones of a pavement. It is found in the alveoli of the lungs. It is also found in the lining of the heart (endocardium), lining of blood vessels and lymphatics as endothelium.

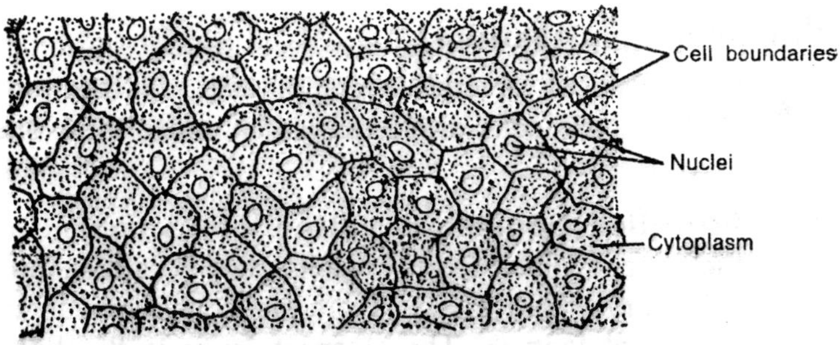

Figure 4. Simple Squamous Epithelium

b) **Columnar epithelium** is single layered cells of tall columnar shaped on basement membrane. Eg: living of alimentary system and consists of mixture of cells. Some absorb the products of digestion and others secrete MUCUS which is a thick, sticky substance secreted by modified columnar cells called GOBLET CELLS. This epithelium is also found in some parts of genito-urinary tract.

c) **Cuboidal or cubical epithelium** : It is a modified columnar epithelium consists of cube-shaped cells joined closely together lying on the basement membrane, found in kidneys and in some glands. Eg: Thyroid gland to secrete hormone.

d) **Ciliated columnar epithelium** : This simple epithelium is having fine hair-like processes called cilia. The cilia consist of microtubules situated on the free surface of the columnar cells. The wave like movement of many cilia is to propel the contents of the tubules. Eg: lining uterine tubes, uterus, respiratory passages, and central canal of spinal cord.

The movement of cilia in the respiratory tract prevents mucus, dust etc. entering the lings. In the fallopian tubes, the ciliary movement conveys the ovum into the uterus.

Compound epithelium

It consists of several layers of cells. In this type of epithelium, the cells are arranged in more than one layer.

1. **Stratified Squamous epithelium** is present on the surface which requires protection from mechanical injury. Five to six layers are considered to be the usual feature. The deepest layer is the basal cells and they are columnar. The intermediate layers are polyhedral cells which gradually becomes typically of squamous epithelium. Eg: 1. Keratinised stratified squamous epithelium, lining skin; 2. Non keratinised stratified squamous epithelium lining the oesophagus.

2. **Stratified Cuboidal epithelium** : Consists of several layers of cells of which the superficial ones are cuboidal and the rest are polyhedral. Eg: ducts of sweat glands and in the male urethra.

3. **Stratified Columnar epithelium** : The deeper layers consist of polyhedral cells, only the surface layer possesses columnar cells.

4. **Transitional epithelium** : It is a stratified epithelium having the capacity of being stretched to a considerable extent. In the unstretched condition, it is five to six layers thick, the surface cells are

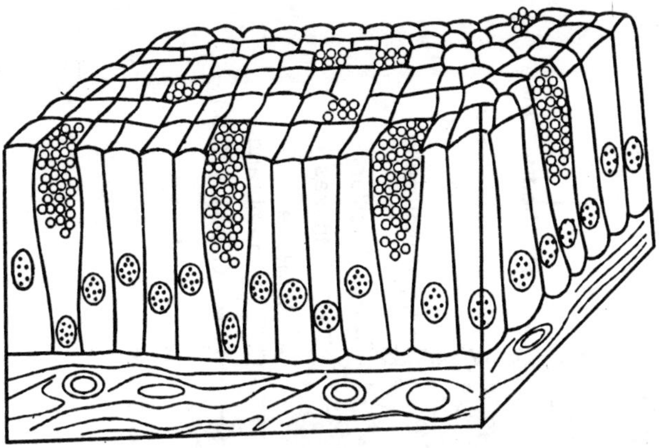

Figure 5. Columnar epithelium

umbrella shaped, the intermediate cells are pear shaped, the basal cells are columnar. For ex: found in the lining of urinary bladder, parts of ureters and urethra.

5. **Pseudo-stratified epithelium** : Name suggests being stratified but actually is of the simple type. All cells touch the basal lamina but all of them may not reach the surface, because some cells are taller than others although both are columnar, the nuclei of the cells are situated at different levels which is responsible for the erroneous impression of stratification.

Functions of epithelium

1. Mechanical protection as in the case of the skin, which prevents mechanical injury to the deeper tissues.
2. **Conservation of moisture:** Stratified epithelium prevents loss of water from the body.
3. **Absorption** : Single layered or simple epithelium has the property of absorption, the end products of digestion in this case.

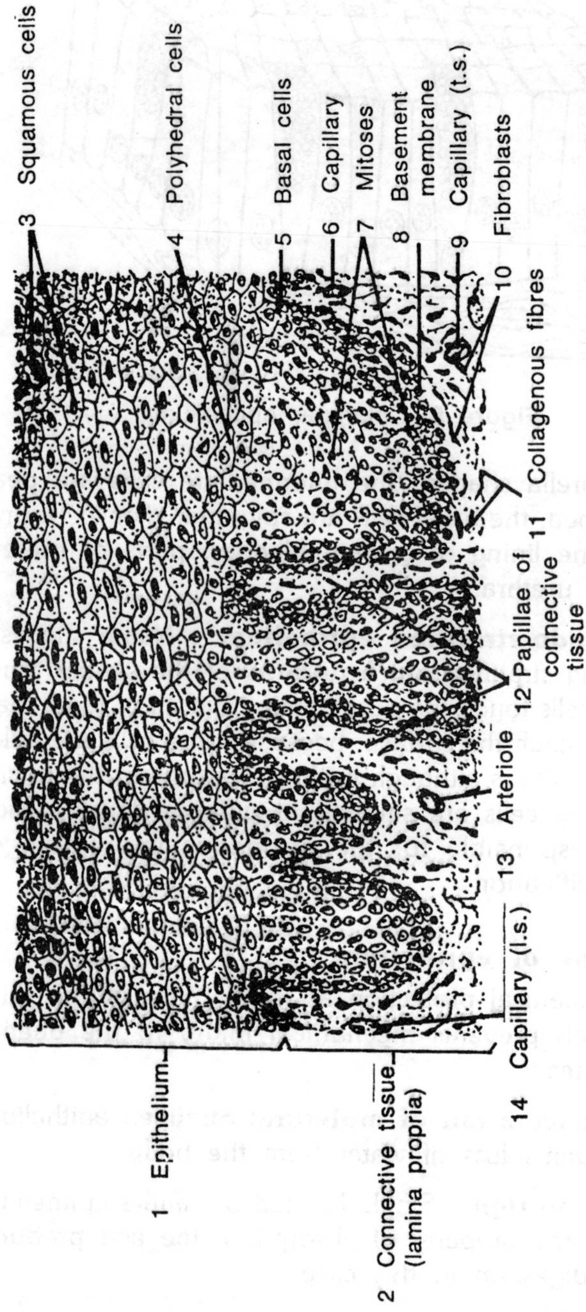

Figure 6. Stratified Squamous epithelium

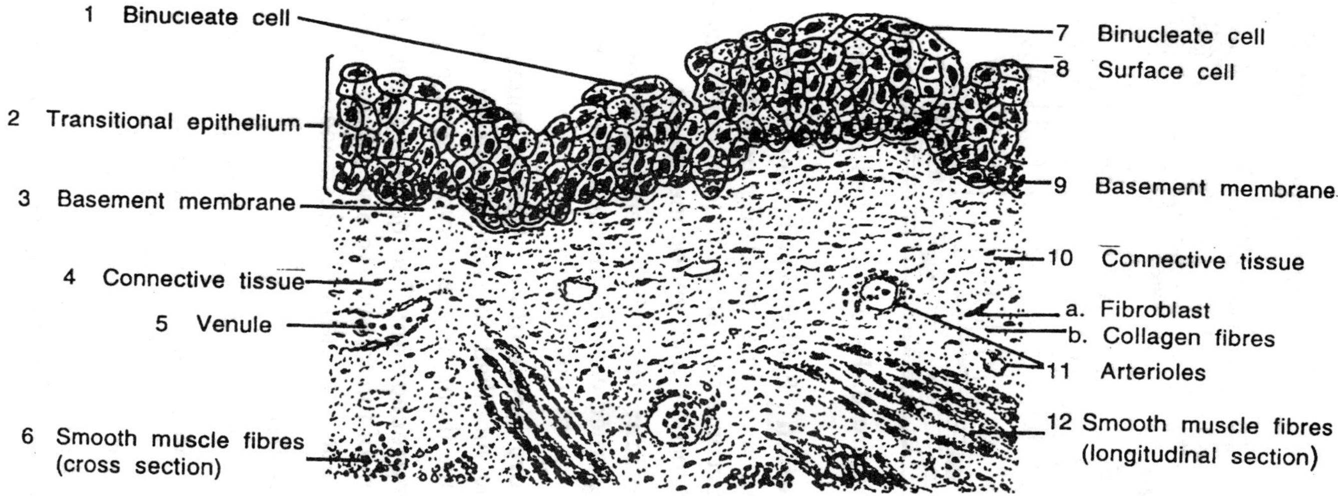

Figure 7. Transitional epithelium

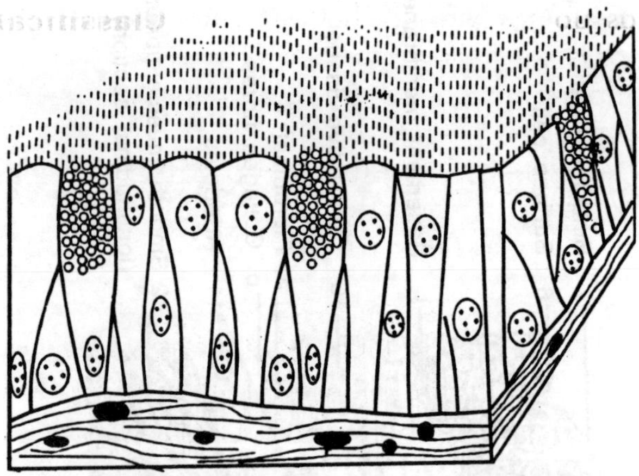

Figure 8. Pseudo-stratified epithelium

4. **Secretion :** Epithelial cells may become specialised to form unicellular glands Eg: goblet cells, they may also become specialised to form multinuclear glands Eg: exocrine and endocrine glands.

5. **Excretion:** The tubular epithelium of the kidney is concerned with the function of excreting the waste products of metabolism.

6. **Sensory perception :** Certain epithelial cells are greatly modified to receive sensory impulses and transmit them to the nervous system.

7. **Chemoreception:** The gustatory cells of the epithelium of the tongue are also sensory receptors but they react to chemical substances.

Cell connections:

There are different types of epithelial cell connections.

1. **Tight junctions:** They completely encircle each cell and form a permeability barrier between cells. They are found in the lining of the intestines.

2. **Desmosomes:** They are mechanical links that function to bind cell membranes together.

3. **Gap junctions:** They are small channels between cells that allow small molecules and ions to pass from one epithlial cell to an adjacent epithelial cell. In this way, gap junctions are involved with intercellular communications. Most epithelial cells possess gap junctions.

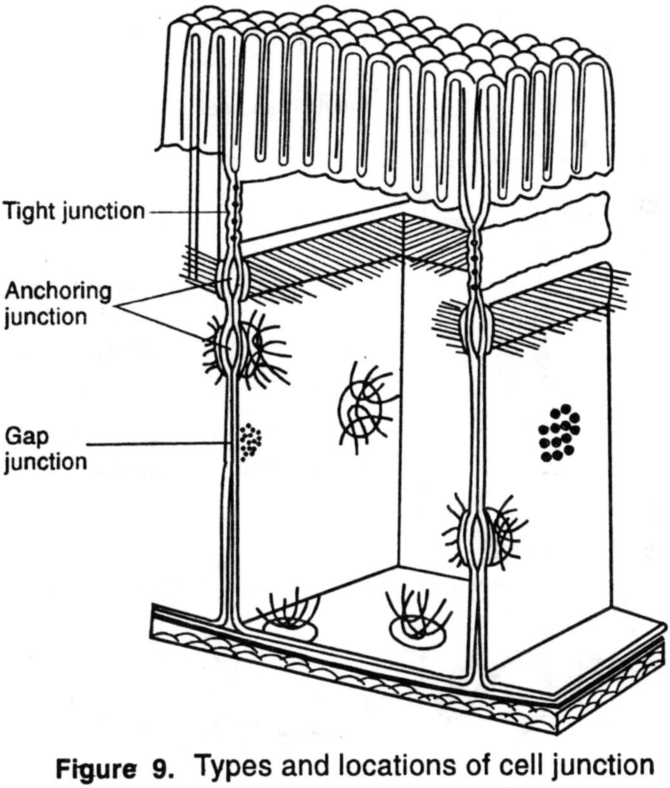

Figure 9. Types and locations of cell junction

Glands

Glands are defined as collection of epithelial cells specialised for secretion to serve many purposes. a) keeps a surface moist, b) provides lubricant for frictional surfaces. c) enzymes for digestion and d) hormones for control and regulation of body functions.

Classification of Glands

Two basic types of glands are found in the body exocrine and endocrine. Exocrine glands are those that possess ducts through which the secretion is expelled into the lumen of an organ. Eg: parotid glands, the intestine, or to the exterior as in the case of sweat,

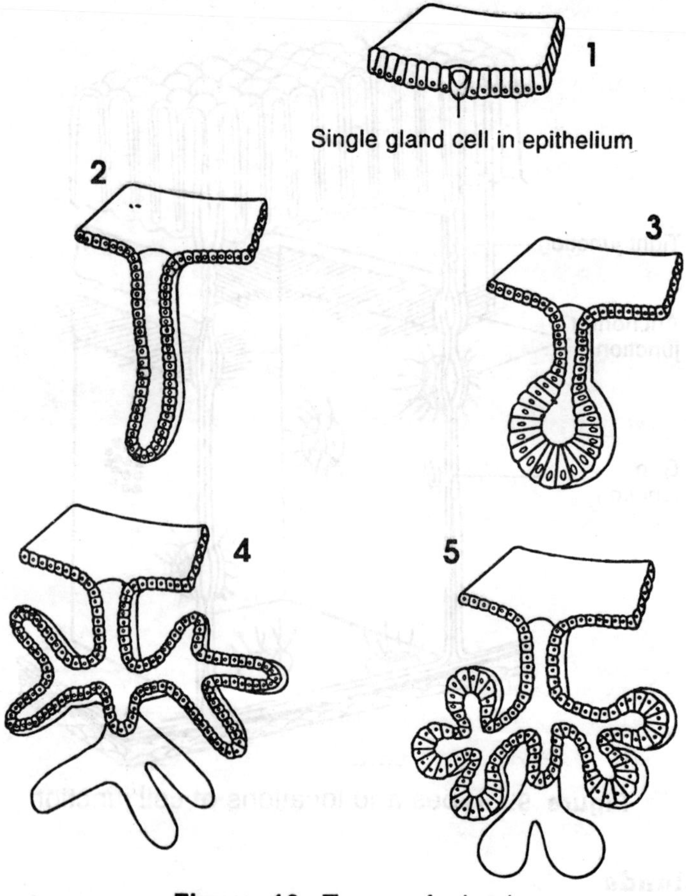

Figure 10. Types of glands

1 Unicellular (Eg. goblet cells in mucous membranes).
2. Simple tubular (Eg. sweat glands and stomach glands).
3. Simple acinar or alveolar end in a saclike structure (Eg. sebaceous glands).
4. Compound tubular (Eg. duodinal glands).
5. Compound acinar or alveolar (Eg. pancreas).

sebaceous and mammary glands. Endocrine glands do not possess a duct system, hence they are also known as ductless glands. Their secretions are taken into the vascular system through the blood vessels. A gland may have an exocrine as well as an endocrine part. Eg: Pancreas. Such gland is called an Heterocrine gland.

Membranes

A membrane is a thin layer of tissue that covers a structure or lines a cavity. Most membranes are composed of epithelium and the connective tissue on which the eipithelium rests.

Types of membranes

1. **Mucous membranes**

   They line the cavities of the digestive, respiratory, excretory and reproductive tracts. Many but not all, mucous membrances have goblet cells that secrete mucus.

   Function : Protection, absorption and secretion.

2. **Serous membranes**

   They are found in the peritoneum, pleura and pericardium They secrete serous fluid which lubricates the surfaces.

3. **Synovial membranes**

   They line the cavities of freely movable joints except over the articular cartilage. They secrete synovial fluid which lubricates the cartilage at the ends of bones during their movements and nourishes the cartilage covering the bones at joints.

4. **Cutaneous membrane**

   i.e. Skin

The Connective tissues

The connective tissues of the body form a type of basic tissue which is designed to withstand various types of mechanical stress and strain and which bind, connect and support tissues including its own kind.

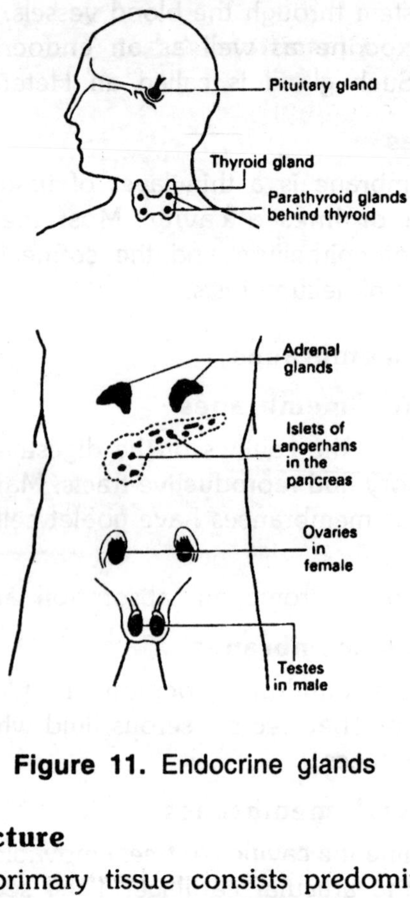

Figure 11. Endocrine glands

Basic structure

Other primary tissue consists predominantly only cells, hence they are soft and jelly like and are thus, liable to bend or be torn under physical duress. Connective tissue while having a cellular component, also possesses an intercellular substance which is non living. The character of the intercellular substance is variable. In blood it is completely fluid, in other types it consists of fibres embedded in a homogenous ground substance known as the Matrix. The density of connective tissue mainly depends on the concentration of the contained fibres.

Connective tissue can be vary hard and rigid due to the deposition of mineral salts in the intercellular substance as in the case of bone.

Classification of Tissues

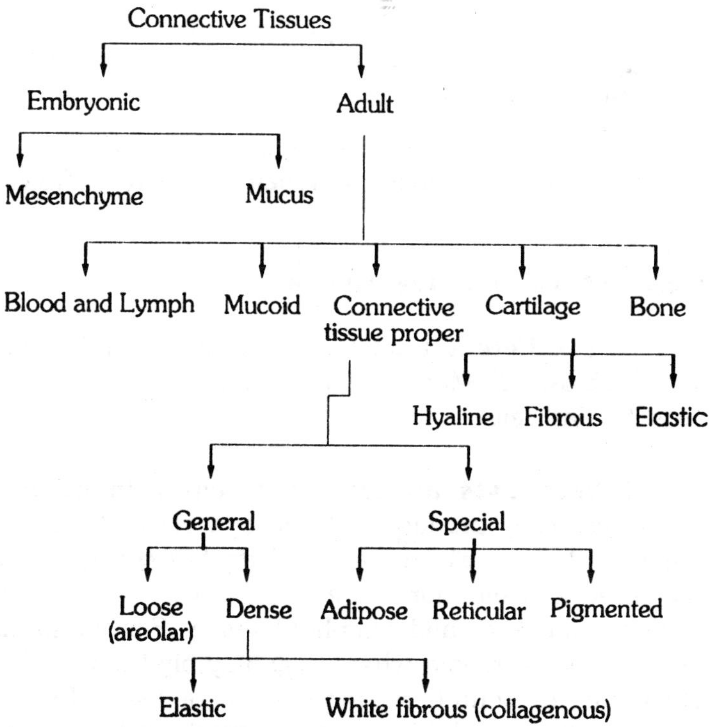

Functions of Connective tissues

The functions of connective tissues are manifold depending on its types.

1. **Mechanical** : It provides support for the body. Bones and cartilage are primarily concerned with providing a frame work for the body. Loose connective tissue binds and connects different types of tissues. Eg: Skin with muscle or muscle with bone. It also holds together different groups of the same tissue as in case of muscle fibre.

2. **Nutrition:** The ground substance or matrix of connective tissue holds large amounts of water in which are dissolved electrolytes. It is thus, that water balance is maintained in tissues and cells are provided with nutrition.

3. **Defence:** The wandering cells of connective tissue act as defence forces of the body. They are responsible for phagocytosis and development of immunological reactions.

4. **Repair:** Fibroblasts present in connective tissue are the agents involved in repair of tissues following injury.

Cells of Connective tissue

The different types of cells involved include, 1. Fibroblasts 2. Macrophages 3. Plasma cells 4. Mast cells 5. Fat cells.

Fibroblasts are large flat cells with irregular processes. They produce collagen and elastic fibres and a matrix of extra cellular material. Very fine collagen fibres are called Reticulin fibres, are found in very active tissue, such as, the liver and lymphoid tissue. Fibroblasts are active in tissue repair, where they may bind together the cut surface of wounds or form granulation tissue. In some glands, a type of fibroblast called reticular cells, produce fine fibrous strands called Reticulin and are associated with phagocytosis.

Macrophages are irregular shaped cells with granules in the cytoplasm. Some are fixed that is attached to connective tissue fibres. Some are motile. They are actively phagocytic. Their activities resemble the monocytes of defence system. Eg: Monocytes in blood, phagocytes in the alveoli of lungs, Von kupffer cells in liver sinusoids, microglial cells in central nervous system.

Plasma cells are derived from B-Lymphocytes. They synthesise and secrete specific antibodies into the blood in response to the presence of foreign material such as microbes. Cells synthesise and release proteins are known as Gamma globulins (Antibodies).

Mast cells are similar to basophil leucocytes. They are found in blood vessels, and under fibrous capsule of some organs. Eg: liver and spleen. They produce Heparin, Serotonin and Histamine, which are released when the cells are damaged by disease or injury. Histamine is involved in local and general inflammatory reactions and may be associated with the development of allergies and hypersensitivity. Heparin prevents coagulation of plasma which may aid the passage of protective substances from blood to affected tissues.

Areolar tissue: This is the most generalised of all connective tissues. The matrix is described as semisolid with fibroblasts, widely distributed with elastic and collagen fibres. It is found in almost every part of the body connecting and supporting other tissues. Eg: under the skin, around muscles, supporting blood vessels and nerves, in the gastrointestinal system, in the glands supporting secretory cells.

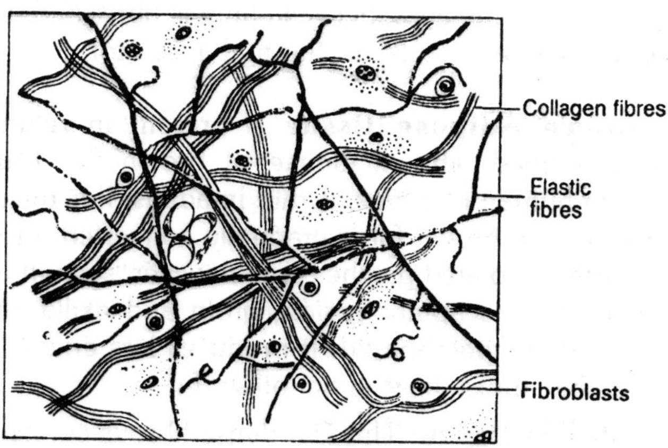

Figure 12. Areolar tissue

Adipose tissue (fat cells): Adipose tissue consists of fat cells, containing fat globules in a matrix of areolar tissue. These cells are distributed mostly under the skin and also with organs like heart, kidneys and mesentery. There is more accumulation of this tissue in females which give shape to the body and also secondary characteristics. Females can tolerate more cold than males. Fat cells act as insulating to the body. They vary in size and shape according to the amount of fat they contain. They are of two types, white and brown.

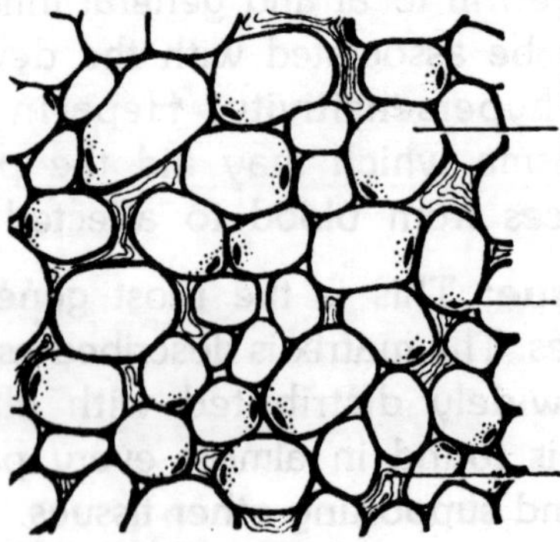

Figure 13. Adipose tissue

White Adipose tissue makes about 25% of body weight in well-nourished adults. It is found supporting the kidneys and the eyes, between muscle fibres and under the skin, where it acts as thermal insulator.

Brown Adipose tissue is present in relatively small quantities. The incidence of brown fat, though present in human embryos, is rare in adults. It is believed that embryonic brown fat is gradually converted into the white variety. Isolated patches are, however, seen in adult life at the inter scapular region, groin and axilla where brown tissue is metabolised. It produces less energy and considerably more heat than other fat.

Fibrous tissue: This is a dense fibrous connective tissue made up mainly of closely packed bundles of collagen fibres, with very little matrix, and very few cells lying in rows between the bundles of fibres and developed from fibroblasts.

Collagen or white fibres: They are known as white fibres because in unstained preparation they are distinguished from elastic fibres as being colourless. Under low magnification, collagen fibres are seen to run a wavy coarse in bundles. The thickness of a bundle depends on the number of fibres it contains. Individual fibres do not branch. The basic unit of a collagen fibre is a microfibril. This is composed of tropocollagen molecules. It forms the tendons and ligaments. It also forms the dura mater, the outer layer of pericardium, the fascia and the fibrous covering of certain organs.

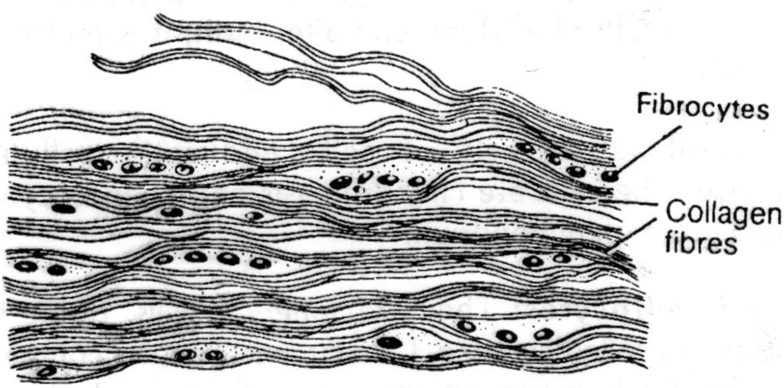

Figure 14. White fibrous tissue

Elastic tissue or Yellow elastic tissue is capable of considerable extension and recoil. There are few cells and the matrix consists mainly elastic fibres. Fibres run singly and in unstained preparations, they are seen as highly refractile. The broken ends recoil and curl up. It is found in the walls of the blood vessels, in the bronchi and alveoli of lungs.

Reticular tissue: It consists of fine interlacing reticular fibres and reticular cells. It forms the framework of certain organs. For Ex: Spleen and lymph nodes.

Functions of fibrous tissues

1. Forming ligaments which bind bones together.
2. Outer protective covering of some organs. Eg: the Kidney, lymph node, spleen and the brain.
3. Forms tendons of muscle that attaches to bones.
4. Protective layer for the bone and cartilages.

Mucoid tissue is a jelly like tissue. It is seen in the umbilical cord of child at birth. It is also found in the vitreous humour of the eye ball.

Cartilage

Cartilage is a type of specialised dense connective tissue meant for lending support and bearing weight. In embryonic life, the skeletal system is represented by cartilage. In latter foetal life and after birth, it is replaced by bones.

Cartilage consists of cells and inter cellular substance. The cells are chandroblasts and chandrocytes derived from perichondrium.

Chondrocytes: They are spherical cells, reside in small spaces called lacunae. Usually, each lacuna contains 2-4 cells. Such group or cartilage cells are called cell nests. The cytoplasm is rich in glycogen and fat. Young cartilage cells are known as chrondroblasts. They show cytoplasmic processes which are branching. The tropocollagen and mucoprotein which form the intercellular substance are formed in the cartilage cells.

The perichondrium is the covering of the cartilage. The intercellular substance contains cartilage cells, fibres and amorphous ground substance or matrix. They are of 3 types - according to the types of fibres and the amount of amorphous substance present in intercellular material. They are, hyaline, elastic and fibro cartilages.

1. **Hyaline cartilage :** It is glossy, bluish white translucent in appearance. It is widely distributed in the foetus and in the adult. It is the weakest of the three types of cartilage. It is found at the following sites :

   a) Costal cartilages

   b) Nasal, tracheal, bronchial and some of the laryngeal cartilages

   c) Articular cartilages.

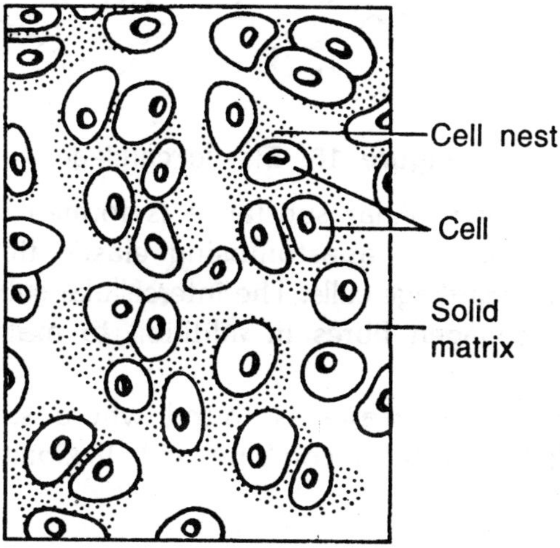

Figure 15 Hyaline cartilage

2. **Elastic cartilage :** This type of cartilage is found where flexibility is needed and the part requires the ability to come back to its normal shape after deformation. This cartilage is present in

   a) External ear (PINNA)

   b) Epiglottis.

   c) Corniculate, cuneiform and apices of the aretynoid cartilage of the larynx.

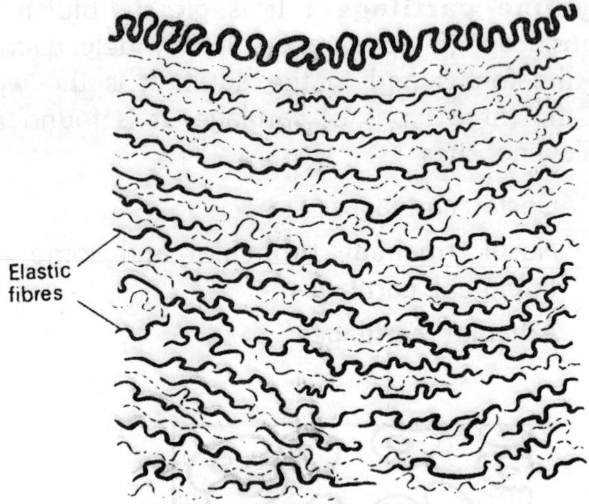

Figure 16. Elastic cartilage

The intercellular substance is formed by network of branching and anastomosing elastic fibres, dense around the cartilage cells. The intercellular substance also contains collagen fibres in addition to matrix.

3. Fibro cartilage is found where strength and rigidity have to combine with flexibility and it is

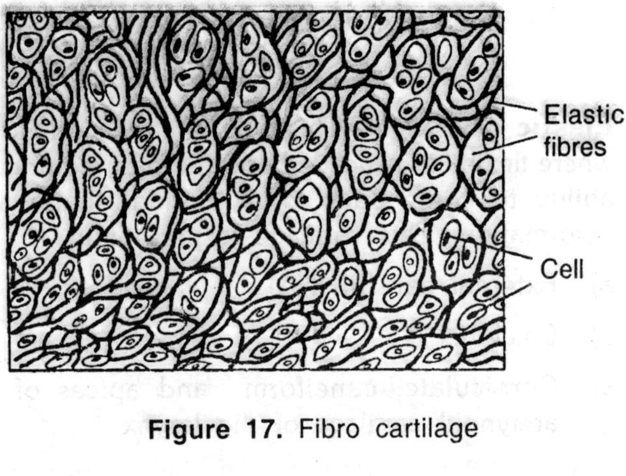

Figure 17. Fibro cartilage

adapted to withstand shearing forces. It is the strongest of the three types of cartilage. Fibro cartilage is present in

a) Intervertebral discs
b) Pubic symphysis
c) Articular discs between the bones of the knee joint called semilunar cartilages.
d) in some ligaments.

In this cartilage, there is abundance of collagen fibres. The amorphous type of intercellular matrix is present everywhere, but less in between bundles of collagen fibres where cartilage cells are also present. The number of cartilage cells are fewer than in hyaline cartilage and are, usually, arranged in rows between the fibre bundles.

Perichondrium

This is present as a peripheral sheath except in articular cartilage. Perichondrium consists of 2 layers, an outer fibrous layer and an inner chondrogenic layer. The chondrogenic layer is formed by relatively undifferentiated cells which are derived from mesenchyma. These cells give rise to chondroblasts by mitosis.

Bone

Bone is another type of specialised dense connective tissue which contains mineral deposits in the intercellular ground substance. It is hard resilient and has a tensile strength which approaches that of cast iron. At the same time it is lining and capable of remodelling itself under conditions of altered stress and other physical force.

Functions

1. It gives internal frame work and thus, gives shape and form to the body.

2. It transmits body weight.
3. It provides attachment to muscles.
4. Two or more bones form joints for movements.
5. It provides protection to important viscera, organs of thorax, cranium etc.
6. It forms major calcium deposits of the body.
7. Bone marrow has got haemopoietic function.
8. Major locomotor system.

Structure

It has cellular component and a ground substance. The types of cells are, osteoblasts, osteocytes and osteoclasts. They represent different functional states of same cell type. The ground substance consists of organic and inorganic elements. Organic elements are densely organised bundles of collagen fibres, situated on ground substance. Inorganic elements make up about 65% of bone tissue and consist mostly of calcium salts, 85% of bone calcium is calcium phosphate, about 10% is calcium carbonate. These mineral salts exist in crystalline and amorphous forms.

$Ca_{10}(PO_4)_6(OH)_2$.

Gross structure

On cut section of bone, 2 types of bone tissue are recognised, dense or compact and spongy or cancellous tissue. The dense bone has an outer covering called periosteum. It is regenerative in fracture of bones. If a long bone is split longitudinally it reveals that the 2 ends including the adjacent parts of the shaft consist of spicules or trabecula running in different directions and anastomosing with each other to form a lattice work. This lattice work has inter communicating spaces and contains marrow. This is spongy or cancellous bone. It is covered by compact bone, In the middle of shaft, usually, a space will be there, called medullary cavity.

Almost all long bones possess a gross structure described above. Flat, short and irregular bones have a cancellous texture covered by a thin layer of compact bone. The bones of vault of skull are composed of an inner and an outer thick layers of compact bone. These layers enclose a layer of cancellous bone called **Diploe.**

Microscopic structure of bone

Compact bone: The structure of compact bone centres around a number of neuro vascular canals running almost parallel to long axis of the bone. These are known as **Haversian canals** and each contains capillaries and nerves. Each Haversian canal is surrounded by lamellae of bone tissue which appear as concentric rings of 3-7 layers thick. On an average, there are 6 lamellae around each canal. Between these lamellae are small spaces known as Lacunae. This space contains bone cells or osteocytes. Each such unit consisting of Haversian canal, surrounding lamella, lacunae with osteocytes are known as Haversian system or Osteon. The two Haversian canals are connected by a transverse canal known as Volkmann's canal.

Periosteum: Forms an outer covering of all bones except in the regions which are covered by articular cartilage. It is also absent around sesamoid bones. Structurally, periosteum consists of 2 layers, an outer fibrous and an inner osteogenic layer. The fibrous layer is relatively cellular and consists of dense connective tissue and a few fibroblasts. The histologic osteogenic layer is variable, when active bone formation goes on, it consists of multilayered osteoblasts. In the resting stage, these cells assume spindle shaped bands of collagen and elastic fibres. From the under surface of the periosteum these fibres are seen to penetrate into lamella of bone but never into the haversian system. These fibres are called **Sharpey's fibres.**

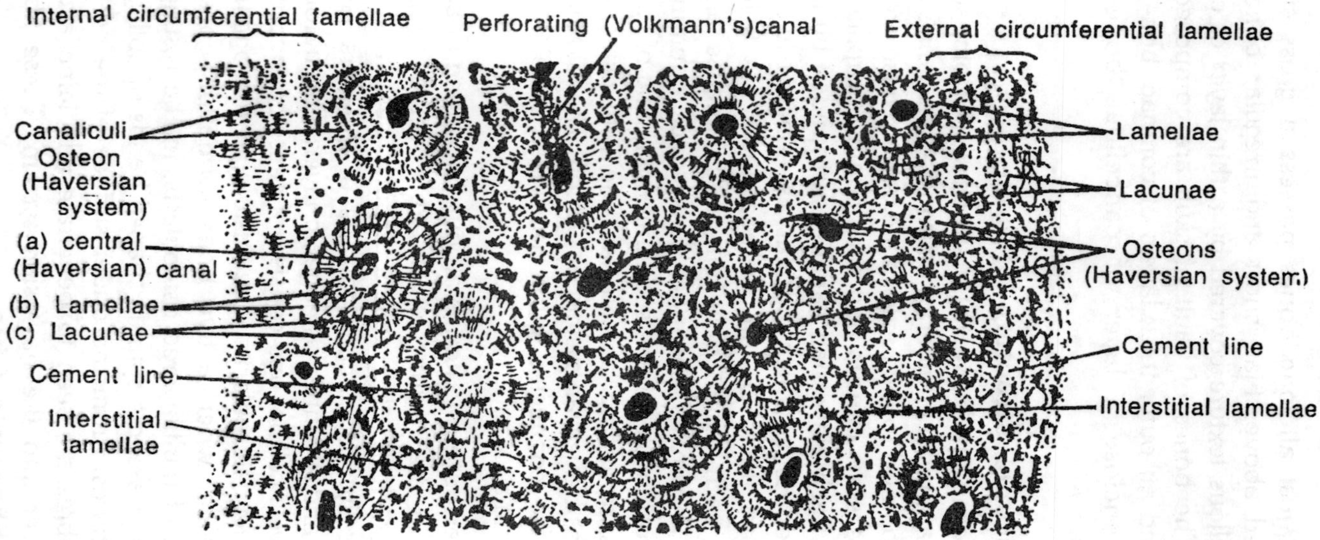

Figure 18 Compact Bone

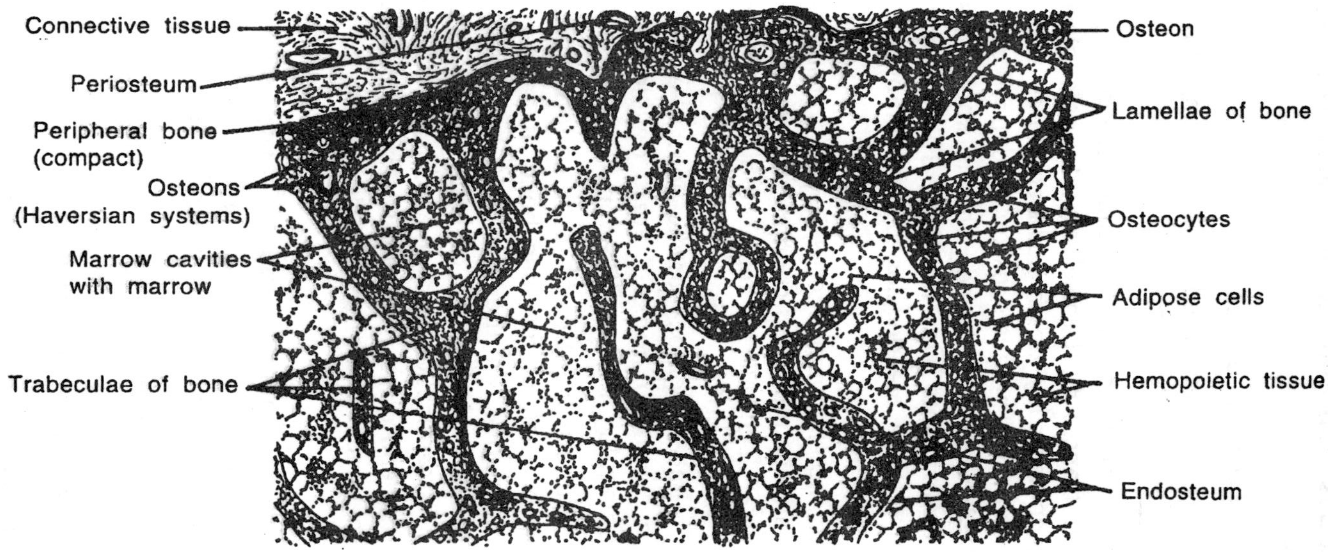

Figure 19 Cancellous Bone

Endosteum: is the inner lining of medullary cavity of bones.

Development of bones

Bones are developed from intra membranous or intra cartilaginous substance.

1. The mesenchymal cells acquire osteogenic properties and transform themselves into osteoblasts. The osteoblasts lay down collagen fibres and ground substance. There is subsequent deposit of minerals, intercellular substance. This is known as **Intra membranous Ossification.** The flat bones and the clavicle are developed from intramembranous ossification.
2. The mesenchymal model is first transformed into a cartilage model by chondrification and thereafter, the cartilage cells are replaced by osteoblasts which lay down bone. This is known as Endochondrial or Intracartilaginous ossification. The long bones and short bones are developed from intracartilaginous ossification.

A primary centre of ossification appears in Diaphysis or shaft of the long bone. It appears during embryonic period, in the uterus. A secondary centre appears after birth in ends of long bone ie, epiphysis centre. This ossification continues towards the shaft and towards the end of each epiphysis. The hyaline cartilage covers the ends of bone. This is known as articular cartilage.

Between diaphysis and epiphysis is a layer of cartilage known as epiphyseal cartilage. As long as this cartilage remains, growth in the length of bone is possible.

The epiphyseal end of the diaphysis is known as metaphysis.

Muscle Tissue is described in Unit 4.

Nervous Tissue is described in Unit 5.

THE BODY AS A WHOLE

Cavities of the body

The cavities are made up of bones or muscle and bones to protect important systems or organs.

1. **Cranial cavity:** It is mainly formed by skull bones and contains brain and its covering. It also contains the pituitary gland and pineal body.

2. **Thoracic cavity** is situated in the upper part of trunk and it is made up of bones, ribs and intercostal muscles, sternum in front, vertebral column in back side, 12 pairs of ribs and 11 pairs of inter costal muscles. Contents are lungs and heart and its blood vessels, pleural space around the lungs, pericardial cavity around the heart, the thoracic duct, the thymus gland, thoracic aorta, oesophagus, inferior vena cava, the vagus nerve and the azygos vein.

Boundaries of thoracic cavity

Superior	-	The structures forming the neck
Inferior	-	The diaphram
Anterior	-	The sternum, front portion of ribs with intercostal muscles.
Posterior	-	The thoracic vertibrae with their intervertebral dics, back portion of ribs with thier intercostal muscles.
Sides	-	Sides of ribs with their intercostal muscles.

3. **Abdominal cavity:** This is the largest cavity in the body. Superiorly, the diaphragm separates it from thoracic cavity. Inferiorly, the pelvic cavity is continuous with this cavity. Anteriorly is the flat muscles of anterior abdominal wall. Posteriorly are

the vertebral column and muscles forming the posterior abdominal wall.

Contents : Gastro intestinal system with accessory organs. Eg: liver, spleen, gallbladder, pancreas, spleen, kidneys and adrenals.

4. **Pelvic cavity:** It is roughly funnel shaped, situated in lower end of abdominal cavity, mainly, formed by bony structure with hip bones, sacrum, coccyx and the muscles of the pelvic floor.

Contents

In females	:	The urinary bladder and the ureters, pelvic colon and rectum, uterus and its ligaments, fallopian tubes and ovaries.
		Pelvic blood vessels, lymphatic vessels, glands and nerves
In males	:	The urinary bladder and the ureters, pelvic colon and rectum.
		The prostate gland, seminal vesicles, vas deferens and ejaculatory ducts
		Pelvic blood vessels, lymphatic vessels, glands and nerves.

Applied anatomy

Neoplasms or tumors: It is the abnormal growth of tissues of any system are called neoplasms or tumors. There are two types, Benign and Malignant tumors. The rate of growth of cells is more rapid in malignant tumors, comparatively less rapid in benign tumors. Benign tumor causes pressure effect on surrounding organs, where as, malignant tumors has characteristic local spread and to other systems, like, to central nervous system or to lungs or vertebrae spread through lymphatic system or vascular system.

Cachexia: It is the condition of progressive weakness due to loss of appetite, wasting and anaemia, associated with malignancy. The severity is usually, indicative of the stage of development of malignant tumor.

Questions

1. Draw a diagram of a cell and name its parts.
2. Name the characteristics of cells.
3. Describe the mitosis and meiosis.
4. Describe the various types of epithelium.
5. List the different types of connective tissues.
6. List the properties of muscle.
7. Describe the nerve cell, with a diagram.
8. List the various types of tissue membranes with an example of each.
9. Write short notes on:
   a) Cell junctions
   b) Gland
   c) Thoracic cavity.

UNIT 3

Skeletel System

The Skeletal system consists of the framework of bones and cartilage that protects organs and permits movement.

Classification of bones according to their shape

1. Long bones eg: limb bones, finger bones.
2. Short bones eg: carpel bones of the hand and tarsal bones of the foot.
3. The flat bones eg: sternum and bones of vault of the skull.
4. Irregular bones eg: the vertebral column.
5. Pneumatic bones of the skull have the air spaces.
6. Sesamoid bones, eg: patella and pisiform.

Blood supply

Bone is highly vascular, the blood vessels are

1. Nutrient artery enters in the middle of the bone and supplies most of the bone marrow, innr portion

of compact bone of the diaphysis and metaphysis. It sends branches into Haversian canals.

2. Periosteal artery, supplies periosteum. This layer has very high blood supply. From this layer, regeneration of bone takes place normally or after fracture of the bones.

3. Epiphysial artery supplies the epiphysial plates or ends of the bone.

Regeneration of bone

Bone is matured by 20-24 years, then all the secondary centres fuse with corresponding parts of the bones. If damage or fracture of bone occurs, the new bone formation from the periosteum takes place by means of osteogenesis and chondrogenesis from periosteum, to form soft and hard callus, then union of fracture end takes place and fuses completly. It depends upon age. In children fusion takes place in short period, whereas in adult and elderly person, takes a little longer period from 2 to 3 months.

1. **Long bones:** These are found in limbs. Each long bone consists of a shaft and two ends. Long bones act as levers in the body for locomotion.

2. **Short bones** : Are seen in bones of the carpus and tarsus. They are made up mostly of cancellous bone tissue and covered by a thin layer of compact bone. They are light and strong.

3. **Flat bones:** They consist of two layers of dense bone tissue with intervening layer of spongy bone. They are strong bones, which form the skull. Another flat bone is scapula, it affords large area for the attachment of muscles.

4. **Irregular bones** are the vertebrae and some of the bones of the face.

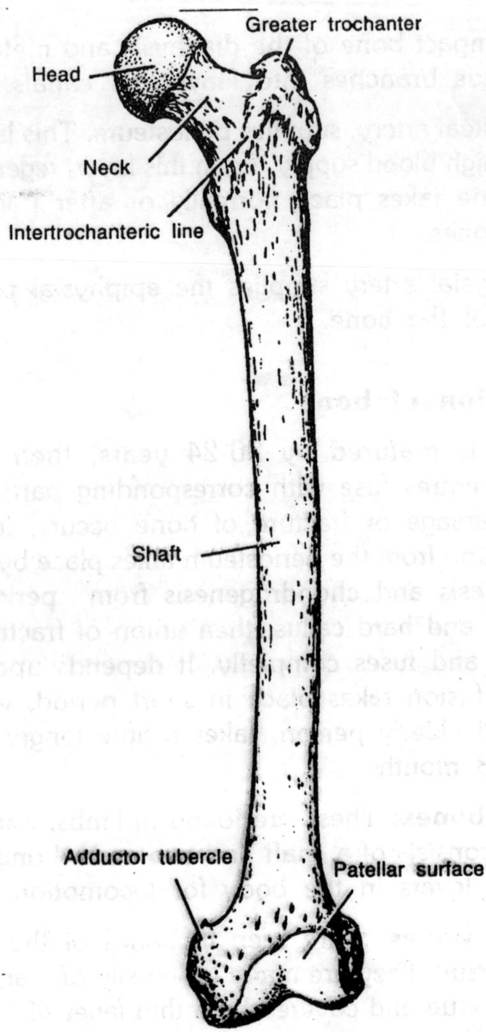

Figure 20. Long bone

5. **The Sesamoid bones:** These are developed in the tendons of muscles. The patella of knee joint is example of this type.

Skeleton consists of 200 bones and it is classified as axial and appendicular skeleton.

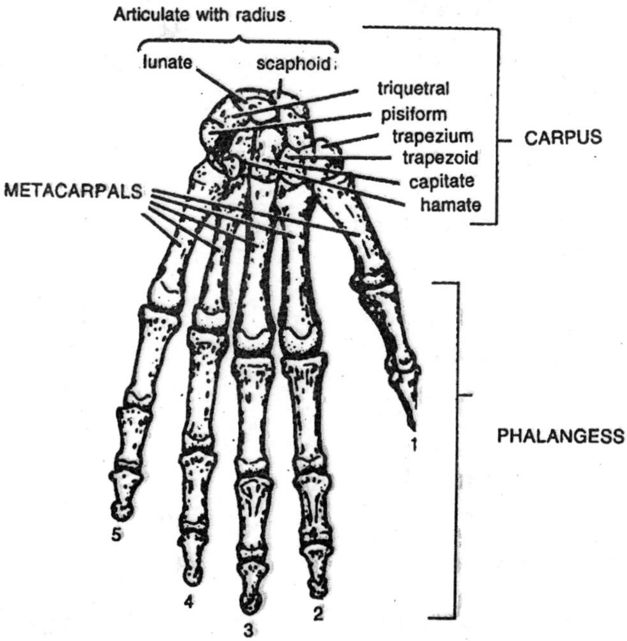

Figure 21. Short bone

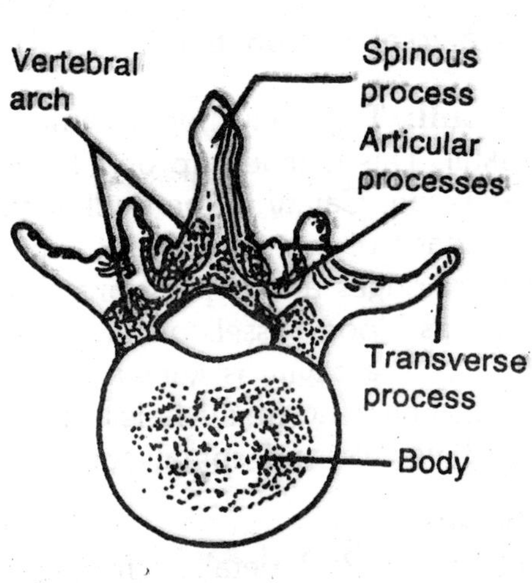

Figure 22. Irregular bone

Axial Skeleton

It consists of	No. of bones
Skull	
Cranium	8
Face	14
Vertebral Column	26
Sternum	1
Ribs	24
Hyoid bone	1
Total	**74**

Appendicular Skeleton

Upper Limbs	32 x 2 = 64
Lower Limbs	31 x 2 = 62
Total	**126**

Bones of Axial and Appendicular skeleton = 74 + 126 = 200

In addition to this, there are 3 small bones in each ear making a total of 206 bones.

The Skull: The bony frame work of the head is called the skull. This is made up of calvaria or skull cap and facial skeleton. Cavity in the skull is called cranium. The upper surface of cranial cavity is vault of the skull, and marked by ridges and depressions to accommodate the brain and its blood vessels on the inner surface, the lower surface of the cavity is known as the base of the skull. It is perforated by many holes for the passage of nerves, blood vessels and spinal cord.

Cranial bones

1. Occipital, 2 Parietal, 1 frontal,
2. Temporal, 1 Sphenoid, 1 Ethmoid.

1. **Frontal bone** is bone of the fore head. It forms part of the orbital cavities and the prominent ridges above the eyes are the supraorbital margins. Inside the bone, there are two air filled cavities or frontal air sinuses lined with ciliated mucous membrane. They open into the nasal cavities. Posteriorly, this bone joins with parietal bones by coronal suture. It also joins with sphenoid, zygomatic, lacrimal, nasal and ethmoid bones by fibrous joints or sutures

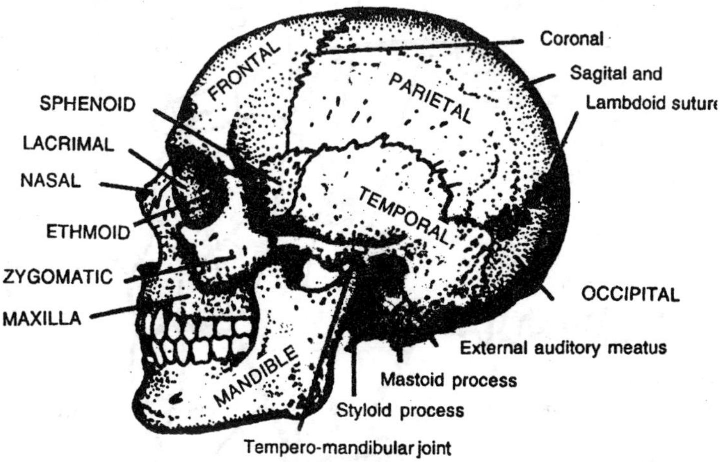

Figure 23. Frontal bone (Skull)

2. **Perietal bones:** These bones form the sides and roof of the skull. Both bones articulate each other in the median plane as sagittal suture, with occipital bone as lambdoidal suture and with temporal bone as squamous suture. The inner surface is concave and grooved by the brain and blood vessels. It lodges middle meningeal artery. Rupture of this artery during head injury, bleeds into the cranial cavity causes pressure on the soft brain.

3. **Temporal bones:** There are two bones one on either side of the skull. Each bone consists of a number of parts,

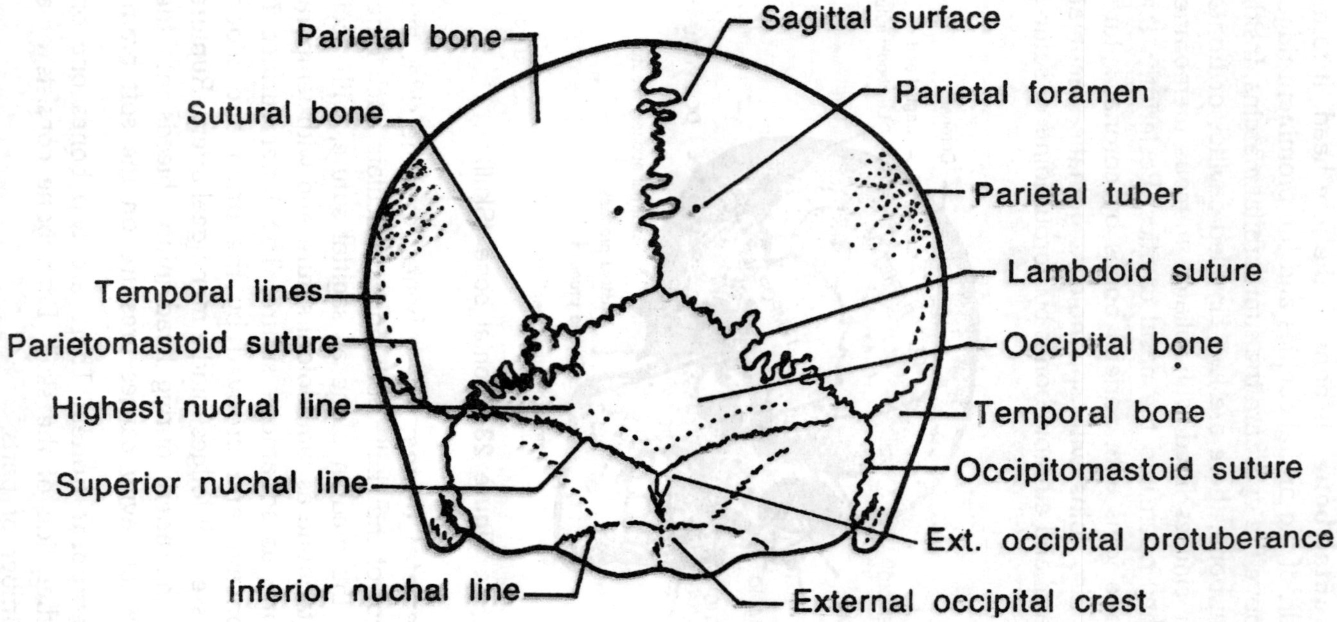

Figure 24. Sutures seen on the skull when viewed from behind

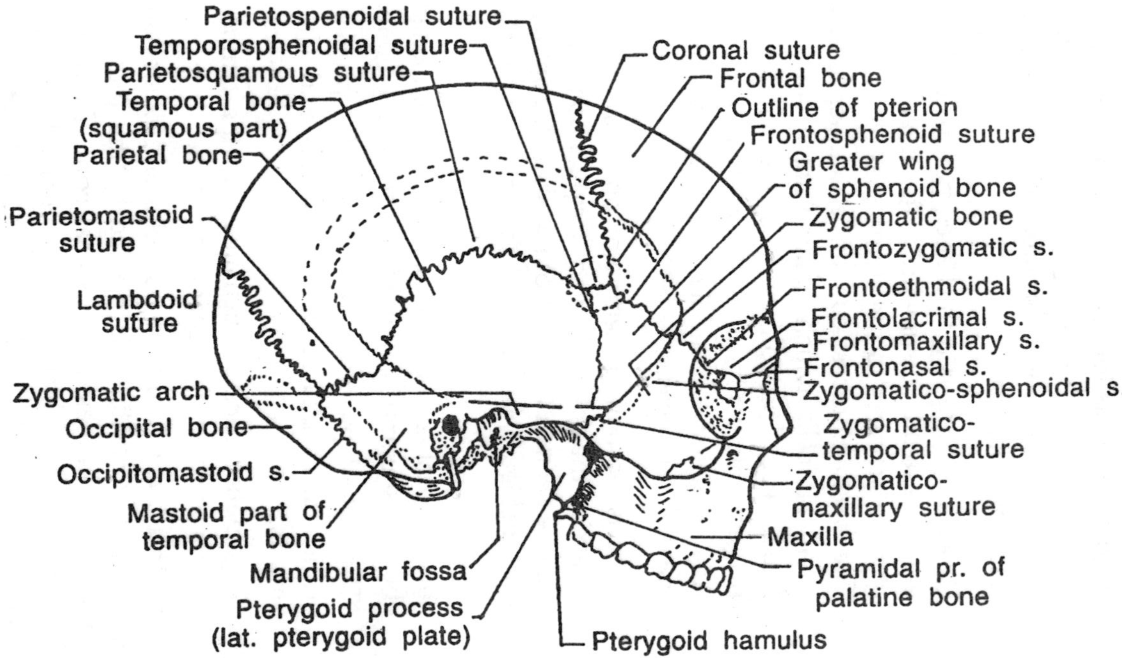

Figure 25. Sutures seen on the lateral aspect of the skull

a) Squamous part is thin and fan shaped. It projects upwards and gives origin to temporalis muscle. From this, the zygomatic process or zygoma projects forwards to join the zygomatic bone and this forms zygomatic arch. Behind and below the root of this process, is the external auditory meatus.

b) Mastoid process is a thickened part behind the ear. It extends downwards. Its outer surface gives attachment to the sterno-mastoid muscle. The mastoid process contains a number of very small air cells which communicate with the middle ear. The epithelium of the middle ear or tympanic cavity lines the mastoid air cells. Any infection of middle ear, may spread to mastoid air cells.

c) Petrous portion of temporal bone is wedged between the sphenoid and occipital bones and can be seen in the base of the skull. It contains the cochlea, vestibule and semi circular canals.

d) The tympanic portion forms the major part of the external acoustic meatus which is completed by the squamous part of the temporal bone.

e) The styloid process is a long slender process which gives attachment to muscles and ligaments.

f) Zygomatic process articulates with the temporal process of the Zygomatic bone.

4. **Occipital bone** forms the posterior and lower part of the cranial cavity. It is pierced by the foramen magnum for the passage of spinal cord. There are masses of bone which form the condyles which articulate with atlas to form atlanto-occipital joint. Above each condyle there is a foramen known as the posterior condylar foremen. The basilar part of the occipital bone articulates with the body of the

spenoid bone in the formation of occipito-sphenoidal joint. On the outer aspect on either side of the midline, there are two elevations known as superior and inferior nuchal lines for the attachment of muscles.

5. **Sphenoid bone:** It is shaped like a bat with wings stretched. It consists of a body and 2 greater and 2 lesser wings and two pterygoid plates. The body of the sphenoid posteriorly articulates with the basilar part of the occipital bone. On either side, three foramina are present namely foramen rotundum, foramen ovale and foramen spinosum It forms the middle portion of the cranial cavity. On its superior surface of the body, there is a little saddle-shaped depression, the Hypophyseal fossa (Sells tursica) in which the pituitary gland is situated. The body contains large air sinuses whihch open into the nasal cavities.

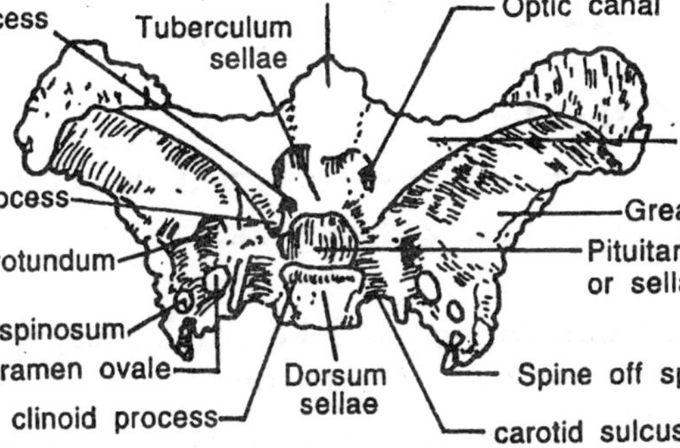

Figure 26. Sphenoid bone

6. **Ethmoid bone:** It is a spongy bone which occupies the anterior part of the base of the skull. It consists of 2 lateral masses or labyrinths composed of the ethmoidal air cells, which communicate with the nasal cavity. The ehtmoid bone consists of a

perpendicular plate and a cribriform plate. The perpendicular plate forms the upper part of the nasal septum. The cribriform plate forms the roof of the nasal cavities and has numerous small foramina through which nerve fibres of the olfactory nerves pass upwards to join the olfactory bulbs. The labyrinths form lateral wall of nasal cavities and from that pass two projections called upper and middle conchae or turbinated processes.

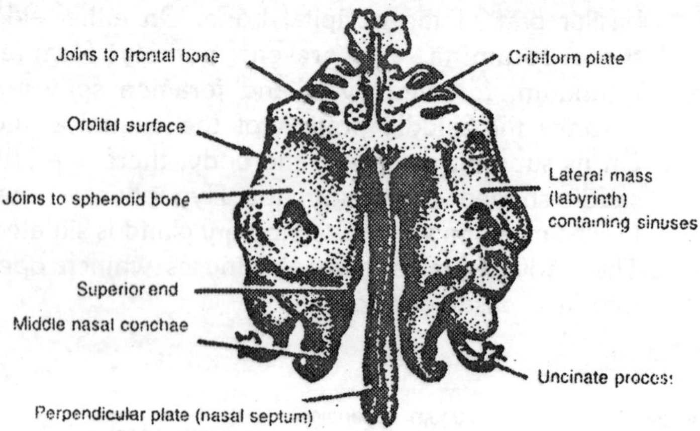

Figure 27. Ethmoid bone

Bones of the face

Skeleton of the face is formed by 14 bones.

2 Nasal bones, 2 zygomatic or cheek bones, 2 Maxillae

2 Palatine bones, 2 lacrimal bones, 2 inferior conchae, 1 mandible, and 1 vomer

1. **Zygomatic bones** form the cheek and part of the floor and lateral walls of the orbital cavities. The temporal process of the zygotic bone articulates with the zygomatic process of the temporal bone and forms zygomatic arch. Superiorly it articulates with the frontal bone. Inferiorly and medially it articulates with maxilla. Posteriorly it articulates with the sphenoid bone.

2. **Maxilla or upper jaw bone:** These 2 bones fuse in the median plane to form the upper jaw which contains upper teeth. It forms the anterior part of the roof of the mouth and lateral wall of the nasal cavities and part of the floor of the orbital cavities. On each side, the bone, contains large air space called maxillary air sinus (antrum of Highmove) Both sinuses open into the nasal cavities. The muscosa of nasal cavities is continuous and also line the maxillary air sinuses.

3. **Palatine bones:** They are "L" shaped bones. They form the roof of the mouth and the floor of the nose.

4. **Lacrimal bones** form lacrimal fossa and part of the orbit at the inner angle of the eye. The fossa is continuous down as lacrimal duct, through which, lacrimal fluid drains into the nasal cavities.

5. **Nasal bones** form the bridge of the nose.

6. **Inferior conchae:** A pair of bones articulates with the lateral wall of nose. These are the largest projections in the nasal cavities. The superior and middle conchae are projections from the ethmoid bone.

7. **Vomer** forms the lower part of the bony partition in the nose.

8. **The Mandible :** This is the only movable bone which forms the lower jaw and contains lower teeth. It consists of a body with alveolar ridge and a ramus which projects upwards almost at right angles to the posterior end of the body. The body and ramus meet to form the angle of the jaw. The ramus continues above as 2 processes, the coronoid process in front and condyle of the jaw or head of mandible behind. The condyle articulates with the temporal bone to from the tempero mandibular joint. The body has a foramen called mental foramen for the

passage of inferior dental nerve. The mandible may be depressed and elevated as in opening and closing the mouth; even, it may be protruded, retracted and moved slightly from side to side as in mastication.

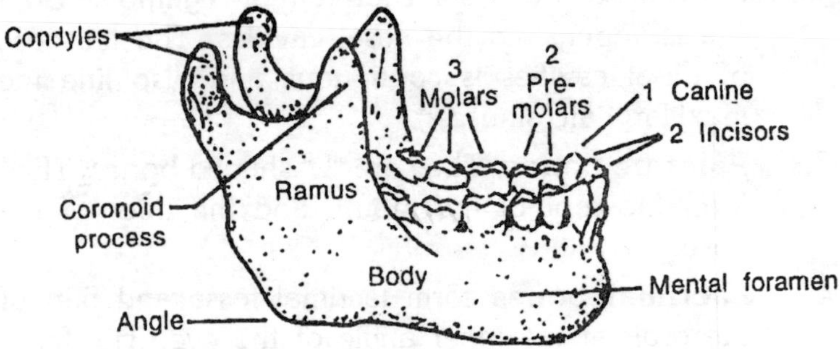

Figure 28. Mandible bone

9. **Hyoid bone:** It is an horse-shoe shaped bone lying in median plane of soft tissue of neck just above the larynx and below the mandible. It is attached to the styloid process of the temporal bone by means of stylo mandibular ligament and it gives attachment to the muscle of the tongue.It does not articulate with any other bone.

Nasal cavity: The bony frame work of the nose is formed by facial bones, is composed of 2 cavities about the middle of the face, seperated by thin nasal septum which extends from the palate up to the frontal bone. These cavities communicate with the paranasal air sinuses, i.e., frontal, ethmoidal, maxillary and sphenoidal air sinuses.

Air sinuses of the skull or paranasal air sinuses: These are the air spaces around the nose and present in the skull. They contain air and lined by the same mucus membrane of nose. The air sinuses communicate with the nose.

Infection from the nose may spread into the air sinuses causing sinusitis.

Sinuses

1. Frontal.
2. Maxillary.
3. Ethmoid.
4. Sphenoid.

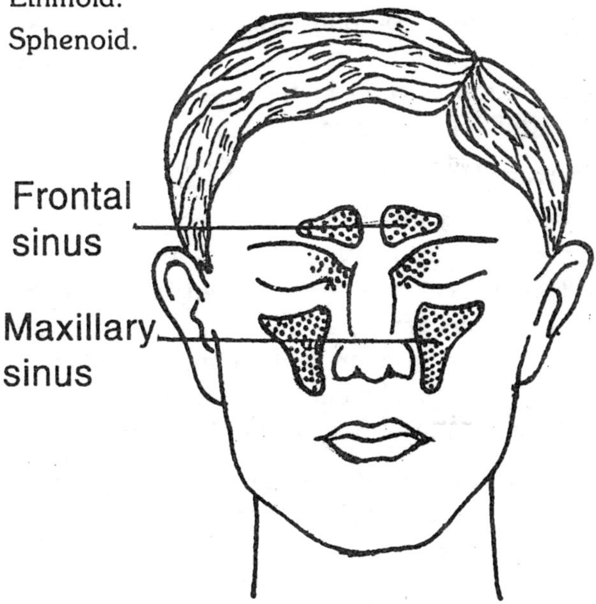

Figure 29. Air Sinuses

1. **Frontal air sinuses:** They are situated in frontal bone, one each side at the roof of the nose, opens into middle meatus of the nose.
2. **Maxillary air sinuses:** They are pair of sinuses, situated in maxillary bone, communicates into the middle meatus. Commonly, these sinuses are prone to infection. The accumulation of fluid in these sinuses causes headache.
3. **Ethmoid air cells:** There are smallest air spaces which communicate with the middle and superior meatus.

4. **Sphenoid air sinuses:** Usually, they are pair of sinuses situated in the body of the sphenoid bone and open into spheno-ethmoid recesses.

Function of air sinuses

1. To give resonance to the voice.
2. To lighten the bones of the skull.

Infection of paranasal air sinuses, causes severe headache usually, maxillary or frontal when there is accumation of fluid in the sinuses. The fluid is drained by artificial puncture.

Fontanelles of the skull

Ossification of the skull bones of an infant is not complete at birth. When 2 or 3 more bones meet, there will be space, this gap is filled with membranes. This membranous gaps are called fontanelles. At birth of child, 2 fontanelles are present in median plane, one is the posterior fontanelle between parietal and occipital bones. It fuses within 2-3 months after birth.

Another is the anterior fontanellae which is in between frontal and two parietal bones. It is the largest,

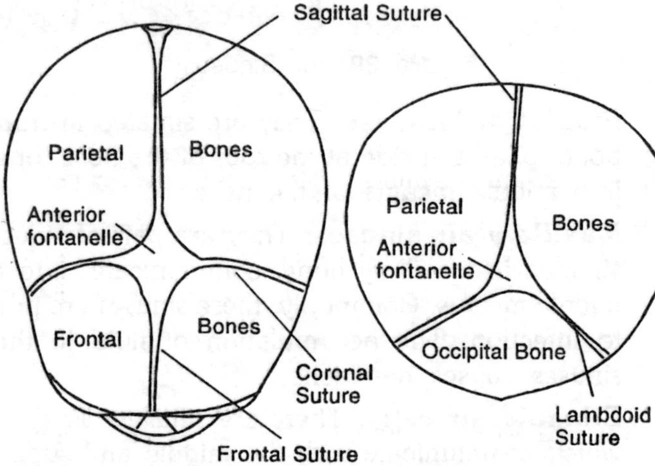

Figure 30. The Fontanelles

may be 1-1½ inches in diameter. This closes by 1-1½ years after birth. Its clinical importance is that any intracranial pressure raises, one can make out by its bulging or putting fingers on the anterior fontanelle.

Sutures of the skull

Joints between two or more skull bones are called sutures. They are firmly fixed fibrous type of joints. There is no movement in these sutures. Some important sutures are,

1. Coronal suture is in between the frontal bone and the 2 parietal bones.
2. Sagittal suture is in between 2 parietal bones along the top of the skull.
3. Lambdoid suture is in between the occipital bone and 2 parietal bones.
4. Squamous suture is in between the parietal bone and temporal bone.

Applied anatomy

Head injuries are common in all road and traffic accidents. The vault of the skull or base of the skull or both may be fractured.

First thing is to observe the head,

1. C.S.F coming out from nose or ear,
2. Bleeding from nose, ear or mouth,
3. External bleeding,
4. Internal bleeding : This we cannot observe. This can be assessed by level of consciousness. Because internal bleeding compress any part of brain, it causes sensory or motor loss of any region of the body.

Any type of head injury should be attended to immediately according to site of damage to the skull. Otherwise either of internal or external bleeding causes death. So, if we give first aid and treatment in time, the patient may survive.

Sequelae following head injuries are numerous and these include,

1. Altered level of consciousness,
2. Motor damage, leading to paralysis.
3. Sensory loss of the body and so on.

To treat head injuries, one should be having full knowledge of anatomy and physiology of the skull and its contents.

The Vertebral column

It is the axial column of different vertebrae. In between the vertebrae, the column is supplemented by fibro-cartilage. The adult column measures about 60-70 cms (24-28 inches) in length. There are 33 vertebrae.They are as follows :

7 Cervical vertebrae to form skeleton of neck region.

12 Thoracic vertebrae to form thoracic vertebral column.

5 Lumbar vertebrae to form lumbar vertebral column.

5 Sacral vertebrae to form sacrum.

4 Coccygeal vertebrae to form coccyx.

Characteristics of a typical vertebra

1. The body of each vertebra is situated anteriorly. The size varies with the site. They are smallest in the cervical region and becomes larger body towards the lumbar region. The body contains nucleus pulposis.

2. **The neural arch:** It encloses large vertebral foramen containing spinal cord and its coverings. This arch is formed by 2 pedicles that project backwards from the body, 2 laminae are expanded plate structures that project to form pedicles towards medial side. Where the pedicles and laminae unite on lateral side, continues as transverse processes

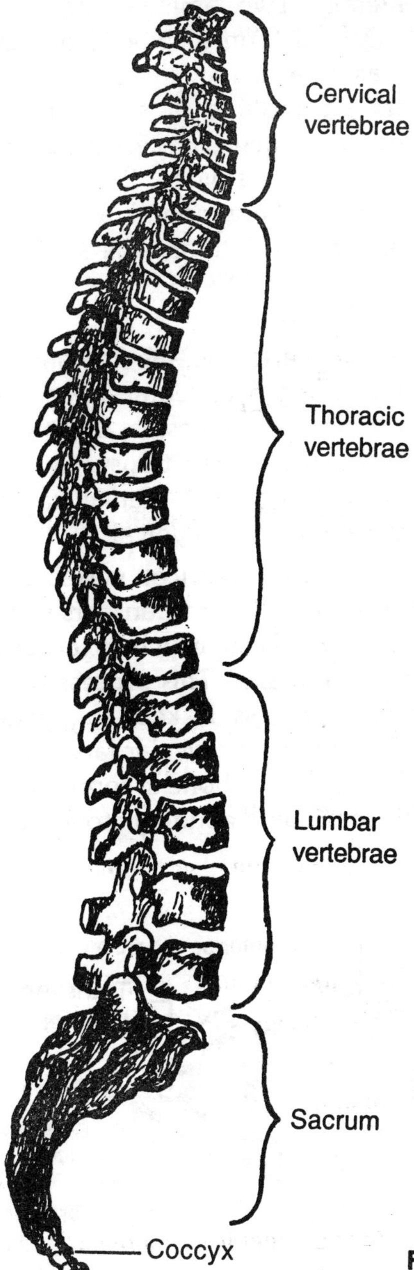

Figure 31. Vertebral column

that project laterally. Two laminae meet in median plane posteriorly and form a spinous process. The neural arch has 4 articular surfaces, 2 superior articular facets articulate with superior vertebra, then the 2 inferior articular facets articulate with inferior vertebra. In between 2 pedicles of 2 vertebrae is called intervertebral foramen. They transmit spinal nerves with its spinal ganglion.

CERVICAL VERTEBRAE

There are 7 cervical vertebrae, the first one is called atlas, 2nd is axis, remaining 5 vertebrae have the same character. In all the transverse processes, these vertebrae are having foramen. Each is called transverse foramen. It transmits vertebral artery to the cranial cavity. The first two cervical vertebrae are atypical.

The Atlas is the first cervical vertebra and it consists of ring of bones with 2 short transverse processes . The anterior part has a facet which is occupied by the odontoid process of the axis. This process represents the body of atlas.This process is kept in position by transerse ligament. The superior articular facet articulates with the condyles of the occipital bone to form the atlanto-occipital joint. In this joint, only nodding movements take place.

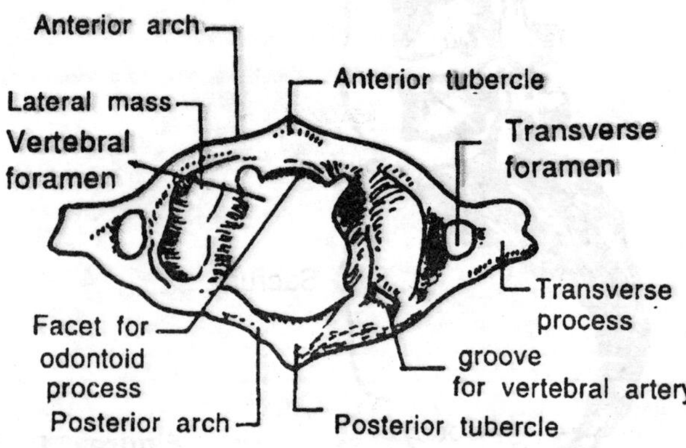

Figure 32. The Atlas

The Axis is the 2nd cervical vertebra. The body is small and its upward continuation is called odontoid process or DENS. The superior articular facet articulates with atlas to form atlano-axial joint. This is a pivot type of synonial joint. In this joint rotation of head takes place.

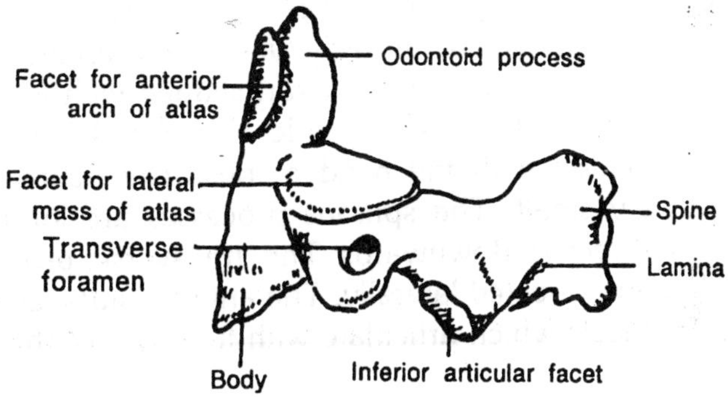

Figure 33. The Axis

The 7th cervical vertebra or vertebra prominence. The spine of seventh cervical vertebra is

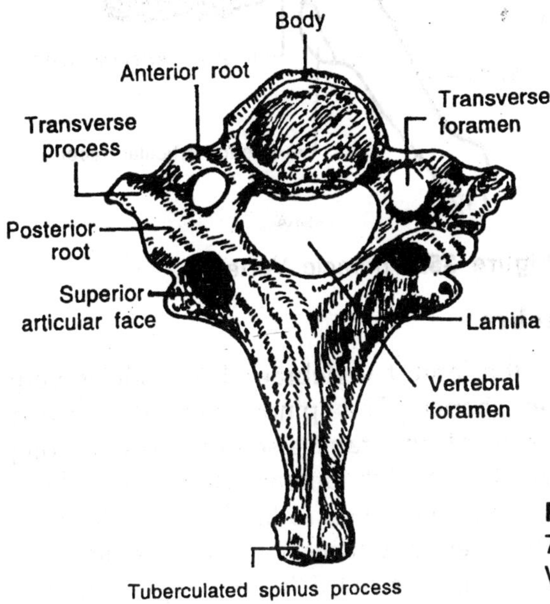

Figure 34. 7th Cervical Vertebra

undivided and most prominent on the back of the neck in the midline. Whereas spines of other cervical vertebrae (3rd, 4th, 5th and 6th) are bipid or divided into 2 parts.

The Thoracic vertebrae

The thoracic vertebrae are larger than the cervical vertebrae and they increase in size as they bow downwards. A typical thoracic vertebra presents some special features. The body is heart-shaped with superior and inferior facets on either side above and below for the articulation with the head of ribs. The neural arch is relatively small. The spinous processes are long and each is directed downwards The transverse processes are long and directed laterally. The anterior surfaces have articular facets which articulate with tubercles of the ribs.

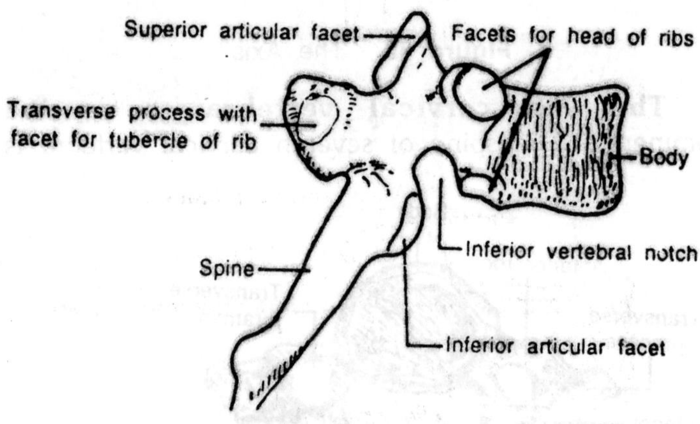

Figure 35. Thoracic Vertebra

Lumbar vertebra

These are the largest vertebrae. The body is very large and kidney shaped. The spinous process is broad and directed backward, the transverse processes are long and directed laterally. The 5th lumbar vertebra articulates inferiorly with sacrum to form sacro-lumbar joint. In older age the 5 lumbar vertebra fuses with sacrum to form sacralization and compress the 5 lumbar spinal nerves and causes severe pain along that nerve root and patient complains low back pain at sacral region, because of sacralization. The aetiology of the fusion is not known.

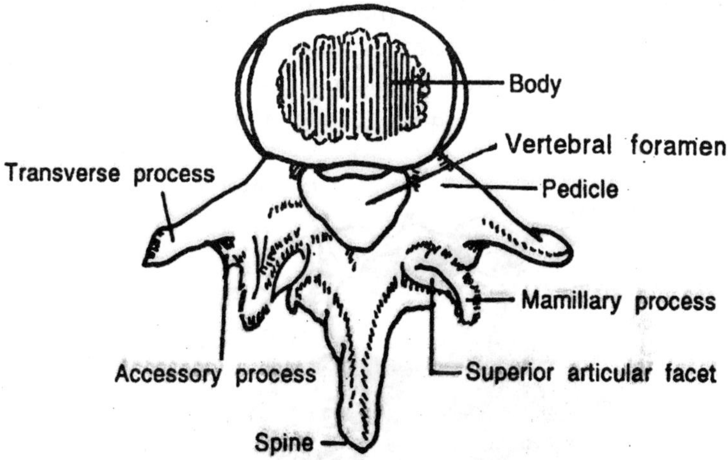

Figure 36. Lumbar Vertebra superior aspect

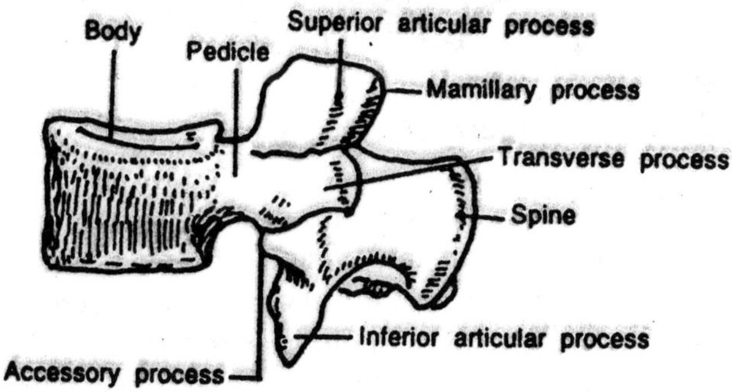

Figure 37. Lumbar Vertebra lateral view

The Sacrum is a triangular bone formed by the fusion of 5 sacral vertebrae. It articulates on either side with hip bones to form sacro-iliac joint. Below it articulates with coccyx to form sacro-coccygeal joint. This joint is more movable in female. The sacrum with 2 hip bones and coccyx form pelvis or pelvic cavity. The base is formed by the 1st sacral vertebra, whereas, apex is formed by the 5th sacral vertebra. The anterior border of the base is called sacral promontary. The anterior surface of the sacrum is concave and shows four transverse ridges which mark the fusion of the sacral vertebrae. The sacrum is having the sacral canal, containing terminal portion of spinal cord and its covering, the sacral and coccygeal nerves.

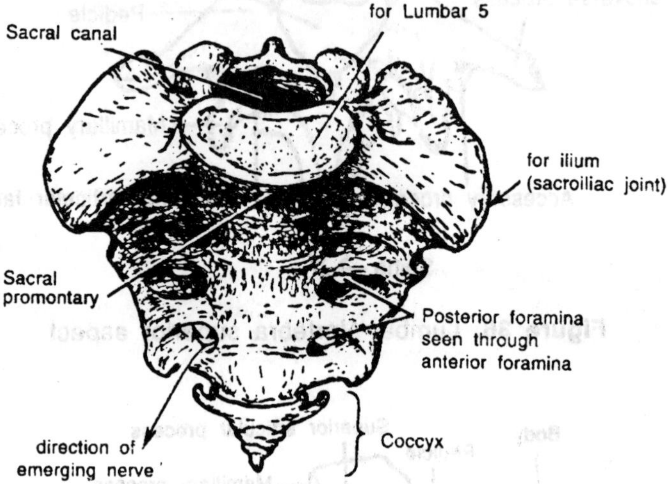

Figure 38. The Sacrum

The Coccyx: It is composed of 4 rudimentary vertebrae fused to form into a single bone. It articulates above with the sacrum to form the sacro-coccygeal joint. The tip of the coccyx gives origin to external anal spincter. In lower animals, the coccygeal vertebrae are continuous as tail. In human beings some times, coccyx bone may contain 5-6 coccygeal vertebrae having characteristic of rudimentary tail.

THE CURVES OF THE VERTEBRAL COLUMN

When looked at the side of the vertebral column it presents 4 anterior posterior curvatures, 2 primary and 2 secondary.

The growing foetus in the uterus lies curled up, so that, the head and the knees are more or less touching. This position shows anterior C - shaped primary curvature. The secondary, the anterior convex cervical curvature develops when the child can hold up his head i.e., about near 3 months and the seconday convex lumbar curve develops when the child can stand and try to walk i.e., about 12-18 months. The anterior concave thoracic and sacral primary curvatures are retained.

The joints of the vertebral column

They are cartilagenous joints formed by intervertebral discs placed between body of each two vertebrae, strengthened by ligaments, running in front the anterior longitudinal ligament and behind the posterior longitudinal ligament. These ligaments run throughout the entire length of the column. Masses of muscle on each side of vertebral column aid in the stability of the spine.

Ligamentum flava

It connects the laminae of adjacent vertebrae. Ligamentum nuchae and the supra spinous ligament connect the spinous processes extending from occiput to the sacrum.

Movements of the vertebral column

The movements between the individual vertebrae are very limited. The movements of the column, as a whole are ...

Flexion - forward bending

Extension - backward bending

lateral bending to each side

rotation to right and left.

There is more movement in the cervical and lumbar regions than elsewhere.

Functions of the vertebral column

1. Strong central long axis to the body to support body weight.
2. Vertebral canal, strong bony canal for spinal cord and its coverings.
3. Between pedicles there are inter vertbral foramina to transmit spinal nerves, blood vessels and lymphatic vessels.
4. It supports the skull.
5. As the column is formed by numerous individual bones a certain amount of movement is possible.
6. Intervertebral discs act as shock absorbers to protect the brain and spinal cord.
7. Upper limbs and body weight is transmitted to the lower limbs.
8. Protects the thoracic and abdominal viscera by forming posterior wall of the trunk.

The thoracic cage

The skeleton of the thorax is made up of ribs and

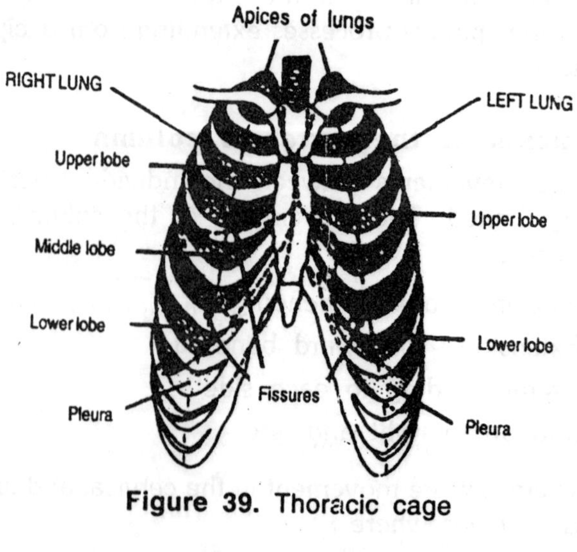

Figure 39. Thoracic cage

cartilages and sternum. The thorax is a cone-shaped cavity broader below than above, and longer behind than in front, formed by the 12 thoracic vertebrae at the back, the sternum in front and the 12 pairs of ribs at the sides.

The sternum or breast-bone is a flat bone divided into 3 portions, the manubrium sterni, the body and the xiphoid process.

1. The manubrium sterni is a triangular shaped bone placed above the body of the sternum. It articulates with clavicles on either side on upper lateral margins to form sterno-clavicular joints. In between the 2 sterno-clavicular joints on upper margin forms the lower limit of suprasternal notch or jugular notch. Under the sternal end of clavicle on lateral margin on either side, it articulates with the costal cartilages of 1st rib. Below the manubrium sterni, it articulates with louis, at this angle, the 2nd rib articulates.
2. The body is long and narrow and notched on each side for articulation of 3, 4, 5, 6, and 7th ribs. Below it articulates with xiphoid process.
3. The xiphoid process is the tip of the bone. It is cartilaginous in young but ossified on older persons. It gives attachment to diaphragm, the linea alba and muscles of the anterior abdominal wall.

RIBS

There are 12 pairs of ribs. They form the bony lateral walls of thoracic cage and articulate posteriorly with the thoracic vertebrae. The upper 7 pairs are attached to the sternum anteriorly by means of their costal cartilages, these are the true ribs. The lower 5 pairs are false ribs. Of these 8, 9 and 10, form costal arches and indirectly articulate with the sternum. The remaining 11 and 12 pairs are called floating ribs because the anterior ends are free in the anterior abdominal wall muscles. Posteriorly they articulate with 11th and 12th thoracic vertebrae.

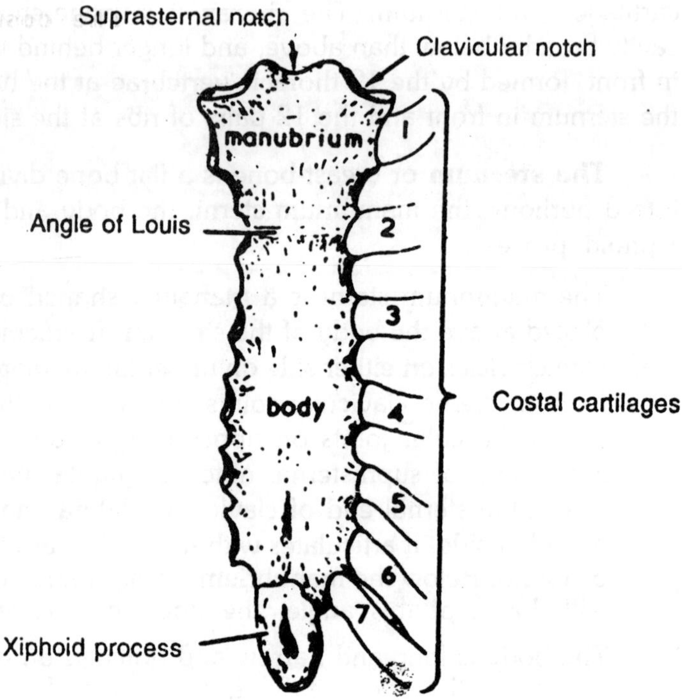

Figure 40. The Sternum

Characteristics of rib

It is a long curved bone. It has 2 ends, anterior and posterior, in between the ends are shaft, neck and head. The posterior end articulates with corresponding thoracic vertebra. On the posterior aspects of neck, there are 2 tubucles, one is medial. It is an articular tubercle and articulates with the facet on anterior surface of the transverse process of the vertebra. The non articular tubercle gives attachment of ligaments. The anterior or sternal end has a depression for the attachment of the costal cartilage. The shaft is thin and flat, having the internal surface and external surface. In the inner surface below, there is a subcostal groove which lodges intercostal vessels and nerve.

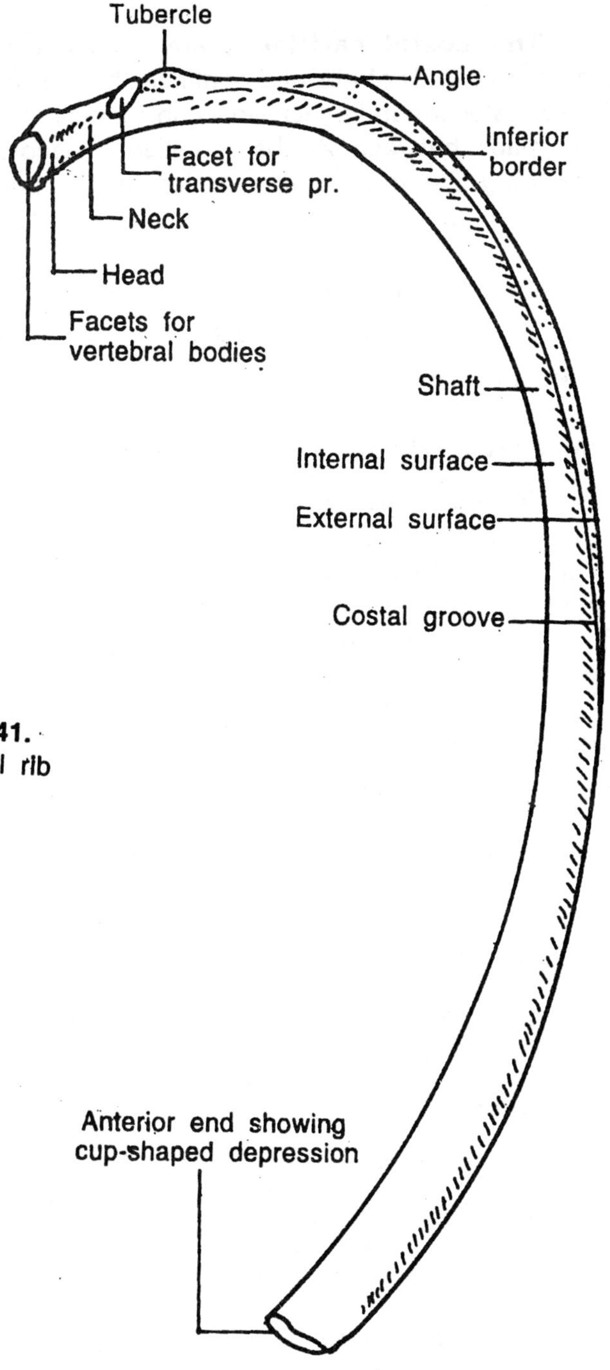

Figure 41.
A typical rib

The costal cartilages are hyaline cartilages at the anterior ends of ribs and connects the ribs to sternum. These costochondral joints allow considerable movements. The space between 2 ribs is called intercostal space containing the intercostal muscles, which help during respiratory movements.

Thoracic Vertebrae

The 12 thoracic vertebrae are already described under the vertebral column.

The Pelvic girdle or Bony pelvis

Pelvis is formed by 2 hip bones or innominate bones with sacrum and coccyx. They articulate with sacrum to form the sacro-iliac joints. The sacrum articulates below with coccyx to form the sacro-coccygeal joint. The 2 hip bones articulate in the median plane to form pubic symphysis joint. The pelvis is divided into the true pelvis or pelvic basin which lies below the brim and the false pelvis formed by the iliac bones extending above the brim. The inlet of true pelvis is the brim formed by crest of

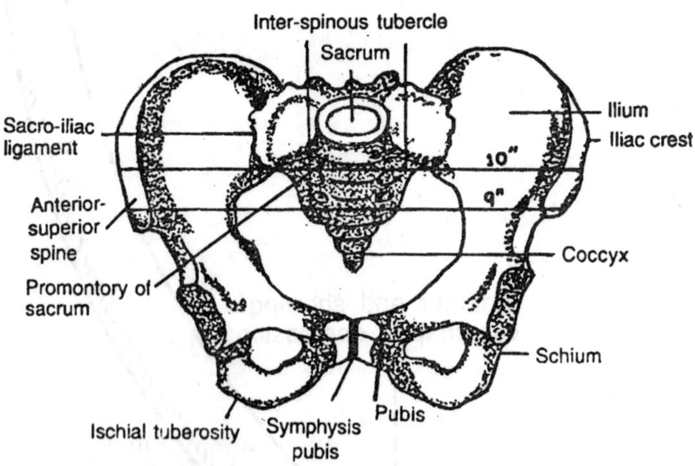

Figure 42. The Female Pelvis

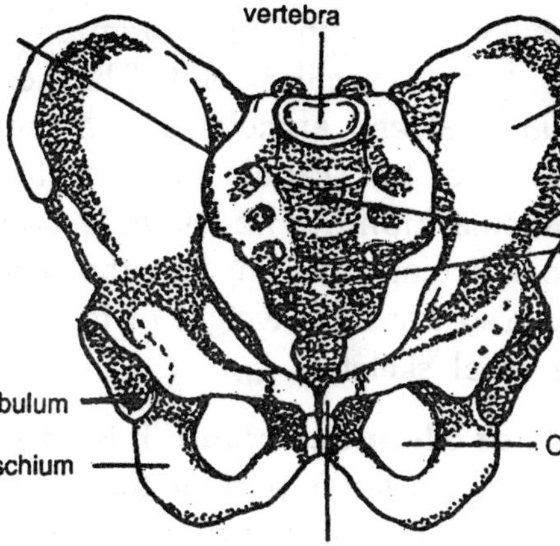

Figure 43. The Male Pelvis

the pubic bones, ilio-pectineal line (both sides) and sacral promontary. The outlet is bounded by the coccyx and ischial tuberosities.

APPENDICULAR SKELETON

The appendicular skeleton consits of the shoulder girlde with upper limbs and pelvic girdle with the lower limbs. The skeleton of the upper limb is connected to axial skeleton by shoulder girdle. This girdle is made up of clavicle and scapula.

Each upper limb consists of 32 bones.

1. Clavicle
2. Scapula
3. Humerus
4. Ulna and Radius
5. 8 carpal bones
6. 5 meta-carpals
7. 14 phalanges.

1. **The Clavicle or collar bone** is a long bone placed horizontally, having a double curve, a shaft and two extremities. The sternal end articulates with the manubrim sterni to form the sterno-clavicular joint. The acromial end or laternal end articulates with the acromion process of the scapula to form the acromio-clavicular joint. The clavicle connects the appendicular skeleton with the axial skeleton and also transmits weight of the upperlimb to the axial skeleton.

2. **Scapula or Shoulder blade:** It is a flat triangular bone, forms posterior part of the shoulder girdle and lies at the back of the thorax. For examination point of view, it has 2 surfaces, 3 borders, 3 angles, and 2 processes.

Surfaces: The anterior or subscapular surface gives origin to the subscapular muscle. The posterior or dorsal surface is divided by the spine of the scapula into supra spinatus and infra spinatus surfaces giving origin to the same named muscles.

Borders are medial border, upper border and lateral border.

Angles

The lateral angle forms into glenoid cavity which articulates with the head of the humerus to form the shoulder joint. The superior angle is the meeting point of upper and medial borders. The inferior angle is the meeting point of medial and lateral borders.

Processes

The coracoid process is a projection from the upper border of the bone. The acromion process is continuous laterally with the spinous process.

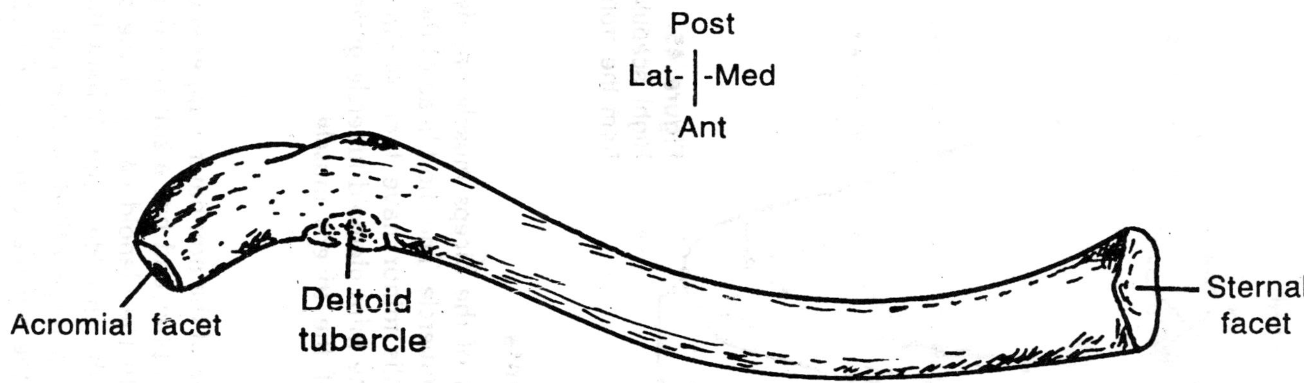

Figure 44. Right Clavicle seen from above

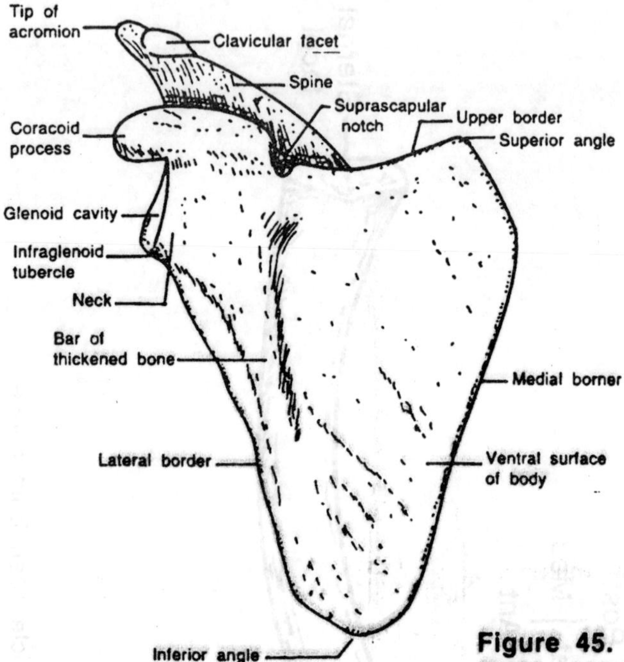

Figure 45. Right scapula, seen from the front

Muscle attachments

The long head of the biceps muscle has its origin in the supra glenoid tubercle. The short head of the biceps muscle and pectoralis minor have their origin in the corocoid process. The infra glemoid tubercle gives origin to the long head of the triceps muscle.

HUMERUS

It is a long bone of the arm having upper end, shaft and lower end. The upper end has a soft rounded head which articulates with the glenoid cavity of the scapula in the formation of the shoulder joint. Where the head meets the shaft has a ridge called anatomical neck. It gives attachment to the articular capsule of the shoulder joint. In front of the upper end of the shaft has the lesser

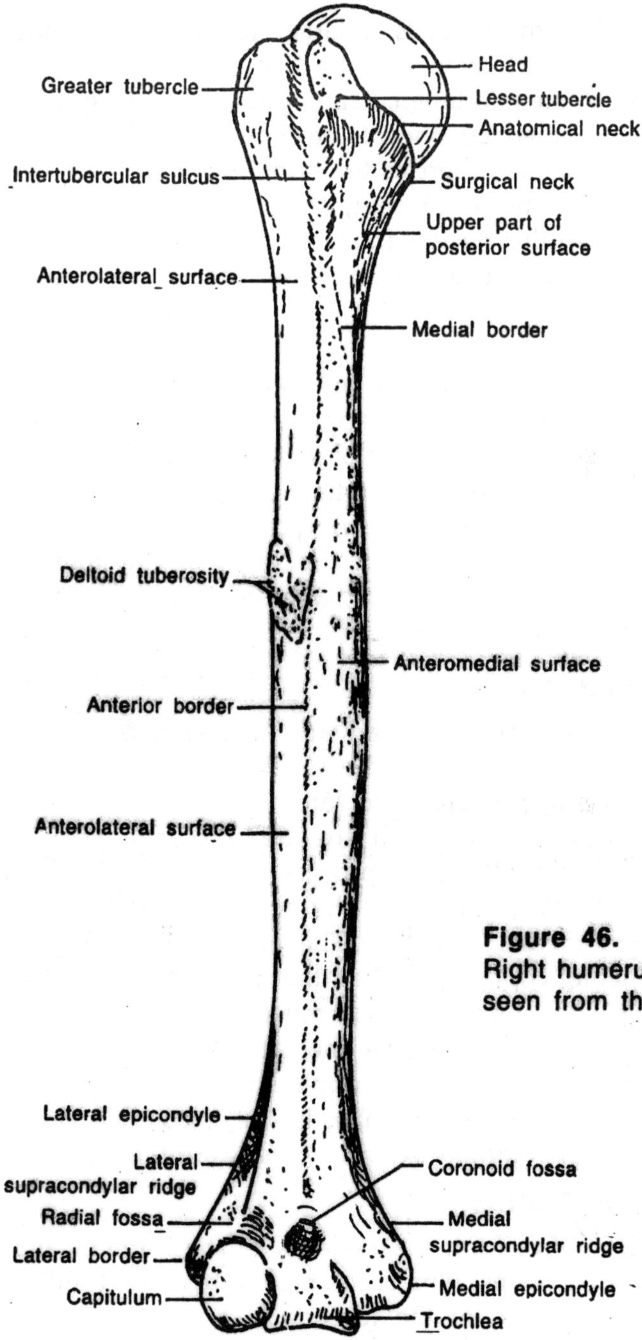

Figure 46.
Right humerus,
seen from the front

tubercle. Postero-lateral is a larger tubercle called the greater tubercle. In between the 2 tubercles, there is a deep groove, the intertubercular groove or bicipital groove which is occupied by one of the tendons of the biceps muscle. Below the tubercles the bone becomes narrower called surgical neck. In that, the circumflex nerve is rotated. When this neck is fractured the circumflex nerve is damaged and the deltoid muscle becomes paralysed.

Shaft

The shaft is rounded in transverse section and becomes flattened when it approaches the lower end. A rough tubercle on the lateral surface is called Deltoid tubercle, to that there is insertion of Deltoid muscle of the shoulder region, that gives roundness to the shoulder. On the posterior surface at the level of the deltoid tubercle, there is a spiral or radial groove and it contains the radial nerve.

Lower end

The lower end is broad and flat, articulates with the radius and ulna to form the elbow joint. The articular surface of the trochlea articulates with the ulna. The capitulum articulates with the head of the radius. Posteriorly, the olecranon process of ulna fits into the olecranon fossa of humerus. The non articular parts are lateral and medial condyles. The most prominent part on the medial condyle is called the medial epicondyle.It gives origin to common flexor muscles of the forearm. The posterior surface of the medial condyle is related with ulnar nerve. The most prominent process on lateral surface of lateral condyle is called lateral epicondyle which gives origin to common extensor muscles of the forearm.

Ulna and Radius

Both bones form the skeleton of the forearm and both are long bones, ulna is the medial bone and radius is the lateral bone of the forearm.

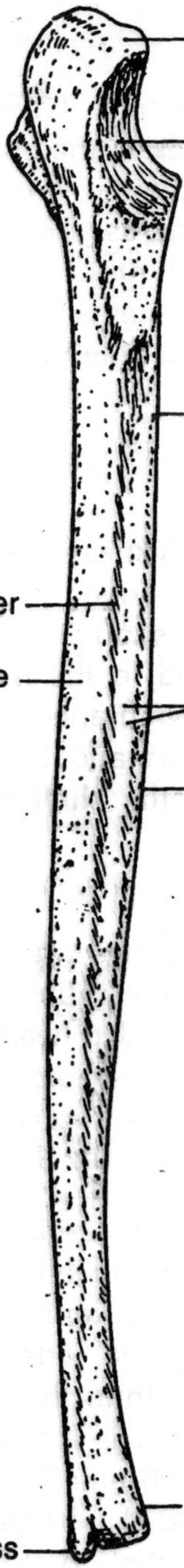

Figure 47. Right Ulna, seen from behind

Ulna

Is a strong and thick bone having upper and lower ends. In between the ends is the shaft. The upper end has posteriorly the olecreanon process which fits into olecreanon fossa of humerus. The anterior surface of upper end has coronoid process which fits into the coronoid fossa of the humerus. The trochlear process articulates with the trochlea of humerus to form the elbow joint.

Shaft

Is thick, tapers its thickness towards the lower end. Its anterior surface gives origin to flexor muscles and the posterior surface gives origin to extensor muscles. Its later border is attached to the medial border of the radius by interosseous membrane. The posterior border is completely subcutaneous and it can be palpated to diagnose the fracture of the shaft of ulna.

Lower end

It is small and articulates with the ulnar notch of radius to form the inferior radio-ulnar joint. On its posterior surface a small rounded head is present. Postero-lateral to the head is the styloid process.

RADIUS

It is a long bone having a shaft and two ends. The upper end is small and round and presents the head. The head articulates with the capitulum of the humerus in the elbow joint. The medial side articulates with the radial notch of the ulna to form the superior radio-ulnar joint. Below the head there is a small constricted part known as neck, and posterio-medial to neck there is a rough tuberosity called radial tuberosity. The tendon of the biceps brachii is inserted to that tuuberosity.

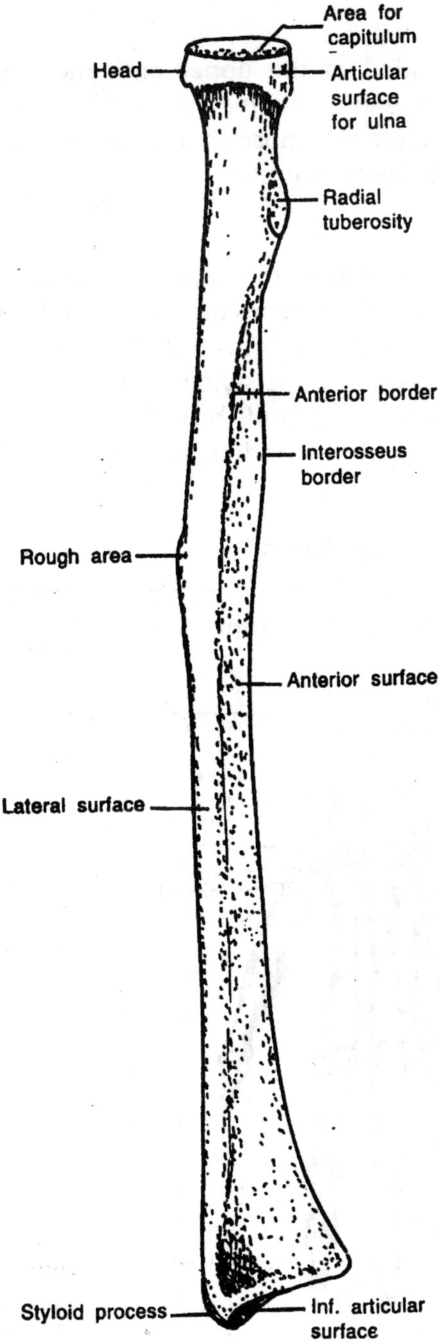

Figure 48. Right Radius, seen from the front

Shaft

Is more rounded at the upper end and widened as it nears the lower end and curved outwards. Its anterior surface gives origin to flexor muscles. The posterior surface gives origin to extensor muscles.

Lower end

Is more expanded than the upper end. It articulates with the carpal bones to form the wrist joint. On its anterior surface one can feel the radial pulse and on its posterio lateral aspect is the styloid process that forms the floor of the anatomical snuff box. At the wrist joint, the inferior surface of the radius articulates with the scaphoid and lunate bones.

Bones of wrist and hand

The bones of the hand are arranged in groups, the carpus are short bones that form the wrist joint. The

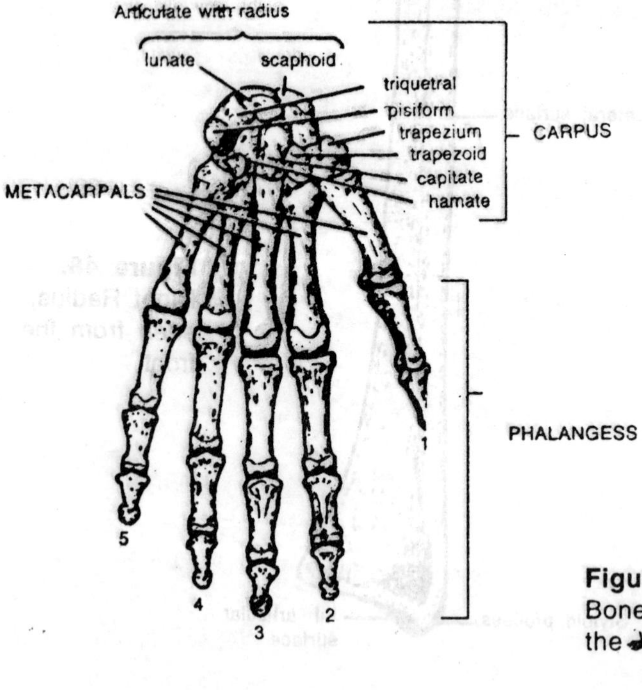

Figure 49. Bones of the Wrist

metacarpals form the skeleton of the palm of the hand and are long bones. The phalanges are long bones of the finger or digits.

The Carpal bones are 8 in number and arranged in two rows. The proximal row from lateral to medial has scaphoid, lunate, triquetral and pisiform. The distal row, has traprzium, trapezoid, capitate and hamate.

Metacarpal bones: These five bones form the palm of the hand. They are counted from the thumb to medical side numbering five bones. The proximal ends articulate with carpal bones to form the carpo-meta carpal joints. The distal ends articulate with phalanges to form the meta-carpo phalangeal joints.

Phalanges: They are 14 in number, two phalanges for thumb, the proximal and distal phalanges, for other fingers, there will be 3, called, proximal, middle and distal phalanges. In between phalanges articulation is called as interphalangeal joints. The two joints in the finger is called proximal and distal interphalangeal joints.

The Skeleton of the lower limb

The bones of the lower limb are connected with the trunk by means of the pelvi girdle. Each lower limb consists of 31 bones.

1	Hip or innominate bone	1	patella
1	Femur	7	Tarsal bones
1	Tibia	5	Metatarsals
1	Fibula	14	Phalanges.

The Innominate or Hip bone is a flat bone, situated on the lateral side bone of the pelvis, with opposite hip bone forms the pubic symphysis. On lateral surface there is a cupshaped depression called the acetabulum. Here all the 3 parts of hip bone fuses and this is the articulation for the head of the femur to form the hip joint. The 3 parts are called, anteriorly the pubis, laterally the ilium and posterio-inferiorly the ischium.

The Ilium has 2 surfaces and 2 borders connected by iliac crest. The inner surface forms false pelvis and gives origin to iliacus muscles. The outer or gluteal surface gives origin to gluteal muscles.

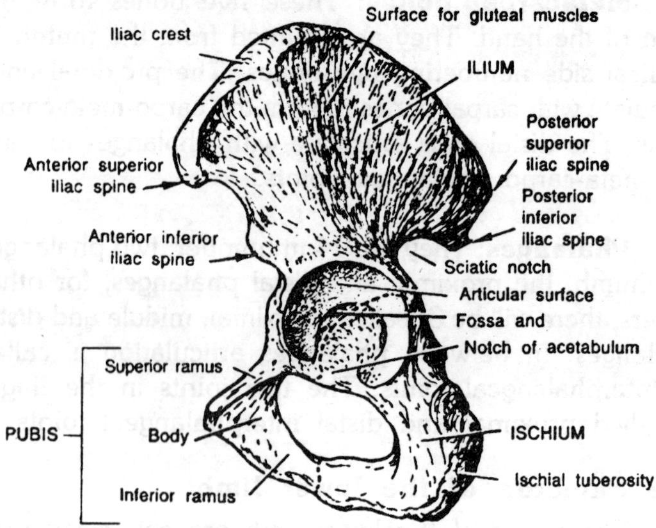

Figure 50. Innominate bone

Borders: The anterior border has the upper limit by anterior superior iliac spines. This border gives attachment to inguinal ligament and the posterior inferior iliac spine forms the lower limit and gives attachment to ligament of the hip joint. The upper limit of the posterior border is called posterior superior iliac spine. On the skin there is a dimple. Corresponding to this spine continuous down the lower limit is called the posterior inferior iliac spine. This border descends down and meets the posterior border of ischium. Between these two bones there is a big notch called greater sciatic notch, through that, sciatic nerve comes out of the pelvis to enter on the posterior surface of the thigh. Superiorly between the 2 borders there is the iliac crest which forms the upper limit of the pelvis and this can be felt easily.

The Pubis: It consists of a body and 2 rami. The body forms anterior boundary of pelvis. The superior ramus meets the ilium in the acetabulum. The inferior ramus meets the ramus of the ischium. Between two rami is the obturator formen. The body meets with opposite body of pubis to form the public symphysis.

The ischium is the thickest and strongest portion of the bone. Posterio-inferiorly is the ischial tuberosity, that transmits weight to the chair in sitting posture. On the posterior border, the ischial spine separates the greater and lesser sciatic notch, when this bridges by ligament, then is called as corresponding foramens.

The obturator foramen is a oval foramen lying below the acetabulum bounded by rami of pubis and ischum. It is filled with obturator membrane. In its anterio-medial part there are obturator canals, which transmit obturator vessels. They pass into the medial compartment of the thigh.

The Acetabulum is a deep cup-shaped cavity formed by all the three portions of the hip bone and articulates with the head of the femur to form the hip joint. The articular surface in the hip is horse-shoe shaped. The margin of the cup has a notch called acetabular notch. Its notch margin gives attachment to ligamentum teres of the head of femur. It carries blood vessels to the head of the femur.

FEMUR

The femur is the strongest and longest bone of the thigh. Below it articulates with the tibia and the patella to form the knee joint. This long bone has an upper extremity, the shaft and the lower extremity.

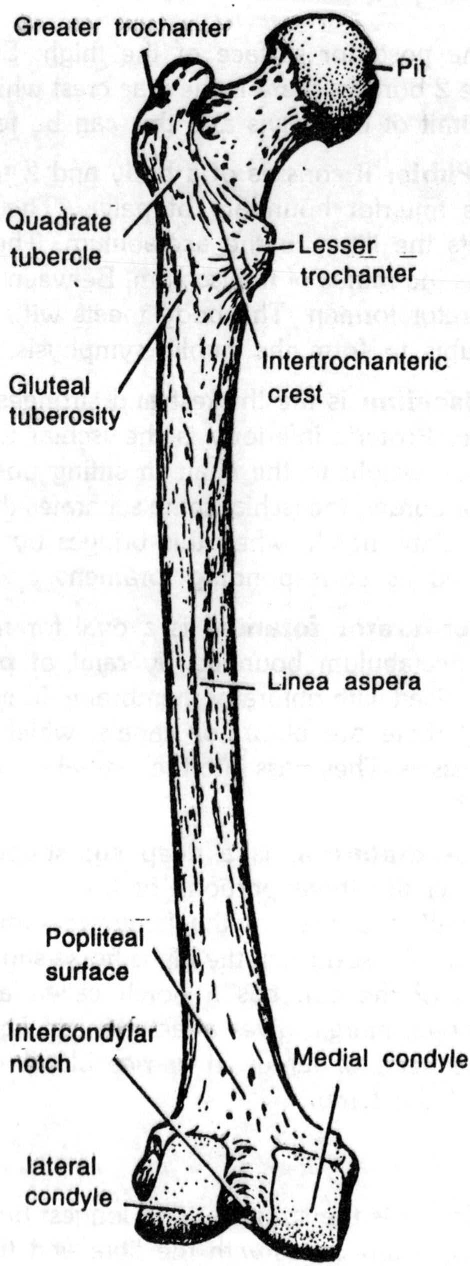

Figure 51. Femur

The upper extremity: It has the head and neck, the head articulates with the acetabulum of the innominate bone to form the hip joint. At the summit of this is an avoid depression, a roughened part for the attachment of ligamentum of teres. Below the head is the oblique neck. The neck makes an angle of about 125°C, where it meets the shaft. The lateral side has the greater trochanter and medially has the lesser trochanter. On the anterior surface of neck meets the shaft called inter trochanteric line, where as the posterior surface where it meets the neck is called inter trochanteric crest. In the middle of inter trochanter there is a quadrate tubercle.

The shaft is cylindrical, smooth and rounded. The rough crest on posterior surface is called linea aspera which gives attachment to muscles. The shaft is covered by thick muscles. The shaft has 3 compartments of thigh.

The lower extremity is wider and presents two condyles, an inter condylar notch and patellar surface. The medial condyle and lateral condyle are very prominent and articulate with the tibial condyles to form the knee joint. On the corresponding surface of each condyles, there are prominences called medial epicondyle and lateral epicondyle.

The inter condyler notch separates the condyles behind. The cruciate ligaments are attached between the 2 surfaces of the notch. The inter condylar notch is separated anteriorly by patellar surface and posteriorly by poplitial surface. The poplitial surface is on the back at the lower end of the shaft above the condyles.

Patella or knee cap

It is roughly triangular, it is a sesamoid bone developed in the tendon of the quadriceps extensor muscles of the thigh. The base faces superiorly, and the apex points downwards. The posterior smooth surface articulates with the patellar surface of the femur but it does not enter into the formation of the knee joint. The anterior rough surface can be felt.

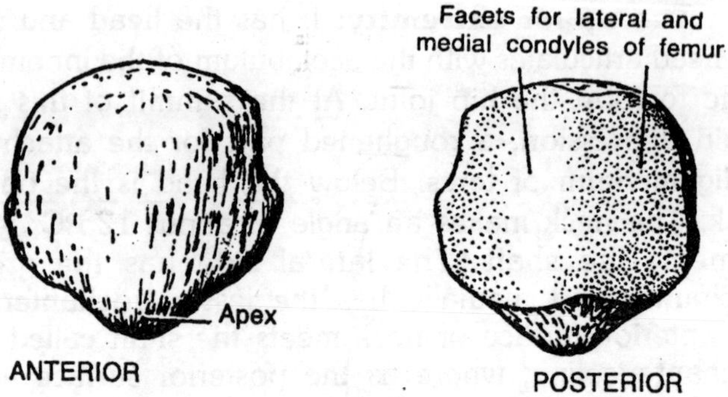

Figure 52. Patella or knee cap

TIBIA

The tibia or shin bone is the medial strong bone of the leg. It is a long bone having an upper end, the shaft and the lower end.

The upper extremity presents the medial and lateral condyles. Both condyles form an expanded portion which articulates with the corresponding condyles of the femur to form the knee joint. The posterior surface of the lateral condyle presents a facet for the articulation of fibula to form the superior tibio-fibular joint. Both condyles measure about 10 cms. There is a tibial tubercle. Below the condyles in the centre is the tibial tuberosity, to that ligamentum of patella is inserted.

The shaft on cut section is triangular, its anterior border is prominent and subcutaneous, the medial surface is completely subcutaneous. The posterior surface gives origin to flexor muscles eg: gastrocnemius and soleus.

The lower extremity: It is smaller when compared to the upper end. It enters into the formation of the ankle joint. On the medial side there is an expanded area known as medial malleolus. On the lateral side it articulates with the tibia to form the inferior tibio-fibular joint.

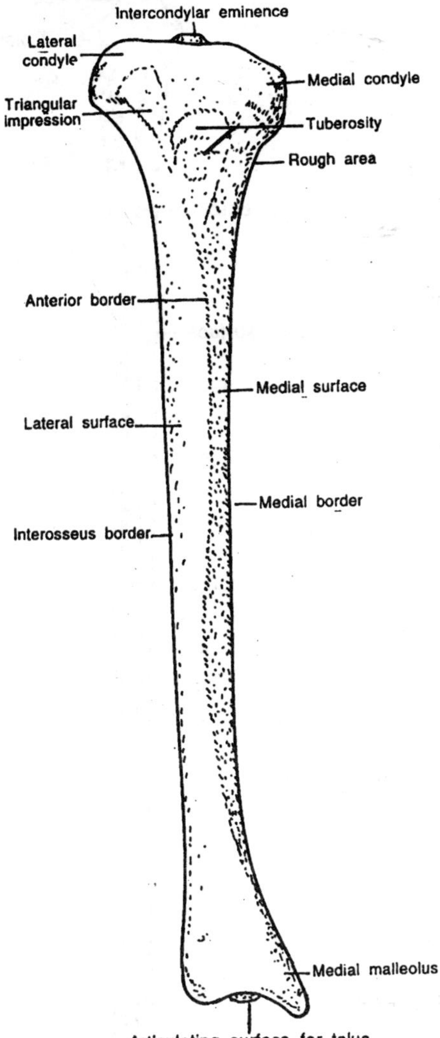

Figure 53. Right tibia, anterior aspect

FIBULA

It is the lateral bone of the leg. It is a long bone having an upper end, a shaft, and the lower end. On the upper extermity a little expanded end is called the head which articulates with the tibia to form the superior tibiofibular joint. The head can be felt on the lateral side just below the knee joint.

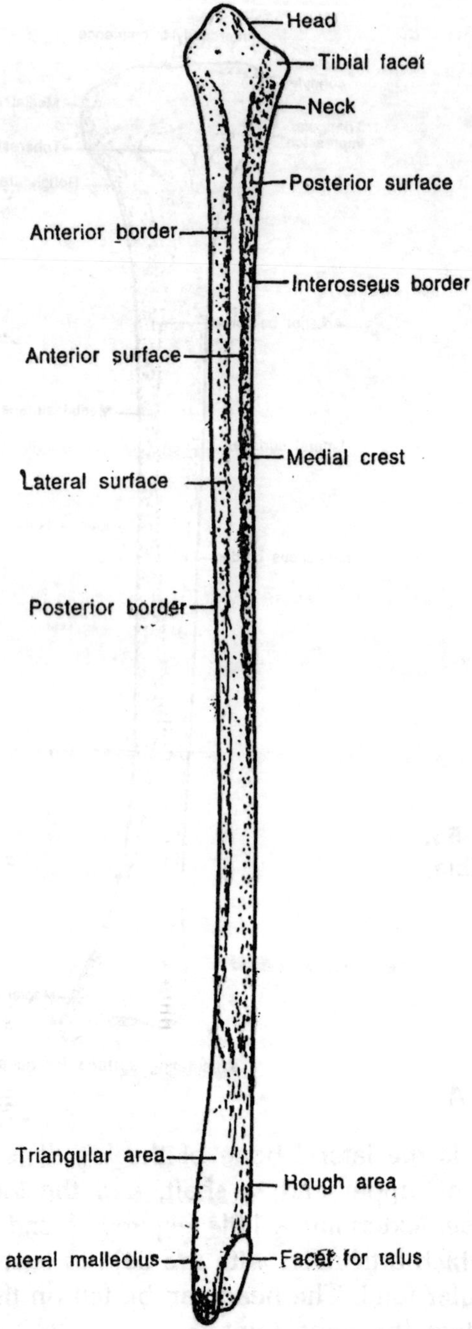

Figure 54. Right fibula, seen from the front.

The shaft: It is a long slender bone which gives origin to the 3 compartment muscles.

The lower extermity is prolonged and expanded downwards as lateral malleolus. It can be felt near the ankle joint. The lower extremity articulates with the fibula in the formation of the inferior tibulofibular joint.

Bones of the foot

There are seven tarsal bones. The talus articulates with the tibia and fibula to form the ankle joint. They articulate anteriorly with meta tarsal bones to form the skeleton of the foot (tarso-metatarsal joints). The tarsal bones are:

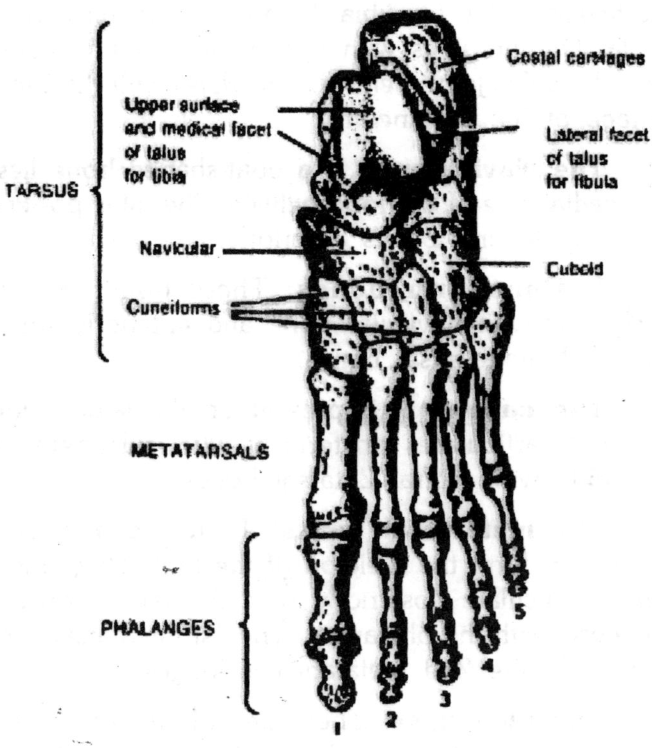

Figure 55. Bones of the left foot

1 Calcaneum

1 Talus

1 Navicular

3 Cuneiform bones (medial, intemediate and lateral

1 Cuboid

The Calcaneum: It is the largest of the tarsus. It forms the heel of the foot. This can be palpated easily. The heel is a transmitting point of weight. On its posterior surface is the insertion of the tendon of Achilles or tendo calcaneous. It articulates superiorly with the talus. In front, it articulates with the cuboid bone.

The talus: It is the highest point of the foot, where it articulates with the tibia. Laterally it articules with the fibula. On the sides with two malleoli it articulates to form the ankle joint, below it articulates with the superior surface of the calcaneum.

The Navicular: It is a boat-shaped bone lies on the medial side of the foot, between the talus posteriorly and 3 cuneiform bones anteriorly.

3 Cuneiform bones: These bones articulate posteriorly with navicular bone and anteriorly with the medial 3 meta tarsal bones.

The cuboid: It is present on the lateral side of the foot, articulates posteriorly with calcaneum and anteriorly with lateral 2 tarsal bones.

The metatarsal bones: There are 5 metatarsal bones that form the skeleton of the foot. They are long bones, articulate posteriorly with the tarsal bones and anteriorly with the phalanges. The 1st metatarsal is short and thick, the 2nd metatarsal is longest.

The phalanges: There are 14 phalanges in the toes and they are arranged as in the finger of the hand. They are much shorter than the fingers.

THE ARCHES OF THE FOOT

The arches maintain the concavity inferiorly to transmit the weight to the ground and protect blood vessels. There are 4 arches of the foot, 2 longitudinal and two transverse arches.

Medial longitudinal arch: This is the highest of the arches. It is formed by the calcaneum, the navicular, 3 cuneiform and 3 medial metatarsal bones.

The lateral longitudinal arch is formed by the calcaneum, the cuboid and two lateral metatarsals.

Transverse arches: These run across the foot. There are 2 arches. The transverse arch is formed by the tarsal bones. Another transverse arch is formed across the heads of the metatarsals. The stability of the arches is maintained by the

1. attachment of ligaments
2. long flexor tendons
3. short muscles of the foot and plantar aponeurosis
4. shape of the tarsal bones.

THE JOINTS

A joint or articulation is the name applied to describe the site at which two or more bones come together. The term arthrology is applied to the study of joints. They are classified as

1. The fibrous joints (immovable joints)- synarthroses
2. the cartilagenous joints (slightly movable joints)- amphiarthroses
3. the synovial joints (freely movable joints)- diarthroses

1. Fibrous joints or synarthroses: It is immovable in which no movements between the bones are possible. For eg.,

(i) Sutures or joints of the skull bones, the coronal suture is in between the frontal and two parietal bones, the sagittal suture runs between uniting 2 parietal bones, the lambdoid suture is in union between both parietal bones and the occipital bone.

(ii) **Gomphosis** or peg and socket joints, for eg., teeth in their alveolar sockets.

(iii) **Syndesmosis :** The bones of articulation are connected by membrane eg: inferior tibio fibular joint.

(iv) Primary cartilaginous joints are found between the diaphysis and epiphyses of the long bones before fusion of the epiphysical line.

2. Cartilaginous joints or Amphiarthroses: They are the slightly movable joints. The joint surfaces are separated by an intra articular disc a) secondary cartilaginous joint of the **pubic symphysis:** where intra articular disc intervenes between 2 pubic bones.

   b) The inter vertebral joints: The inter-vertebral disc is in between 2 bodies of vertebrae.

   c) The joint between the manubrim sterni and body of the sternum

3. Synovial joints (freely movable joints) or Diarthroses: These joints are freely movable. There are several varieties in the synovial joint.

Characters of the synovial joint

All the synovial joints have certain characteristic points.

1 Articular or hyaline cartilage covers the bony ends that forms the joints.

2. Articular capsule or fibrous capsule binds two bony ends.

3. The ligaments support the external articular capsule.
4. Synovial membrane lines the inner surface of articular capsule.
5. Synovial membrane secretes fluid called synovial fluid which helps for lubrication of the joint.
6. Small sacs of synovial fluid or burase are present around the joint, to act as cushions to prevent friction between bone and ligament or tendon.

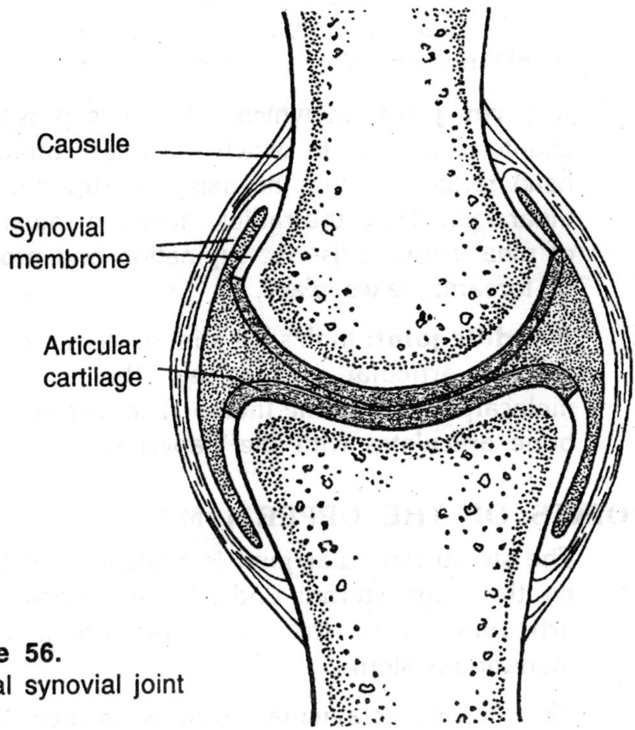

Figure 56.
Typical synovial joint

Types of synovial joints

1. **Plane joint or gliding joint** in which two flat surfaces of bones articulate with each other. Eg., joints between tarsal and carpal bones.

2. **Ball and socket joint,** eg., the shoulder joint and hip joint, in shoulder joint, the ball is the head of the humerus and socket is glenoid cavity. This joint permits movement in all directions.

3. **Hinge joint,** eg., elbow and knee joint, these allow the movements of flexion and extension in one plane. Inter phalangeal joints are hinge joints.

4. **A condyloid joint** is almost same as hinge joint but it is so adopted to permit movement in two planes eg: a) wrist joint b) temporo-mandibular joint. The movements possible in this joint are flexion, extension, abduction and adduction and slight circumduction but not rotation.

5. **A pivot joint,** in which rotation is possible eg: atlanto-axial joint in which the atlas carrying the head rotates around the axis and superior radio-ulnar joint. Here the radius moves in radial notch of ulna in one axis i.e., supination and pronation of forearm, takes place.

6. **A saddle joint:** In this the joint space has concave-convex articular surface eg: the first carpo-metacarpal joint of the thumb. The first metacarpal bone articulates with the trapezium.

JOINTS OF THE UPPER LIMB

1. The sterno-clavicular joint is a plane joint formed by the large sternal end of the clavicle which articulates with the clavicular notch of the manubrium sterni.

2. The Acromio-clavicular joint is formed by the acromial end of clavicle articulating with acromion process of the scapula.

3. The shoulder joint or the humero-glenoidal joint is a ball and socket of the synovial variety. The head of the humerus forming one-third of a sphere

articulates with the glenoid cavity of the scapula. The cavity is deepened by the attachment of fibro-cartilage, the glenoidal labrum. The bones are united together by loose articular capsule, supported by ligaments and musculo-tendinous cuff. The loose articular capsule is attached below to the surgical neck. The tendon of the long head of the biceps muscle passes through the capsule of this joint. In this joint free movements takes place when compared to the ball and socket of hip joint. The movements are flexion, extension, rotation are internal and external, abduction and adduction and circumduction. This is the most freely movable joint in the body.

4. The elbow joint is a hinge joint of synovial variety. The movements are in one plane. The trochlear notch of the ulna fits into the trochlear surface of the humerus to form the elbow joint. The head of the radius articulates with the capitulum of the humerus to form humero-radial joint. The movements in this joint are only flexion and extension. The carrying angle of the elbow: when the forearm is fully extended in supination there will be an angle on lateral side of elbow joint, between the long axis of arm and the long axis of forearm. The angle is about 170°, this is due to the obliquity of the articulating surfaces.

5. The Radio-ulnar joints: These joints are between two opposite borders of radius and ulna connected by interoseous membrane. There are two joints, one is the superior-radio-ulnar joint where the head of the radius articulates with radial notch of ulna. The movements are supination and pronation of the forearm. Supination means the hand faces anteriorly, pronation means the palmar surface of hand faces posteriorly where the radius moves over the ulna. Another joint is the inferior radio ulnar joint.

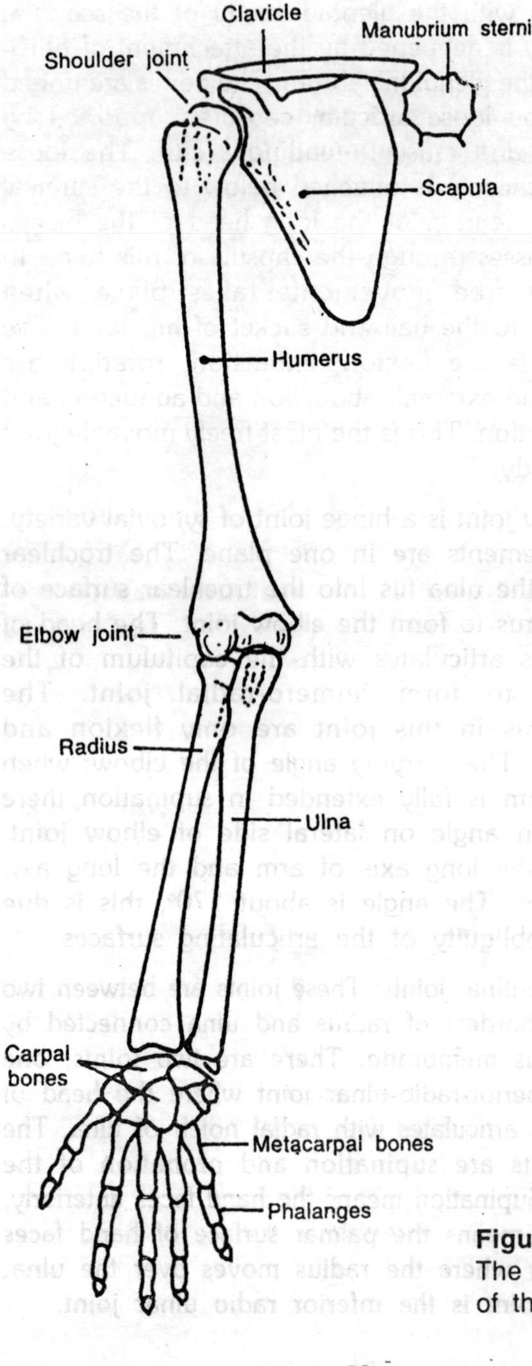

Figure 57. The joint of the upper limb

6. The wrist joint or Radio-carpal joint: It is the condyloid joint of the synovial variety. It is formed between the convex border of proximal row of carpal bone and concavity of the radius. The movements in this joint are flexion, extension and abduction and adduction. Circumduction also occurs.

7. Joints of hand and digits

   a) **The carpal joints:** It is the plane or gliding joint of the synovial variety.The articulating surface is between the promiximal and distal row, and also between two adjacent surface of carpal bones. The movement is only gliding.

   b) **The carpo-metacarpal joints** formed between the bases of metacarpals and anterior surface of distal row of carpal bones. The carpo-metacarpal joint of the thumb is a saddle joint. It is formed between the base of 1st meta carpal bone and trapezium. The inter meta carpal joints are formed between the bases of meta-carpals.

   c) **The metacarpo-phalangeal joints** are the condyloid joints of the synovial variety. The heads of the metacarpals articulate with the bases of the proximal phalanges. The movements are flexion, extension, abduction and adduction.

   d) **The interphalangeal·joints:** They are hinge joints of the synovial variety. These joints are formed between the·2 phalanges. In the thumb there is only one interphangeal joint where as in other fingers there are 2 interphangeal joints that is proximal and distal inter-phalangeal joints. The movements are flexion and extension.

JOINTS OF THE LOWER LIMB

1. **The hip joint** is a ball and socket joint of the synovial variety. The head of the femur fits into the acetabulum of the innominate bone. The articular capsule is thickened by 3 strong ligaments, the ilio femoral, pubiofemoral and ischiofemoral ligaments. This gives additional support to the joint. This is the strongest joint in the body. The movements at the hip joint are flexion, extension, abduction and adduction, medial and lateral rotation. The combination of all these movements is called circumduction.

2. **The knee joint:** It is a modified hinge joint of the synovial variety. The movements take place only in one axis.(i.e. flexion and extension) This joint is formed by the condyles of the femur, and superior surface of the condyles of the tibia. The patella is placed on the patellar surface of the femur and acts as a gliding joint. It does not take part in the formation of the knee joint. The intra articular structure is made up of the medial and lateral semi lunar cartilages. Between the corresponding condyles there are cruciate ligaments called the anterior cruciate ligament and the posterior cruciate ligament which bind the femoral and tibial condyles. The articular capsule is very extensive and is strengthened by expansions from the muscle and ligamentum patella. The movements are flexon and extension, and slight medial rotation. The knee joint possesses the largest synovial membrane which lines the joint stuctures, and forms several burse about the joint.

3. **The Tibio-fibular joints:** These joints are formed by the upper and lower ends of both tibia and fibula. The shafts of both these bones are connected by interosseous membrane. In these joints no movement takes place.

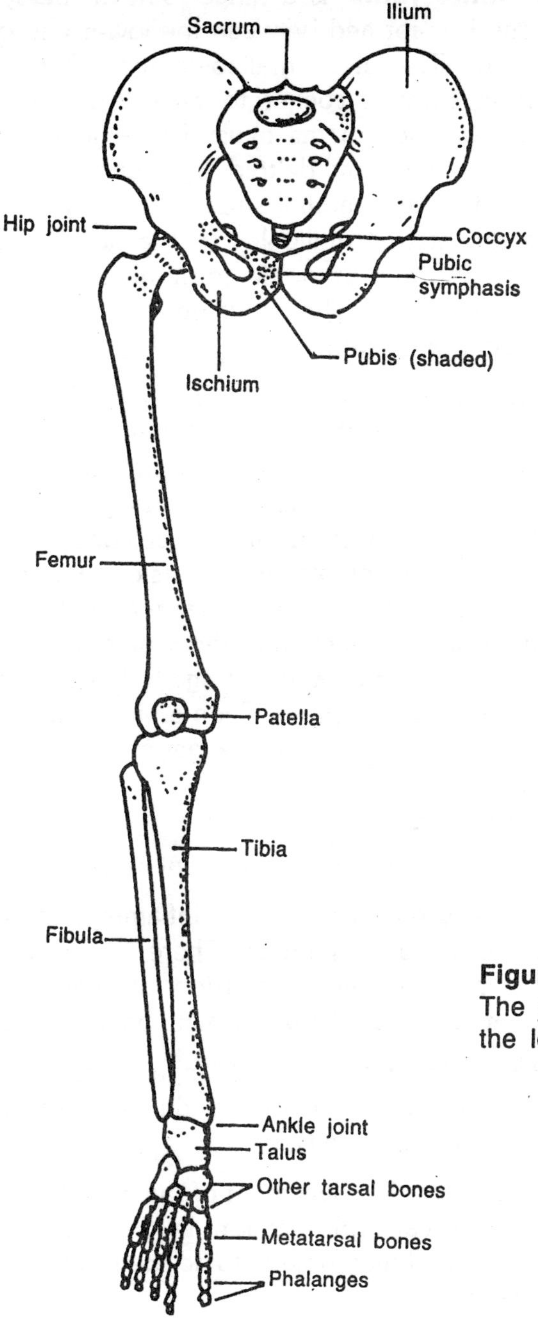

Figure 58. The joints of the lower limb

4. **The ankle joint:** is a hinge joint of the synovial variety. It is formed between the lower end of tibia and talus. The lateral malleolus of the fibula which together form a socket to receive the trochlear surface of body of the talus. The articular capsule is strengthened by deltoid ligament. The deltoid ligament on the medial surface of the joint passes from the medial malleolus to the adjoining tarsal bones. Saprain of ankle joint occurs when this ligament is torn. The movements are dorsiflexion and plantar flexion.

5. **Joints of the foot:** The joints of the foot are named as like in the hand, intertarsal joints, meta-tarso-phalangeal and interphalangeal joints. The movements are very less comparing to the hand. In the sub-talar joint or talo-calcaneo-navicular joint, the movements are inversion and eversion of the foot. Inversion means raising medial borders of the foot and eversion of the foot is raising lateral margin of the foot. Any damage to ligament or torn ligament is called sprain. Then an individual cannot walk, if he tries to walk, he experiences severe pain.

Applied Anatomy

1. **Arthritis:** Infection of any joint is called arthritis.
2. **Rheumatoid arthritis** is the inflammation of either small joints or big joints. There is thickening of articular tissue, with extension of synovial tissue over articular cartilages, which become eroded.
3. **Osteo-arthritis** is an old age disease, or age advancing disease. It occurs due to degeneration of articular cartilages.
4. **Dislocation:** Displacement of the articular surfaces of a joint is called dislocation. Dislocation can occur in any joint. It may be due to accidents or congenital dislocation.

5. **Traumatic injury** to joints.

The trauma will damage the soft tissues, tendons and ligaments round the joint. In dislocations there may be additional damage to intra capsular structures. If the repair is incomplete there may be some loss of stability.

Questions

1. What general functions does the skeletal system perform ?
2. List the constituents of bone and the factors that influence its development.
3. Name the different types of bones. Give one example of each type and describe its structure.
4. State the functions of the skeleton.
5. Describe the thorax, shoulder girdle and pelvis.
6. What is the difference between the male and female pelvis ?
7. Describe femur with a neat diagram.
8. Describe the mandible with a diagram.
9. What are the types of joints found in the human body ? Give one or two examples for each type.
10. Name the sutures of the cranium.

UNIT - 4

The Muscular System

This system is very important to communicate to another person by means of talk, and also your feeling by facial expression i.e., muscles of face, then walking by locomotor muscles of the limbs. Study of muscles is called Myology.

Types					
	1. Voluntary	-	Skeletal	-	Striated.
	2. Involuntary		Cardiac	-	Striated.
			Smooth	-	Non-striated.

Structure

1. **Striated muscles** are under the voluntary control eg., limb muscles. When examined, each is found to consist of a numerous fasciculi separated by fibrous septa passing between the fasciculi from the covering fascia. The fasciculi are made up of a number of fibres. The skeletal muscle is made up of muscle cells. A skeletal muscle fibre is an elongated muscle cell. It has a limiting cell membrane known as Sarcolemma, the cytoplasm enclosed by the sarcolemma is called sarcoplasm, which

contains myofibrils which are the contractile elements. Myofibrils are arranged parallel to the long axis of the fibre. Under higher magnification, each myofibril shows cross striations consisting of alternating dark and light zones. These cross striations are characteristic of a striated muscle. A skeletal muscle fibre is multinucleate. The number of nuclei depends upon the length of the fibre. The alternating dark and light zones seen under the light microscope are caused by a difference in the refractive index. The dark zone is anisotropic and is known as the 'A' band, while the light zone, since it is isotropic, is termed as the 'I' band. A myofibril consists of a number of smaller structures called myofilaments. The compartments of myofirbils are called sarcomeres. They are the basic functional units of striated muscle fibres. According to physical and chemical properties, myofilaments are of three types

1. Thin filaments, their main component is protein actin
2. Thick filaments - formed of protein myosin
3. Elastic filaments are composed of protein titin

There are three types of skeletal muscles fibres

1. Slow oxidative fibres
2. Fast oxidative fibres
3. Fast glycolytic fibres

2. **Cardiac muscle:** The cardiac muscle forms the musculature of the heart called myocardium. The structural organisation of cardiac muscle resembles that of skeletal muscle to some extent only. The main points of difference are that, each muscle fibre (cell) contains a single centrally placed nucleus and each fibre branches and anastomoses with another fibre. This gives rise to a branching and anastomosing system of cylinders. In the spaces

between cells connective tissue cells are present and the fibres in the form of endo-mysium. The blood vessels, nerves and groups of muscle fibres are enclosed by perimysium.

Intercalated discs between cardiac muscle fibres (end to end) are made up of plasma membrane. They contain both gap junctions and desmosomes. Desmosomes afford firm attachments between ells and strengthen the tissue. Gap junctions provide a route for quick conduction of muscle action potentials throughout the heart.

3. **Smooth muscle** consists of fibres which are long and spindle shaped. Each fibre is a cell contains one centrally placed nucleus. Each cell is limited by a cell membrane, the plasmalemma. The cytoplasm is a designated sarcoplasm. Under microscope, fine longitudinal striations are visible. These are the myofibrils. Although they are composed of actin and myosin, cross striations are absent. The smooth muscle lines the respiratory, alimentary and urinary systems. It is also found in blood vessels, iris, ciliary body of eye, arrector pili of hair, follicles and walls of hollow viscera. Their capacity for regeneration is considerable when compared with other muscle tissues.

Properties of muscles

Contractility is the ability of skeletal muscles to shorten with force. When they contract, they cause movement of bones at the joints and also other structures to which they are attatched. Nervous stimuli causes them to contract. This property of muscle is called exitability stimuli from electricity applied direct to the muscle or its nerves will cause the muscle to contract. In medicine nerves and muscles are tested by eliciting the muscle response which might have been affected by disease.

Blood supplies energy in the form of adenosine triphosphate (ATP) for muscle contraction.

After a person dies ATP is not available for muscle contraction, there is no release of cross bridges that have been formed. As a result, the muscles become rigid. This condition is called rigor mortis.

Creatinine phosphate is another high energy molecule that the muscle fibres can store.

ATP is produced by aerobic and anaerobic cellular respiration.

Muscle relaxation occurs as calcium ions are actively transported back into the sacroplasmic reticulum. The returning of muscle length to its original length (recoil) is called elasticity.

MUSCLE Fatigue

Repeated muscle contractions use up ATP faster than it is produced and lactic acid accumulates faster than it can be removed, the muscle then becomes tired and the efficiency of contraction decreases. Rest brings back the production of ATP and at the same time the lactic acid is removed.

Classification of muscle contractions

1. **Isometric (equal distance) contractions:** In this type the length of the muscle does not change. The amount of tension increases during the contraction process. The muscles of the back contracts isometrically and constantly maintains the length of the muscles. In this way the body posture is maintained.

2. **Isotonic contractions:** In this type the amount of tension produced by the muscle is constant during contraction but the length of the muscle decreases. This is seen in the muscles of the arms and fingers when they are moved. There are two types of

isotonic contractions, one is concentric contraction and the other is eccentric contraction.

A combination of isometric and isotonic contractions are seen in most muscle contractions in which the muscle shorten some distance and the degree of tension increases.

Muscle tone : It refers to a sustained, partial contraction of portions of a resting skeletal or smooth muscle. This occurs in response to activation of streth receptors. At any instant, a few muscle fibres are contracted while most are relaxed. This small amount of contraction firms up a muscle without producing movement and is essential for maintaining posture.

Functions of muscle

1. Locomotor for walking.
2. Respiratory eg: the diaphragm.
3. Talking eg: Muscles of vocal cord.
4. Expression of emotion by facial muscles.
5. Propeltion of food in G-I tract is by smooth muscles.
6. Pumping of blood by cardiac muscle.
7. Urination by contraction of smooth muscle of the urinary bladder.

The skeletal muscles are sometimes named according to their shape as deltoid and trapezius, according to the direction of their fibres as rectus abdominis, according to the position of the muscle as pectoralis major, and according to their function, as flexor, extensor abductor and adductor. The muscles are usually attached to two definite points. The more fixed point is named as the origin, and the more movable part is named as insertion. The muscle fibres pass over the joint, so when the muscle contracts the movement takes place on that joint. At insertion point, the size of muscle decreases and ends as tendon. Most of the origin and insertion are attached to bony points. Each group of muscles opposes another are called Antagonist. Flexors are antagonists of extensors,abductors are antagonist to adductors.

Tendons are white glistening inelastic fibrous bands. They bind muscles to bones. Apponeuroses are flattened sheets or bands of fibrous tissue.

Facia : A sheath of fibrous tissue which envelops the body beneath the skin. (Superfical facia). It also encloses the muscles and groups of muscles and separates their several layers or groups. (Deep fascia).

Aponeurosis : A fibrous sheet or expanded tendon, giving attachment to muscular fibres and serving as the means of origin or insertion of a flat muscle. It sometimes also performs the function of a fascia for other muscles.

CHIEF MUSCLES OF THE BODY

1. Muscles that move the head

1. Sternocleidomastoid – Action explained in muscles of neck.

2. Semispinalis capitis – Both muscles extend head, contraction of one muscle rotates it to side opposite contracting muscle.

3. Splenius capitis – Both muscles, extend head; contraction of one muscle laterally flexes and rotates it to same side as contracting muscle.

4. Longissimus capitis	–	Extends head and rotates it to same side as contracting muscle.

2. Muscles of the face

These are the small muscles of facial expression and muscles around the opening on the mouth and eyes.

Zygomaticus major, and minor and so on : These small muscles take origin from the zygomatic bone and is inserted into the skin of the face. When they contract, face shows the feeling of the person, may be smiling, surprise or weeping, so whatever emotions can be shown on the face. Another muscle that controls the opening of eyelids against dust particles or sun's rays, is oribicualris occuli. Around the opening of the mouth, the oribicularis oris controls the opening, closing and use of the lips.

All the face muscles are supplied by 7th or facial nerve. Damage to this nerve causes facial palsy.

The muscles that move the tongue are

1. Genioglossus	–	Depresses tongue and thrusts it anteriorly. (Protraction)
2. Styloglossus	–	Elevates tongue and draws it posteriorly (Retraction)
3. Palatoglossus	–	Elevates posterior portion of tongue and draws soft palate inferiorly on tongue.
4. Hyoglossus	–	Depresses tongue and draws its sides inferiorly.

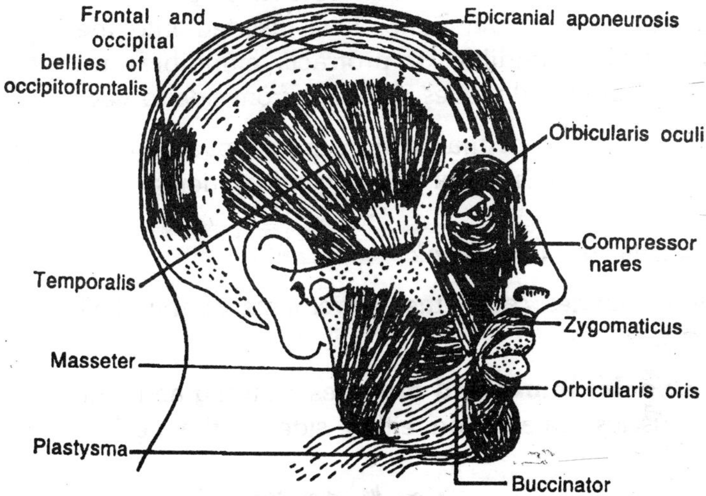

Figure 59. Muscles of the Head and Face

2. Muscles of mastication

They are masseter, temporalis, medial pterygoid and lateral pterygoid muscles.

Masseter : It arises from maxilla and zygomatic arch and is inserted into the angle and ramus of mandible. It elevates the mandible while closing the mouth. It also assists in side to side movements of mandible and protrudes the mandible.

Tamporalis: It is a fan shaped muscle. It arises from the temporal and frontal bones and inserted into the coronoid process and ramus of mandible. It elevates and retracts mandible and assists in side to side movements of mandible.

Medial pteryoid : It arises from the medial surface of lateral portion of pterygoid process of sphenoid bone and maxilla. It is inserted into the angle and ramus of mandible. It elevates and protracts mandible and moves mandible from side to side.

Lateral pterygoid : It arises from the greater wing and lateral surface of lateral portion of ptenygoid process of sphenoid bone. It is inserted into the condyle of mandible. It protracts mandible and opens mouth and moves mandible from side to side.

All the muscles of mastication are supplied by the mandibular division of the trigeminal nerve.

3. Muscles of the Neck

These muscles cause the movements of the skull and neck.

Sternocleidomastoid muscles : Strong and pair of muscles situated on either side of the neck.

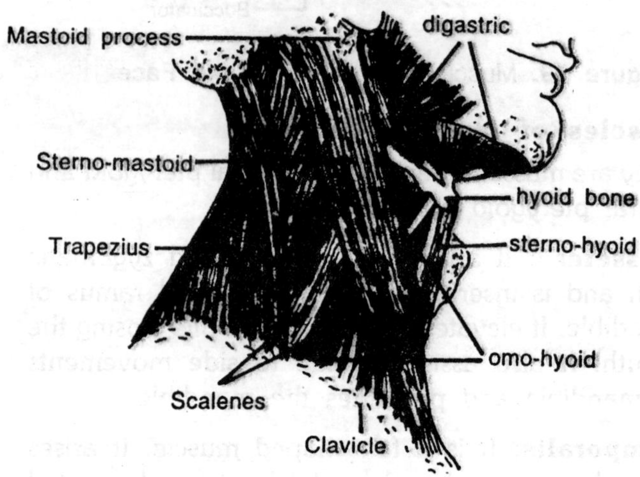

Figure 60. Muscles of the Neck

Each originates from the sternum and clavicle and ascends up and inserted into the mastoid process of the temporal bone. When it contracts on one side, side bending of the neck takes place, when both muscles contract they bend the head downwards. They are supplied by accessory nerve.

Trapezius muscle : It arises from the occipital bone, ligamentum nuchae, spines of seventh cervical and all thoracic vertebrae. It is inserted into clavicle and acromion and spine of scapula. It elevates clavicle, adducts scapula, rotates scapula superiorly, elevates or depresses scapula and extends head. It is supplied by accessory nerve and cervical nerves C_3 and C_4.

The prevertebral muscles : These are small muscles of the neck. Each muscle is connected between the bodies and transverse process of cervical vertebrae. When they contract just flexion of cervical vertebrae takes place.

THE MUSCLES OF THE UPPER LIMB

Scapular movements

The following muscles are attached to the scapula and cause its movement.

1. Trapezius - rotates scapula (elevates and depresses)
2. Levator scapulae - Elevates scapula
3. Rhomboids - Retracts scapula
4. Serratus arterior - Protracts scapula
5. Pectoralis minor - Depresses scapula

Muscles that move the Humerus

1. **Pectoralis major** - It arises from clavicle, sternum and cartilages of second to sixth ribs. It is inserted into greater tubercle and intertubercular sulcus of humerus. It flexes, adducts, and medially rotates the arm. It is supplied by medical and lateral pectoral nerves.

2. **Teres major** - Its origin is from the inferior angle of scapula. It is inserted into intertubercular groove of the humerus. It extends arm and assists in adduction and medial rotation of arm. It is supplied by lower scapular nerve.

3. **Latlissimus dorsi** - Its origin is from spines of inferior thoracic vertebrae, lumbar vertebrae, crests of sacrum and ilium and inferior four ribs. It is inserted into intertubercular groove of humerus. It extends, medially rotates and adducts arm. It is supplied by thoracodorsal nerve.

Rotator cuff muscles: They consist of four muscles. They attach the humerus to the scapula and form a cuff or cap over the proximal humerus. They are

1. **Infraspinatus muscle** - Its origin is from infraspinatus fossa of scapula. It is inserted into the greater tubercle of humerus. it rotates arm laterally and adducts arm. It is supplied by suprascapular nerve.

2. **Supraspinatus muscle:** Its origin is from supraspinatus fossa of scapula. It is inserted into the greater tubercle of humerus. It assists deltoid muscle in abducting arm. It is suppiled by suprascapular nerve.

3. **Subscapularis muscle:** Its origin is from subscapular fossa of scapula. It is inserted into the lesser tubercle of humerus. It rotates arm medially. It is supplied by upper and lower subscapular nerves.

4. **Teres minor:** Its origin is from inferior lateral border of scapula. It is inserted into greater tubercle of humerus. It rotates arm laterally, extends and adducts arm. It is supplied by axillary nerve.

If there is injury to rotator cuff, one or more of these muscles or their tendons may be damaged.

The deltoid muscle covers the shoulder region and gives round appearance to shoulder region. Its origin is from the clavicle and the fibres fuse on the lateral side and descends on upper lateral side of the arm and inserted into the deltoid tuberosity of the humerus. The nerve supply is by the circumflex nerve. The function is abductor of the upper limb at the shoulder joint.

Clinical Anatomy: Intra muscular injection is given to Deltoid muscle. If the needle of the syringe damages the nerve, then there will be paralysis of the Deltoid muscle.

Muscles of the arm: The arm is divided into anterior or flexor and posterior or extensor compartment by deep fascia of the arm.

Flexor compartment: These muscles act on both shoulder and elbow joint as flexor of arm at shoulder and flexor of arm at elbow joint. The muscles are, coraco-brachialis, biceps brachii and brachialis muscles.

The Biceps brachii muscle: It acts on both shoulder and elbow joints, it has 2 heads of origin,

1. The long head arises from the supraglenoid tubercle of scapula.
2. The short head arises from the tip of the coracoid process of scapula.Both heads fuse to form a bulky muscle and tapers to form a tendon downwards and inserted into the radial tuberosity of the radius below the neck of the radius.

Action

1. Flexor of the upper limb at the shoulder joint.
2. Flexior of the fore-arm at the elbow joint.
3. The screwing movement at the superior - radial ulnar joint when the fore-arm is semiflexed.
4. Powerful supinator at the superio-radial ulnar joint when the fore-arm is semiflexed.

Nerve supply: The musculo-cuatenous nerve supplies the biceps and all other muscles of the anterior compartment. Brachialis and brachioradialis muscles also flex the forearm

Extensor compartment: The muscle in this compartment is the triceps bracii. Triceps means 3 heads of origin,

1. The long head arises from infraglenoid tubercle of the scapula,
2. The lateral head arises from the posterior surface of humerus.
3. The medial head arises from the lower posterior surface of the Humerus.

This is the thick bulky muscle that one can feel.

Insertion: It is inserted into the upper surface of olecranon process of the ulna.

Nerve supply: The radial nerve.

Action: Extensor of the fore arm at the elbow joint

Anconeus is another muscle which extends the forearm. It is also supplied by radial nerve.

4. Muscles of the fore arm

The fore arm having two compartments on cross section, the anterior or flexor compartment and the posterior or extensor compartment.

Flexor Muscles : This group of muscles act at the wrist joint, carpo-meta-carpal joints, metacarpo-phalangeal joints and inter phalangeal joints.

Action : Flexion at all the above joints.

Nerve Supply : All the muscles of forearm except flexor carpi ulnaris is supplied by median nerve. Flexor carpi ulnaris is supplied by ulnar nerve.

Extensor Muscles: The extensor muscles act at the wrist joint, the carpo-meta carpal joints, metacarpo-phalangeal joints and interphalangeal joints.

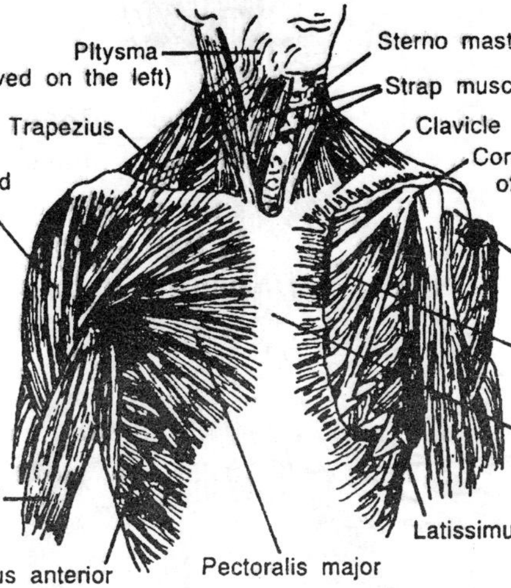

Figure 61. Muscles of neck, chest and arm

Nerve supply: The Radial Nerve.

Trunk Muscles

It is further divided into the muscles of the vertebral column, thorax, abdominal wall and pelvic floor. The diaphragm is in between the thoracic and abdominal cavities.

Back Muscles that move the vertebral column

The back muscles are very strong to maintain erect posture. There are twentyone pairs of muscles that move the vertebral column. They are very complex because they have multiple origins and insertions and there is considerable overlap among them. Two important groups of muscles are explained below.

1. **The erector spinae:** This is the largest muscular mass of the back and consists of three groups of muscles. They arise from vertebrae and pelvis and inserted into superior vertebrae and ribs. They extends the vertebral column.

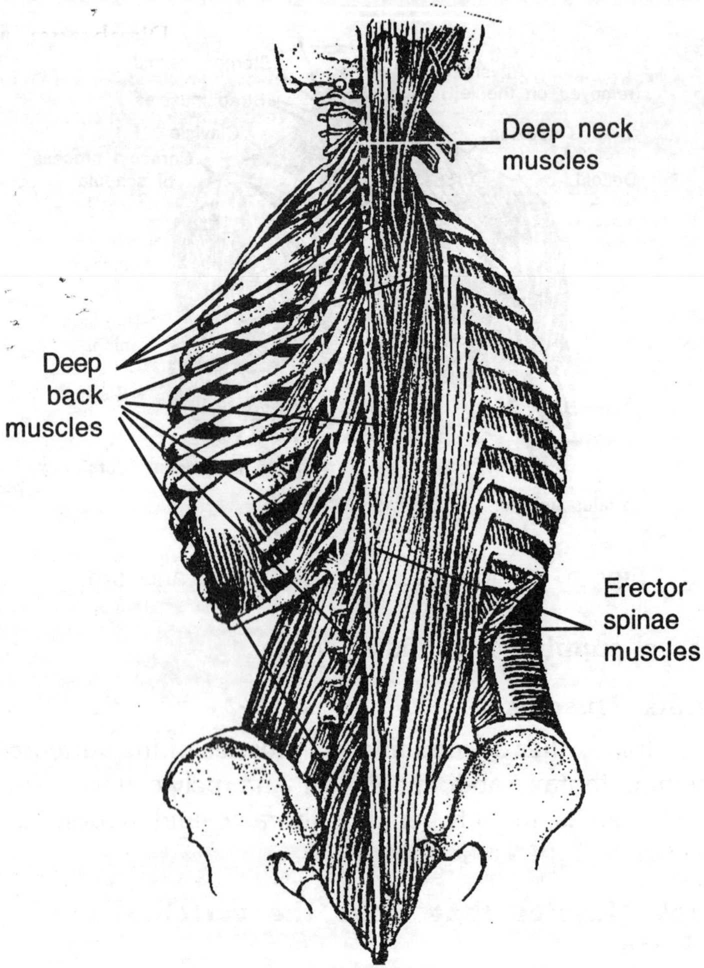

Figure 62. Muscles of the back, seen from a posterior view

2. Deep back muscles. They arise from the vertebrae and inserted into vertebrae. They extend the vertebral column and help bend vertebral column laterally.

The rectus abdominus, external oblique, internal oblique quadratus lumborium, psoas and iliacus muscles also play a role in moving the vertebral column.

Muscles of Respiration

The chest cavity is made up of 12 pairs of ribs. The space in between the ribs is called intercostal space. This space is filled by intercostal muscles. The muscles of respiration are

External intercostal muscles	11 pairs increase the dimension of thorax
Internal intercostal muscles	11 pairs decrease the dimensions of thorax.
Diaphragm	1

Origin and insertion of intercostal muscles are to the adjacent ribs.

Function: Respiratory muscles of the thoracic cavity.

Nerve supply: The intercostal nerves

In asthmatic respiration, the intercostal space is deepened.

Diaphragm

The Diaphragm is a dome shaped musculo - tendinous structure separating the thoracic cavity from the abdominal cavity. It forms the floor of the former and the roof of the later cavity.

It arises from the bodies of lumbar vertebrae by means of crura and from the posterior surface of the xiphoid process and from the inner surface of the lower 6 pairs of ribs and insertion or converge to form central tendinous portion.

Function: In inspiration, contraction of the muscle flattens the dome of diaphragm so enlarging vertical diameter of the thoracic cavity. In expiration, the muscle fibres of the diaphragm relax, the dome rises and as the size of the thoracic cavity is decreased and air is forced out of the lungs.

Diaphragm also assists in the acts of micturition, defaecation and in parturition.

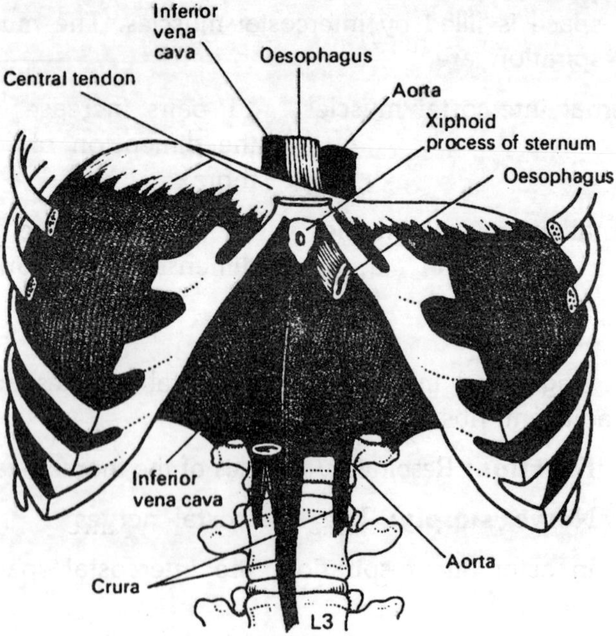

Figure 63. Diaphragm

Openings: There are 3 openings in the diaphragm

1. The aortic opening for the passage of the aorta and thoracic duct which lies behind it.
2. Oesophageal opening through which oesophagus and vagus nerve pass.
3. Caval opening through which inferior vena cava passes.

Relations: Above or superiorly, pericardium and heart, the bases of right and left lungs and their pleural coverings.

Below or inferiorly, the liver, stomach, spleen, supra renal glands and kidneys.

Nerve supply: Phrenic and lower six intercostal nerves.

Muscles of the Abdominal wall

The muscles of the anterior abdominal wall flex and rotate the vertebral column and compresses the abdominal cavity. They also hold in and protect the abdominal organs. Linea alba is the tendinous area of the abdomnal wall that extends from the xiphoid process of the sternum to the symphysis pubis.

1. **Rectus abdominus:** It arises from the pubis and inserted into cartilages of fifth to seventh ribs and xiphoid process. It flexes the vertebral column
2. **External oblique:** It arises from inferior eight ribs. It is inserted into iliac crest and linea alba. Both muscles contract and compress abdomen. Contraction of one muscle flexes and rotates vertebral column.
3. **Internal oblique:** It arises from pelvis and is inserted into the cartilages of inferior three or four ribs and linea alba. It compresses abdomen, flexes and rotates vertebral column.
4. **Transversus abdominus:** It arises from vertebrae, pelvis and ribs. It is inserted into xiphoid preocess, linea alba and pubis. It compreses abdomen.

   They are supplied by brancles of lower thoracic vertebral nerves.

   Quadratus lumborum : It arises from iliac crest and iliolumbar ligament. It is inserted into inferior border of twelfth rib and transverse processes of first four lumbar vetebrae. It acts on the twelfth rib during inspiration and expiration. Contraction of one side bends vertebral column laterally.

Function

1. They give strength to the abdominal wall.
2. They protect abdominal viscera.

Any weakness in the abdominal wall, the contents

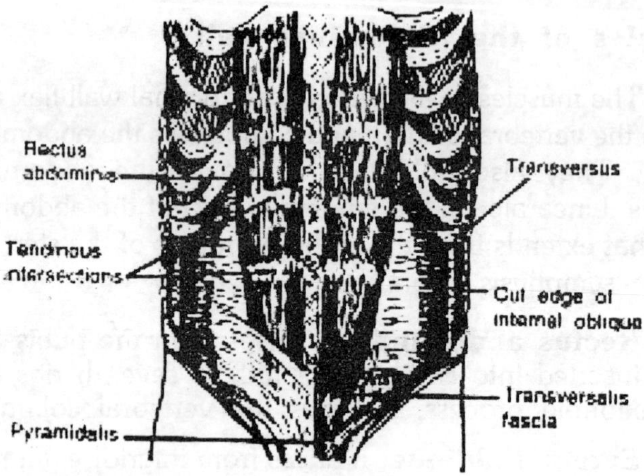

Figure 64. Muscles of anterior abdominal wall

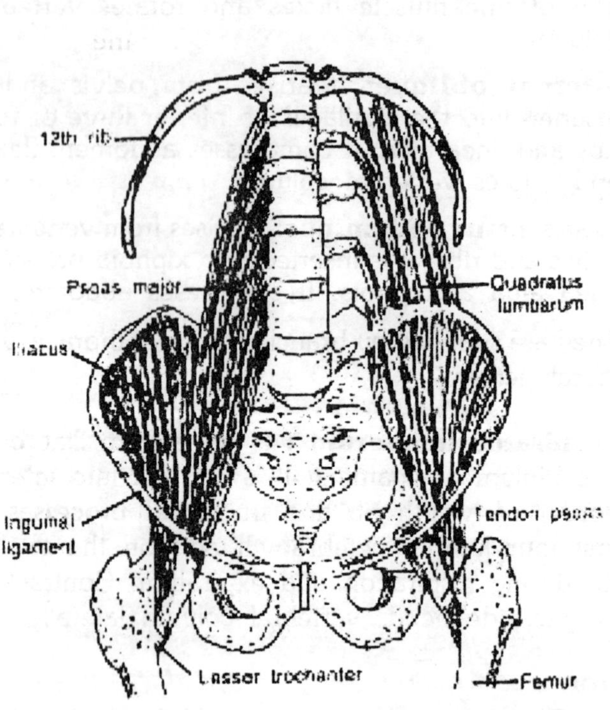

Figure 65. Muscles of the posterior abdominal wall and pelvis which felx the hip joint

protrude out i.e., called hernia. If weakness around umbilicus causes protrusion which is called umbilical hernia.

Inguinal hernia

Some times the abdominal contents pass through inguinal canal. The canal extends between superficial inguinal ring and deep inguinal ring. The canal is just above the inguinal ligament. Protrusion of abdominal content/s at inguinal region or superficial inguinal ring is called inguinal hernia.

Muscles of pelvic cavity — **Levator Ani** / **Cossygeus**

The levator Ani is the muscle at the outlet of pelvic cavity forms the pelvic diaphragm. It is attached to coccyx, ischium and pubis. It is pierced in the median plane.

In male -
1. Urethral orifice.
2. Anal orifice.

In female -
1. Urethral orifice.
2. Vaginal orifice.
3. Anal orifice.

In female this muscle plays an important role in expelling the foetus during parturition. Any damage to this muscle in female causes prolapse of the uterus, and in both sexes prolapse of rectum occurs.

Lavetor ani is divisible into two parts, the puboccygeus muscle and iliococcygeus muscle.

Coccygeus

It assists in raising and supporting the pelvic floor. It resists intra abdominal pressure and pulls coccyx anteriorly after defaecation and parturition (child birth)

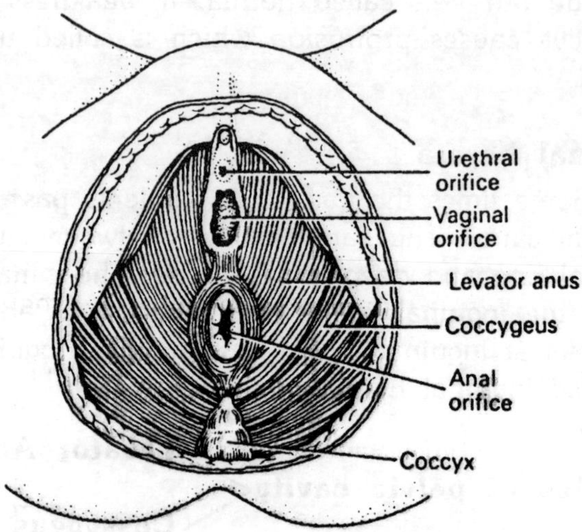

Figure 66. Muscles of the pelvic floor

6. Muscles of the lower limb

The muscles of the lower limb include the muscles of the hip, thigh, leg and foot. They help in locomotion, stability and equilibrium. Any damage to the muscles of the lower limb will change the manner of walking (gait) i.e., pathological walk.

a) Ilio-psoas muscle

It consissts of two muscles, psoas muscle and iliacus muscle.

1. **Psoas muscle :** It arises from the lumbar certebrae. It forms part of the posterior abdominal wall. It is inserted into the lesser trochanter of the femur. It is supplied by 1.2 – 1.3 lumbar nerves.
2. **Iliacus muscle:** It arises from iliac fossa and it is inserted into the tendon of psoas muscle. It is supplied by the femoral nerve.

Both muscles flex and rotate thigh laterally. They also flex the vertebral column.

b) Gluteal Muscles

The gluteal muscles are

1. Gluteus Maximus
2. Gluteus Medius
3. Gluteus Minimus

Gluteas maximus : It arises from the iliac crest, sacrum and coccyx. It is inserted into the iliotibial tract of tensor fascia lata and linea aspera of femur. It extends and rotates thigh laterally. It is supplied by inferior gluteal nerve.

Gluteus medius and Minimus : They arise from ilium. They are inserted into the greater trochanter of femur. They abduct and rotate thigh laterally. They are supplied by superior gluteal nerve.

Usually intramuscular injections are given into the superolateral quadrant of gluteal muscle i.e., to gluteus medius muscle where no damage is done to the sciatic nerve and other nerves and gluteal arteries.

c) Muscles of the thigh

The thigh has three compartments

1. Extensor or Anterior
2. Flexor or posterior
3. Adductor or medial

Extensor muscles: The extensor (anterior) compartment of the thigh has quadriceps femoris muscle. It is made up of 4 muscles i.e., Rectus femoris, 3 vasti muscles. (Vastus medialis, Vastus intermedius and Vastus lateralis) They unite to form a single muscle. The tendon of qudriceps femoris muscle is attached to patella, below this bone, there is a tendon called ligamentum patella which is inserted to the tubercle of the tibia.

Function: Extends the leg at knee joint.

Nerve supply: Femoral nerve.

Sartorius : It is the longest muscle in the body. It arises from the anterior superior iliac spine and inserted into the medial side of the tuberosity of the tibia. It belongs to the anterior compartment even though it flexes the limb. During walking it flexes simultaneously at hip joint and at the knee joint.

Nerve Supply: Femoral nerve.

Flexor (posterior) compartment: This is made of 3 strong muscles called Biceps femoris, semimembranosus and semitendinosus. These are also called the hamstring group.

Function: Flexor of the leg at knee joint.

Nerve supply: Sciatic nerve.

Adductor Compartment: The muscles in this compartment are

1. Adductor longus
2. Adductor brevis
3. Adductor magnus

Function: They are the adductors of the thigh at the hip joint.

Nerve Supply: Obturator nerve.

d) Muscles of the leg

The leg is also having 3 compartments

1. Extensor or Anterior
2. Flexor or Posterior
3. Peroneal or Lateral

Extensor Compartment (Anterior Compartment) has 4 muscles, tibialis anterior, extensor hallucis longus, extensor digitorium longus and peroneus tertius.

Function: Dorsiflexion of the foot at the ankle joint.

Nerve supply: Anterior tibial or deep peroneal nerve.

Flexor Compartment (Posterior Compartment) : This compartment has 2 strata of muscles. they are,

1. Superficial or calf muscles (gastrocnemius)
2. Deep muscles.

Superficial muscles of flexor compartment are very prominent called calf muscles.

They help to propel blood towards the heart. The muscles are two in number.

Flexor compartment consists of gastrocnemius, soleus and plantaris muscles.

Function: Help in walking, running,

All the 3 muscles fuse to form the tendon of Achilles or tendocalcaneous, and inserted into posterior surface of the calcaneum. This tendon can be palpated easily in living anatomy. If this tendon is cut, one cannot walk.

Nerve Supply: By tibial nerve.

Deep muscles of flexor compartment

1. **Popliteus :** It arises from lateral condyle of femur. It is inserted into proximal tibia. It flexes and medially rotates the leg. It is supplied by tibial nerve.
2. **Flexor hallucis longus :** It arises from inferior two thirds of fibula. It is inserted into distal phalanx of great toe.
3. **Flexor digitorum longus:** It arises from posterior surface of tibia. It is inserted into distal phalanges of four outer toes.
4. **Tibialis posterior :** It arises from tibia, fibula and interosseous membrance. It is inserted into second, third and fourth metatarsals, navicular, all three cuneiform bones and cuboid.

All the above three muscles plantar flex and inverts foot. All are supplied by the tibial nerve.

Peroneal (lateral) compartment muscles:

1. **Peroneus longus** : It arises from head and body of fibula and lateral condyle of tibia. It is inserted into first metatarsal and first cuneiform bones.

2. **Peroneus bravis** : It arises from body of fibula. It is inserted into fifth metatarsal bone.

All the two muscles plantar flex and evert foot. They are supplied by superficial peroneal nerve.

ANATOMICAL SPACES

1. **The axilla is a pyramidal** shaped space between the side of the arm and lateral wall of chest wall. The axilla contains the axillary vessels, the axillary lymph nodes and the brachial plexus of nerves. The axilla also contains a prolongation of the breast in the female known as the axillary tail. For any pathology of the breast one should palpate the axillary lymph nodes.

2. **The cubital fossa:** This space is present in front of the elbow joint. It is bounded above by imaginary line between two condyles of humerus. The medial boundary is formed by pronator teres muscle and laterally by brachioradialis muscle. The floor is formed by brachialis muscle. The contents are

    1. Termination of brachial artery.
    2. Beginning of radial and ulnar arteries.
    3. Tendon of biceps.
    4. The median nerve.

3. **The Femoral triangle**: Just below the inguinal ligament is the base, the apex is the meeting place of the sartorius and adductor longus muscle.

Laterally, it is bounded by sartorius and medially by adductor longus muscles. The floor is formed by deep fascia. The roof is formed by skin and superficial fascia.

Contents:

1. Femoral nerve.
2. Femoral vessels and great sephaneous vein.
3. Inguinal lymph nodes.

4 **The sub sartorial (hunter's) canal:** The apex of the femoral triangle is running as passage for vessels and nerve along the front and medial aspect of the thigh to reach the back. It extends to form femoral triangle to the popliteal fossa.

5. **Popliteal fossa:** This fossa is at the back of the knee joint. It is diamond shaped and bounded above by the medial and lateral sides by the hamstring muscles, below by medial and lateral heads of gastrocnemius muscle.

Contents:

1. Popliteal vessels
2. Distal end of sciatic nerve and its divsion
3. Popliteal lymph nodes.

Questions

1. Draw a diagram of a muscle fibre and name its parts and briefly describe.
2. Give an account of the structure and function of the neuromuscular junction.
3. State the function of whole muscle.
4. Describe the diaphragm with a neat diagram.
5. What movements are possible at the shoulder joint? What muscles accomplish these movements?

6. Describe the muscles that move the femur.

7. Write short notes on

   a) Muscles of martication

   b) Muscles of the pelvic floor

   c) The cubital fossa.

   d) Superficial muscles forming the posterior compartment of leg.

UNIT 5

The Nervous system

The nervous system is specilalized to reveive sensations to interpret them and to conduct nerve impulses for action. All mental activitives such as consciousness, thinking, reasoning and judgement etc. are seated in the nervous system. The body's major regulatory and co-ordinating functions are centered in the nervous system. (The other being the endocrine system).

The Nervous system is divided under the following headings.

1. The central nervous system consisting of the brain and the spinal cord.
2. The peripheral nervous system
   31 pairs of spinal nerves.
   12 pairs of cranial nerves.
3. The autonomic nervous system
   Sympathetic system
   Parasympathetic system.

Basic study of the nervous system

The nervous system consists of a vast number of units called Neurons, supported by a special type of

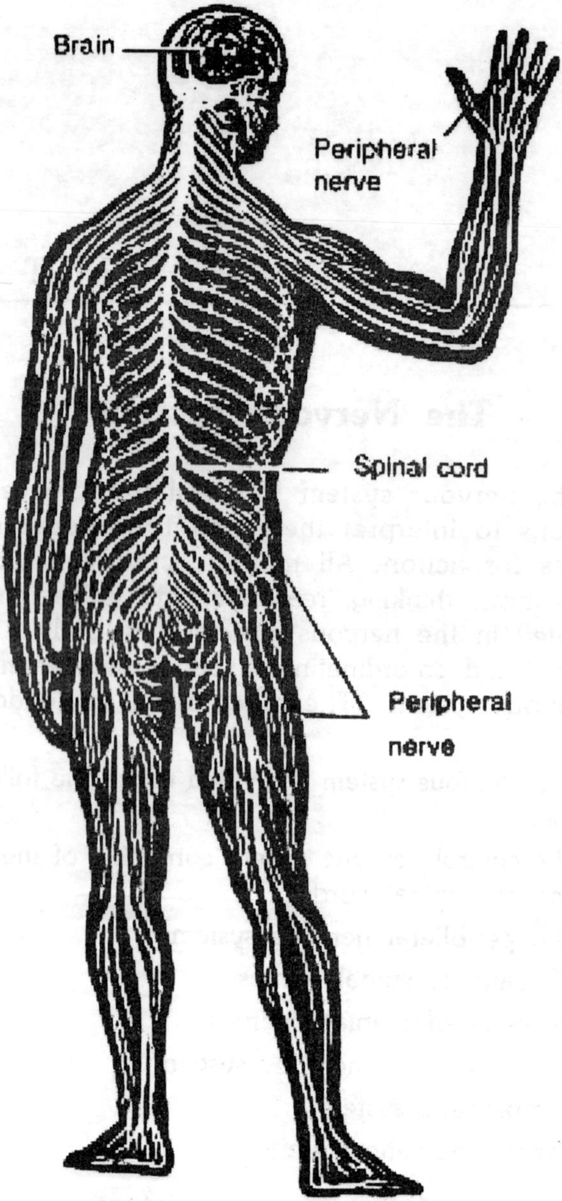

Figure 67. Nervous system

connective tissue, Neuroglia. The unit of the nervous system is a neuron. The types of neurons are

1. Multipolar
2. Bipolor
3. Unipolar.

Neuron : A nerve cell with its processes (axon and dendrites) is called a neuron.

The nerve cell contains a nucleus and cytoplasm which surrounds the nuecleus. The cytoplasm contains organelles such as mitochondria, golgi apparatus and lysosomes. Many neurons contain yellowish brown granuels called lipofuscin pigment, neurofibrils and Nissl bodies. Nissl bodies are the site of protein synthesis. Neurofibrils, composed of intermediate filaments, form the cytoskeleton, which provides support and shape for the cell.

The nerve cells vary considerably in size and shape. The nerve cell can not be seen by naked eye. The nerve cells collect to form grey matter in the central nervous system, and are found at the periphery (cortex) of the brain, inside the brain (in medulla) as islands of grey matter and in the centre of the spinal cord. Out side the central nervous system, they are arranged in groups called 'Ganglia'. Each nerve cell has processes called axon and dendrites. Axon and dendrites are extensions of the nerve cells and form white matter of the central nervous system. In dentrites, the impulse passes towards cell and in axons impulse passes from cell to cell or to tissue. Both are referred to as nerve fibres.

Axons

Each nerve cell has only one axon, carrying nerve impulses away from the cell. The axons are usually longer than dendrities. The length may vary from 10mm to as long as 100 cms.

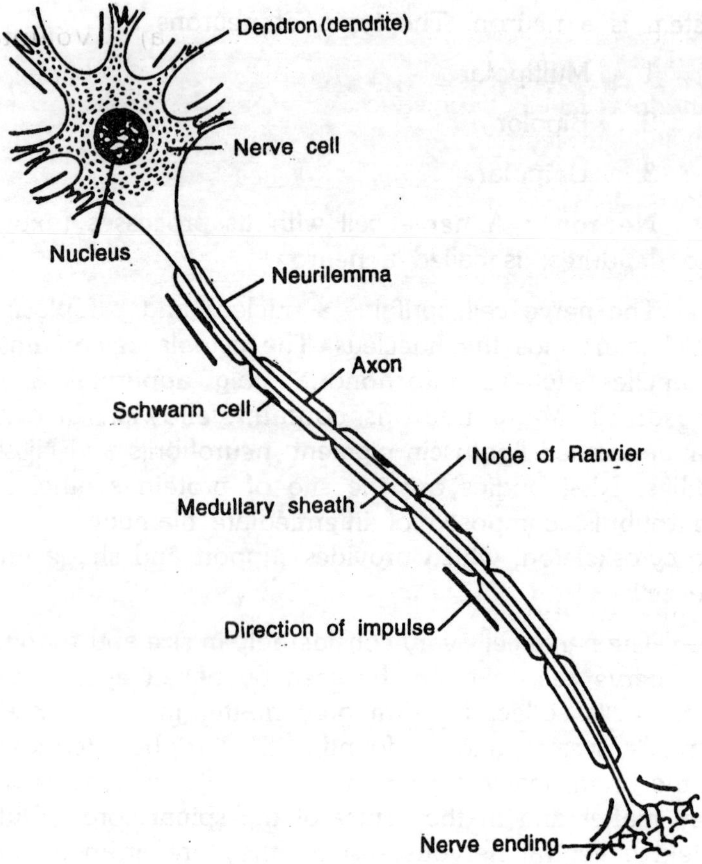

Figure 68. A Neuron

Structure of an axon

It is the extension of cystoplasm (somata) of the nerve cell. The membrane of the axon is called axolemma. Large axons and those of peripheral nerves are divided into myelinated and non-myelinated nerve fibres. The myelinated fibres are surrounded by a myelin sheath. This consists of a series of Schwann's cells, arranged along the length of the axon, so that, it is covered by a number of concentric layers of Schwann cell plasma membrane. Between the layers or plasma membrane, there is a small amount of fatty substance called Myelin. The outermost layer of Schwann cell has a plasma membrane called Neurolemma. Between adjacent schwann cells, the myelin sheath inter digitates called Nodes of Ranvier. Non-myelinated fibres have only Schwann cell plasma membrane covering, where, there is no myelin deposit. Axons of the central nervous system are myelinated by oligodendrocytes.

Dendrites

The dendrites are the processes or nerve fibres which carry impulse towards cell body. They are shorter and branching. Each neuron has many dendrites.

Types of nerves

1. **Sensory or afferent nerves:** These fibres transmit impulses from the periphery of the body to the spinal cord, or to connector neuron of reflex arcs.
    a) Somatic, cutaneous or both senses, originating in the skin, are pain, touch, heat and cold.
    b) Special senses are sight, hearing, smell and taste.
    c) Proprioceptor senses originating from the muscle tendon and joints contribute to the maintainance of equilibrium and posture.
    d) Autonomic afferent nerves originate in internal organs, glands and tissues and are associated with reflex regulation of activity and visceral pain.
2. **Motor or Efferent Nerves:** Motor nerves originate in the brain, spinal cord and autonomic ganglia. They are concerned with

a) Voluntary and reflex skeletal muscle contractions.

b) Involuntary (autonomic) i.e., smooth muscle contractions of G-I tract or Respiratory system.

c) Secreto motor to stimulate glands to secrete.

3. **Mixed nerves:** Both components are present in single nerve called mixed nerves. eg : Spinal nerves contain both motor or sensory fibres.

4. **Termination of nerves:** The sensory nerves, eg in the skin lose their myelin sheath and divide into fine branching filaments, the sensory nerve endings. These endings are stimulated in the skin by touch, pain, heat and cold. The impulse is then transmitted to the brain.

The motor nerves, conveying impulses to skeletal muscles to produce contractions, divide into fine filaments and end in minute pads called Motor end plates where the nerve fibres reach the muscle. In these nerve fibres the myelin sheath is absent. Each muscle fibre is stimulated through a single motor end-plate and one motor nerve has many motor end-plates. The nerve impulse is passed across the gap between the motor end plate and the muscle fibre by the neurotransmitter, Acetylcholine.

A motor unit means a group of muscle fibres with their motor end plates.

The endings at autonomic nerves supplying smooth muscles and glands branch near their effector structure and release a transmitter substance which may stimulate or decrease the activity of the structure.

Properties of nerve tissue

Nerve fibres has 2 characters, one is irritability and another conductivity.

Irritability is the ability to initiate nerve impulse, is exposed to stimuli forms.

1. Outside the body, eg: pain, touch.
2. Inside the body, eg: concentration of carbon-di-oxide in the blood to increase respiratory movements.

Conductivity means the ability to transmit an impulse from

1. One part of the brain to another
2. The brain to skeletal muscles.
3. Proprioceptor impulse to the brain.
4. The brain to organs of the body i.e., smooth muscles of G.I.tract and to glands to secrete.
5. Viscera to brain in association with the regulation of body functions.
6. To brain through sensory nerve endings in the skin are stimulated by temperature, pain and touch.
7. To brain through the special sense organs i.e., eyes, ears, nose and tongue.

SYNAPSE AND CHEMICAL TRANSMITTERS

There is always more than one neuron involved in the transmission of a nerve impulse from its origin to its destination whether it is sensory or motor. There is no anatomical continuity between these neurons, the point at which the nerve impulse passes from one to another, is the synapse. At its free end the axon, of one neuron breaks up into minute branches which terminate in small swelling called pre-synaptic knobs. They are in close proximity to the dendrites, or the cell body of the next neuron. The space between them is the synaptic cleft. At the ends of presynaptic knobs contain chemical transmitters which carry nerve impulses across synaptic clefts. These neurotransmitters are secreted by the nerve cells, actively transported along axons and stored in synaptic vesicles.

The neurotransmitters are, noradrenaline, gamma-aminobutyric acid, and acetylcholine. Other substances, such as dopamine and serotonin may have similar functions.

Neuroglia

The neurons of the central nervous system are supported by connective tissue cells. There are six types of neuroglial cells. Unlike nerve cells, these continue to replicate throughout life. They are macroglial cells namely astrocytes and oligodendrocytes and microglial cells and ependymal cells. The above four types are found in the central nervous system.

1. **Astrocytes**

   These cells form main supporting tissue of the central nervous system. They are star-shaped with branching processes. At the free ends of some of the processes, there are small swellings called 'foot processes'. These cells are found in large numbers near the blood vessels with their foot processes forming a sleeve round them. Astrocytes foot processes and capillary membrane constitute the blood-brain barrier.

2. **Oligo dendrocytes** are smaller than astrocytes.

   They are found

   a) Around the neuron cell walls in the grey matter.

   b) Adjacent fibres in CNS to myelinate.

3. **Microglial cells** are derived from monocytes that migrate from blood into the nervous system before birth. They are found mainly in the area of blood capillaries and act as phagocytes. They clear away debris from dead cells.

4. **Ependymal cells** are epithelial cells. Their shape is cuboidal and columnar and many cells have celia. They line the ventricles of the brain and the central canal of the spinal cord. They form cerebrospinal fluid and assist its circulation.

The other two types of neuroglia are found in the peripheral nervous system (P.N.S.). They are supporting cells.

5. **Schwann cells or neurolemmocytes**

They produce myelin sheaths around the neurons of P.N.S.

6. **Satellite cells** : They support neurons in ganglia of P.N.S.

THE CENTRAL NERVOUS SYSTEM

The brain and the spinal cord are completely covered by 3 membranes, the meninges, lying between the skull and the brain, and between the vertebrae and the spinal cord, named from outside inwards.

Dura mater

Arachnoid mater and

Pia mater

The dura and arachnoid maters are separated by potential space called the subdural space. The space between the arachnoid and piamater, is called subarachnoid space which contains cerebro spinal fluid.

Dura mater: The cerebral dura mater consists of 2 layers of dense fibrous tissue, the outer layer is firmly attached periosteum of the skull called endosteum and the inner layer provides a protective covering to the brain. There is only a potential space between these two layers and this space contains venous sinuses. The inner layer reduplicates to form folds. In between the cerebral hemispheres the fold is called the falx cerebri and between the cerebrum and cerebellum the fold is called Tentorium cerebelli.

Venous drainage from the brain: The blood from the brain drains into venous sinuses found between the dural layers. The superior and inferior sagittal sinuses are in the falx cerebri, the straight and transverse sinuses are in the tentorium cerebelli.

Spinal dura mater: It forms sheath, surrounds the spinal cord, extending from the foramen magnum to the second sacral vertebra. Afterwards it covers the filum terminale and fuses with periosteum of the coccyx. Superiorly, it is the extension of inner dura mater of cranial cavity. It is separated from the periosteum of the vertebrae and ligaments within vertebrae. The space between vertebrae and duramater is called Epidural or Extradural space containing venous anastomotic channels and adipose tissue. It is attached to the margin of formen magnum, and to posterior longitudinal ligaments. These attachments stabilise the dura mater and spinal cord.

Arachnoid mater: This delicate transparent serous membrane lies between the dura and the piamater. It is separated from the dura mater by the sub dural space and from the piamater by the sub-arachnoid space containing cerebro spinal fluid. The arachnoid mater passes over the convolutions of the brain and the inner layers of dura mater in the formation of falx cerebri, tentorium cerebelli, and falx cerebelli. It extends downwards to cover the spinal cord and ends at the 2nd sacral vertebra.

Pia mater: This is a fine membrane closely invests the brain, completely covers the convolutions and dips into each fissure. It is pierced by many minute blood vessels. It continues downwards to cover the spinal cord and at the level of 2nd sacral vertebra. It pierces the arachnoid tube and goes on with the duramater to fuse with the periosteum of the coccyx.

VENTRICLES OF THE BRAIN

Within the brain, there are 4 cavities called ventricles containing cerebro spinal fluid.

Right and left ventricles (lateral)

3rd ventricle and 4th ventricle

The lateral ventricles lie within the cerebral hemispheres, one on each side of the median plane just below the corpus callosum and are separated from each other by a thin membrane, the septum lucidum. They communicate with the 3rd ventricle by inter ventricular formina, a pair of oval openings (foramina of Monro).

The third ventricle is situated below the lateral ventricles between the two parts of the thalamus.

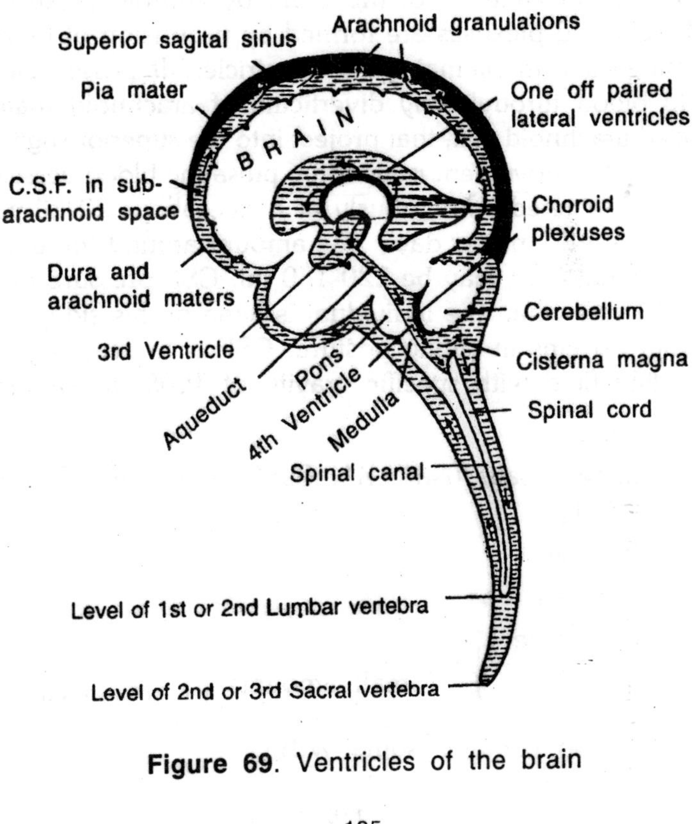

Figure 69. Ventricles of the brain

It communicates with the 4th ventricle through a canal called the cerebral aqueduct (acqueduct of Sylvius).

The 4th ventricle is a diamond shaped cavity situated posterior to the medulla oblongata and posterior to cerebellum. It communicates with the central canal of the spinal cord, and also communicates with the sub archnoid spaces by means of 3 foramina [foramen of Megendie and foramina of Lushka (Paired)]in the roof of the ventricle. Through these foramina only ventricular CSF flows into subarchnoid space around the brain and the spinal cord.

THE CEREBROSPINAL FLUID

Cerebrospinal fluid is continuously secreted into each lateral ventricle of the brain by choroid plexuses. The choroid plexuses are formed by protrusion of blood capillaries with piamater into ventricles. It passes back into blood through tiny diverticula of arachnoid mater called arachnoid villi, that project into the superior sagittal sinus. CSF movement is aided by pulsating blood vessels. CSF is secreted continuously at a rate about 20 ml per hour i.e. 480 ml per day. The amount around the brain and spinal cord may be 120-150 ml. CSF pressure may be 10 cms when the individual is lying on his side, and about 30 cms in sitting posture. CSF is a clear slightly alkaline fluid with specific gravity of 1005. It contains

water

mineral salts (Na^+, K^+, Ca^{2+}, Mg^{2+} and Cl^- and HCO_3)

glucose

Proteins

creatinine }
urea } (Small amounts)

It also contains some W.B.C^S.

C.S.F. is gruadually reabsorbed back into the blood through arachnoid villi. The arachnoid villi project into the dural venous sinuses especially the superior saggital sinus. Normally, C.S.F. is reabsorbed at a rate equal to its production (20 ml/hr or 480 ml/day) and therefore the pressure of C.S.F. is normally constant.

Functions of C.S.F.

1. It supports and protects the brain and spinal cord.
2. It maintains uniform pressure.
3. It acts as cushion and shock absorber.
4. There is inter change of substances between CSF and nerve cells. (nutrients and waste products)
5. It provides an optimal chemical environment for normal neuronal signalling.

THE BRAIN

The brain lies within the cranial cavity. The different parts are

Forebrain - Cerebrum
Thalamus
Midbrain - Midbrain
Hindbrain - Pons
Medulla Oblangata (Brainstem).
Cerebellum

Cerebrum

It is the largest part of the brain and occupies the anterior and middle cranial fossae of the cranial cavity. There are two parts i.e. right and left cerebral hemispheres. Both are connected in the centre by carpus callosum. Both hemispheres are separated by a fold of duramater called falx cerebri. On cross section the superficial part is composed of nerve cells of grey matter (cortex). The deeper part consists of white matter. The outer or external surface of cerebral cortex shows many

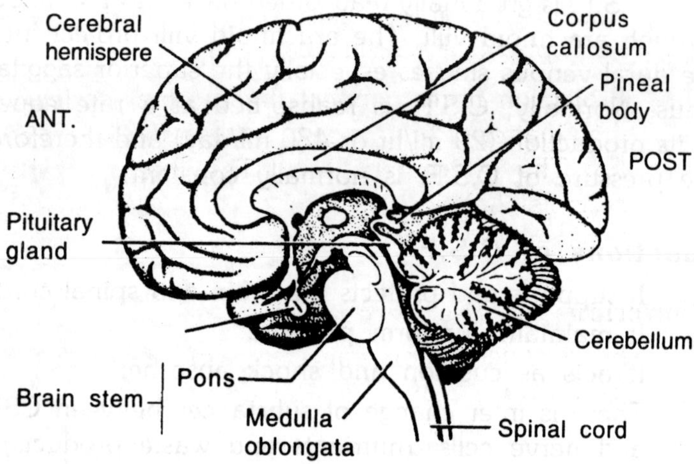

Figure 70. The brain

infoldings. These are separated by sulci or fissures. These convolutions greatly increase the surface area of the cerebrum. The elevations are called as gyri.

For descriptive purpose, each cerebral hemisphere is divided into lobes, which takes the names of the bones of the cranium.

Frontal Lobe
Parietal Lobe
Temporal Lobe
Occipital Lobe

The boundaries of the lobes are marked by sulci. These are, central, lateral and parieto-occipital sulci.

Interior of cerebrum

Inside, it is composed of nerve cells and fibres, and the lobes are connected by masses of nerve fibres or tracts. The afferent and efferent nerve fibres connect the different parts of the brain and spinal cord.

1. Association fibres which connect different parts of the cerebral cortex by means of one gyrus to another gyrus.

2. Commissural fibres which connects the two cerebral hemispheres. (corpus callosum).

3. Projection fibres connect the cerebral cortex with grey matter of brain stem and with the spinal cord. Eg: The internal capsule. The internal capsule consists of projection fibres, and is within the brain between the basal ganglia and the thalamus.

Functions of the cerebrum

1. Sensory perception, pain, temperature, touch, sight, hearing, taste and smell. These are the functions of sensory areas.

2. Initiation and control of voluntary muscle contractions are the functions of motor areas.

3. More complex integrative functions such as memory, emotions, thinking, reasoning, will, judgement, personality traits and intelligence are dealt with by the association areas.

4. The limbic system, together with hypothalamus governs emotional aspects of behavier such as pain, pleasure, anger, rage, fear, sorrow, sexual feelings, docility and affection. Therefore it is called as "emotional" brain.

Areas of the cerebrum

The main areas of the cerebrum are associated with sensory, voluntary motor activity and more complex integrative functions. (mentioned above)

1. **Precentral (motor) area** lies in the frontal lobe immediately anterior to the central sulcus.

The neurons initiate the contraction of voluntary muscles. A nerve fibre from a neuron passes downwards through the internal capsule to the medulla oblangata, where it crosses to the opposite side, then descends in the spinal cord, at the different level in the spinal cord. The nerve impulse crosses a synapse to stimulate a second neuron, which terminates at the motor end-plate of a muscle fibre. The motor area of the right hemisphere of the cerebrum controls voluntary muscle movement of the left side of the body and vice versa. The neuron in the cerebrum is the upper motor neuron and the other in the spinal cord is the lower motor neuron. Damage to either of these neurons may result in paralysis. In the motor area of the cerebrum the body is represented upside down ie., the cells nearest the cortex control the feet and those in the lowest part control the head, neck, face and fingers. (see the figures.)

2. **The premotor area** lies in the frontal lobe immediately anterior to the motor area. The nerve cells are thought to exert a controlling influence over the motor area, ensuring an orderly series of movements. In the lower part of this area just above the lateral sulcus, there is a group of nerve cells known as the motor speech (Broca's) area. This controls the muscle movements necessary for speech. It is dominent in the left hemisphere in the right handed people and vice versa.

3. **The post central (sensory) area** is the area behind the central sulcus. Here are the perception of pain, temperature, pressure and touch, and proprioception of muscle and joints. The sensory area of the right hemisphere receives impulses from the left side of the body, and vice versa.

4. **The parietal area** lies behind the post central area and includes the greater part of the parietal lobe of the cerebrum. Its functions are thought to be associated with obtaining and retaining accurate knowledge of objects.

5. **The sensory speech area** is situated in the lower part of the parietal lobe and extends into the temporal lobe. It is here, the spoken words are perceived. It is a dominant area in the left hemisphere in right-handed people and vice versa.

6. **The Auditory or hearing area** lies in temporal lobe just below the lateral sulcus. These cells receive impulses from the vestibulo-cochlear nerve.

7. **The olfactory or smell area** lies deep in the temporal lobe. It receives impulses from the nose via the olfactory nerves.

8. **The taste area** is thought to lie just above the lateral sulcus in deep sensory area. This area receives impulses from special nerve endings in taste buds in the tongue, mucosa of the checks, palate and pharynx. They are perceived as taste sensation.

9. **The visual area** lies behind the parieto-occipital sulcus and greater part of the occipital lobe. The optic nerve passes from the eye to this area which receives impulses of visual impressions.

Basal ganglia

There are certain small areas of grey matter in the deeper area of each cerebral hemisphere called the Basal ganglia or Nuclei. Two of these are the caudate and lentiform nuclei and together form the corpus striation. The lentiform nucleus is further divided into putamen (lateral portion) and globus pallidus (medial portion). These structures are closely related to another mass of grey matter, the thalamus which lies medially to them. This system of nuclei and fibres are part of the extra pyramidal system and co-ordinates the main voluntary muscle movements. This forms the descending motor path way or the pyramidal system.

Thalamus

It measures about 3 cm (1.2 in.) in length. It comprises 80% of diencephalon. It consists of paired oval massses of grey matter organized into nuclei. An intermediate bridge of grey matter crosses the third ventricle to join the right and left portions of the thalamus.

It is concerned with the reception of sensory impulses from subcortical level and spinal cord and relayed on to the sensory area of the cerebral cortex.

Hypothalamus

It has a number of groups of nerve cells. It is situated below and front of the thalamus, immediately above the pituitary gland. It is connected to the posterior lobe of the pituitary gland by nerve fibres and to anterior lobe by a complex portal system of blood vessels, so indirectly controls the output of hormones. Other functions are to control and integrate the activities of the autonomic nervous system e.g.: control of hunger, thirst, body temperature, heart rate and regulation of diameter of blood vessels. Together with limbic system, it regulates feelings of rage, aggression, pain and pleasure and behavioural patterns of sexual arousal. It regulates the activities of eating and drinking. It also regulates diurnal rhythm and state of consciousness. The suprachiasmatic nucleus of hypothalamus has been called a biological clock.

Electroencephalograph (EEG)

It is the record of the elctrical potentials of the brain derived from leads of the scalp. It is recorded by an electroencephalograph. The EEG displays wavelike patterns known as brain ways. Four kinds of waves can be recorded from normal individuals.

1. Alpha waves – They are present in nearly all normal individuals, when they are awake and resting with their eyes closed. These waves disappear entirely during sleep.

2. Beta waves – They appear when an individual is alert.

3. Theta waves – They normally occur in children and in adults experiencing emotional stress. They are seen in first stage of sleep. They also occur in many disorders of the brain.

4. Delta waves – They are seen in an adult during deep sleep. If they are seen in an awake adult, they indicate brain damage.

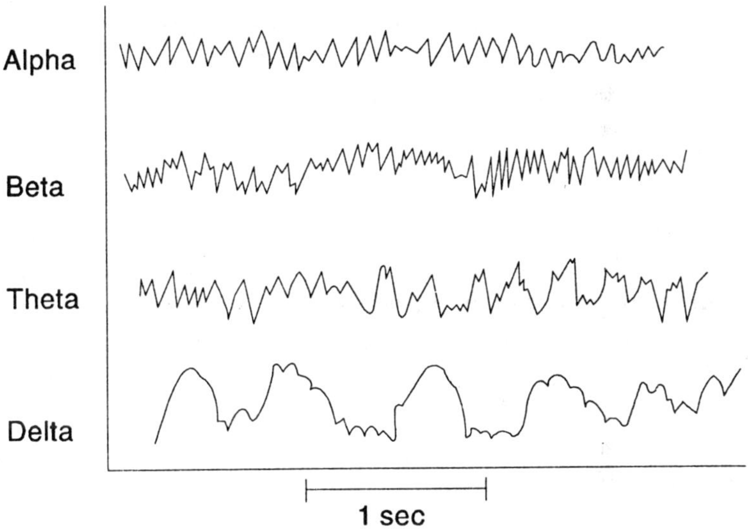

Figure 71. Type of brain waves recorded in an Electroencephalogram (EEG)

EEG is useful in localizing intracranial lesions and brain tumours and distinguishing between diffuse and focal brain lesions in epilepsy. It is also useful in diagnosing brain death.

Limbic System

Limbic system consists of a ring of structures around the brain stem on the inner border of the cerebrum (olfactory cortex and certain deep cortical regions and neuclei of cerebrum) and floor of the diencepholon. The limbic system is connected to and functionally associated with the hypothalamus. By responding to olfactory stimulation. The limbic system initiates responses necessary for survival such as hunger and thirst. Therefore it is sometimes called as visceral brain. It also influences the emotional aspects of behaviour.

The mid brain or mesencephalon

This part of the brain connects the forebrain and hind brain. The mid brain contains cerebral aqueduct, that communicates 3rd with the 4th ventricle for the passage of CSF. It also contains groups of nerve cells and nerve fibres which connect the cerebrum with lower parts of the brain and the spinal cord. These nerve cell groups (substansia nigra) act as relay stations for the ascending and descending nerve fibres. There are dopamine containing neurons in the substansia nigra which degenerate in parkinson's disease.

Tectum is the name given to the posterior portion of the midbrain. It contains corpora quadrigemina (four rounded elevations) which is divided into superior colliculi and inferior colliculi. They are the centres of reflex for movements of the head, and trunk in response to auditory stimuli.

The midbrain also contains the left and right red nuclei which assist the basal ganglia and cerebellum to cordinate muscular movements.

The Pons

It is situated in front of the cerebellum, below the mid brain and above the medulla oblongata. It mainly consists of descending tracts passing between the higher levels of the brain and the spinal cord, a fibrous bridge between the two hemispheres of the cerebellum. There are groups of neurons situated deeply, which act as relay stations and are associated with the cranial nerves.

The pons contains the nucleii of four pairs of cranial nerves namely the trigeminal nerve V (chewing), the abducens VI (certain eyeball movements, the facial) VII (Salivation and facial expression) and few vestibular branches of auditory nerve, VIII (equillibrium).

The pneumotoxic centre and apneustic centre have their nucleii in pons. They help control respiration.

Medulla oblongata

It extends from the pons above and it is continuous below with the spinal cord. It is about 2.5 cms long, and has a pyramid shape. Its anterior and posterior surfaces are marked by central fissures. It is composed of white matter which passes between the brain and the spinal cord and grey matter lies centrally.

The vital centres lie in its deeper structure

1. Cardiac centre
2. Respiratory centre
3. Vaso motor centre
4. Reflex centres of vomiting, coughing, sneezing, swallowing, and hiccuping.

1. **Decussation of the pyramids:** In the medulla the motor nerve fibres descend from the motor area of the cerebrum to the spinal cord, about 75% cross from one side to the other. This means, the motor activity of the right side of the body is controlled by left hemisphere of the cerebrum and vice versa.

2. **Sensory decussation:** Some of the sensory tracts ascending to the cerebrum from the spinal cord, cross from one side to the other in the medulla.

3. **The cardiac centre** controls the rate and force of cardiac contractions. Sympathetic and parasympathetic nerve fibres originating here pass to the heart. Sympathetic stimulation increases the heart beat and parasympathetic stimulation decreases it.

4. **The vaso motor centre:** Controls the diameter of the blood vessels i.e., smooth muscles of small arteries and arterioles to regulate blood flow. Vasomotor impulses pass through the autonomic nervous system. Stimulation may cause either constriction or ditalation of blood vessels. The sources of stimulation of the vaso motor centre are the arterial vaso receptors, body temperature, emotions such as sexual excitement and anger.

5. **The respiratory centre** controls the rate and depth of respiration. Nerve impulse from this centre passes to the phrenic and inter costal nerves which stimulates the contraction of the diaphragm and inter costal muscles. This centre is stimulated by excess of carbon-di-oxide.

6. **Reflex centres:** If there is some irritation in stomach or respiratory system, the sensory impulse passes to the medulla oblongata stimulating the reflex centres which initiates the reflex actions of vomiting, coughing and sneezing.

The following five pairs of cranial nerves have their nucleii in the medulla oblongata. These are the auditory nerve (VIII), the gassopharungeal nerves (IX), the vagus nerves (X), the cranial portion of accessory nerves (XI), and the hypoglossal nerves (XII).

From the right and left lateral surfaces of the medulla olive nucleus projects.

Reticular Formation

Reticular formation consists of a group of nuclei scattered throughout the brain stem (medulla, pons and midbrain). It also extends into the spinal cord and dienceophalon. (A part of the brain consisting primarily of the thalamus and the hypothalamus). The reticular formation has both sensory and motor functions. It receives input from the cerebral cortex and also alerts it to incoming sensory signals. This part of the reticular formation is called the reticular activating system (RAS). It is responsible for arousing from sleep and maintaining consciousness. for ex: We awaken to the sound of an alarm clock, sudden flash lights, to a painful pinch, smelling salts or cold water being splashed on the face. The R.A.S is suppressed by general anaesthetics. Coma results if there is damage to the cells of the reticular formation.

The Cerebellum

It is situated behind the pons and the medulla oblongata, occupying the posterior cranial fossa. It lies inferior to the posterior portion of the cerebrum. It is separated from the cerebrum by the transvere fissure and by an extension of the cranial dura mater called the tentorium cerebelli. It has two hemispheres connected by narrow median strip called the Vermis. The falx cerebelli which is the extension of cranial dura matter is in between the cerebellar hemispheres. Each hemisphere consists of anterior lobe, posterior lobe and floculonodular lobe. The anterior lobe and posterior lobe control subconscious movements of skeletal muscles. The floculonodular lobe on the inferior surface is involved with sense of equilibrium.

The grey matter is superficial and the white matter is deeply placed. The grey matter contains purkinje cells. The cortex has gyri and sucli. The gyri are much smaller than those of the cerebrum. The grey matter is arranged in parallel ridges called folia. The white matter is arranged in tracts called arbor vitae that resemble a branches of a tree. Within the white matter are masses of grey matter called the cerebellar nucleii. These nucleii convey information through nerve fibres from the cerebellum to other brain centres and the spinal cord.

The cerebellum is attached to the brain stem by three pairs of cerebellar peduncles, inferia, middle and superior.

Functions: The cerebellum is concerned with the co-ordination of voluntary muscular movements, posture and equilibrium. They are not under the voluntary control. It co-ordinates activities associated with the maintenance of the balance and equilibrium of the body. The sensory input for these functions is derived from proprioceptors in muscles, tendons and joints, the eyes and the ears. Propriceptive impulses from the joints and muscles indicate their position in relation to the body. Those impulses from the eyes and the semicircular canals in the ears provide information about the position of the head. So impulse from the cerebellum influences the contraction of skeletal muscle to balance and posture is maintained. Damage to the cerebellum will result in uncoordinated muscular movement, staggering gait and inability to walk properly.

Reticular formation is a collection of neurons in the core of the brain stem, surrounded by neural pathways. It has a number of synaptic links with other parts of the braïn. It constantly receives informations being transmitted in ascending and descending tracts.

Functions: Exact functions of reticular system is not known, some may be,

1. Co-ordination of skeletal activity associated with the maintenance of balance.
2. Controls autonomic nervous system.
3. Selective awareness that functions through the reticular activating system.

THE SPINAL CORD

The spinal cord is a part of the central nervous system situated in the vertebral column. It is almost cylindrical in shape, surrounded by meninges and cerebrospinal fluid. It is continuous as medulla oblongata, ends below as conus medullaris and tapers as filum terminale. The caudal end of filum terminale fuses with coccyx. Its length may be 45 cms. It extends from the upper border of atlas to lower border of first lumbar vertebra. Thirtyone pairs of spinal nerves arise along the spinal cord. At the terminal end of spinal cord, there is a group of spinal nerves i.e., lumbar spinal nerves, sacro-spinal nerve, coccygeo-spinal nerve and filum terminale are called the cauda equina.

Structure: On transverse section of spinal cord, it is incompletely divided into two equal parts, anteriorly by shallow median fissure and posteriorly by deep narrow septum, the posterior median septum. Centrally placed is the central canal, which is surrounded by 'H' shaped grey matter which is completely surrounded by the white matter.

Grey matter: It is H shaped in the spinal cord. The two limbs connected by a line i.e., called grey commissure. There is a small opening called central canal. The grey matter has 2 posterior, 2 anterior horns. In addition, there is a lateral column of grey matter in the thoracic part of spinal cord, i.e. in between the anterior and posterior grey horns.

The nerve cells

1. Sensory neurons in the posterior horns receive sensory impulses.
2. Motor neurons (lower motor neurons). They are situated in anterior horns of grey mater and transmit impulses to skeletal muscles.
3. The connector neurons, linking sensory and motor neurons, at the same or different level act as spinal reflex arcs.
4. Autonomic neurons in the lateral column is to supply viscera in the trunk. The anterior grey columns and posterior grey columns are connected to corresponding anterior (ventral) and posterior spinal (dorsal) roots. Both these spinal roots fuse to form

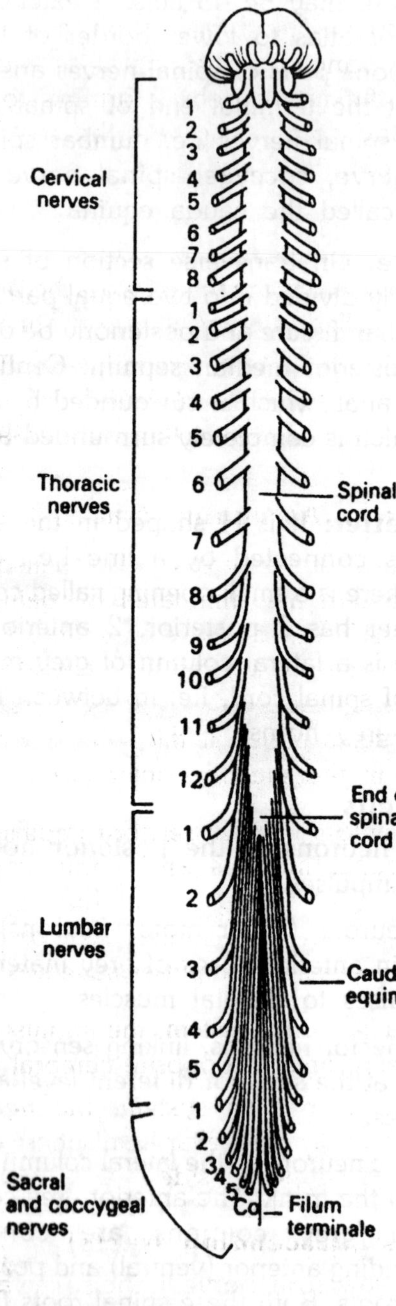

Figure 72. The Spinal cord

spinal nerves. The dorsal spinal roots have ganglia (sensory ganglia). The spinal nerves come out through the intervertebral formina to supply the body. Any compression in the foramen causes sensory or motor loss.

White matter: The white matter of the spinal cord is arranged in 3 columns or tracts, anterior, posterior and lateral. These tracts are mixed type, the one ascending to the brain is called afferent (sensory) fibres. The other descending from the brain is called efferent (motor) fibres. The descending fibres may be from brain to connector neurons, the other to skeletal muscles through the spinal cord, and spinal nerves.

Sensory tracts (Ascending tracts)

1. The cutaneous receptors : The sensory impulses from the skin are stimulated by pain, heat, cold and touch. These impulses pass through a 3 neuron system to sensory area in the opposite hemisphere of the cerebrum. Crossing to other side or decussation, occurs either at the level of entry into the cord or in the medulla oblongata.

2. Proprioceptors : These sensory impulses are from, the tendons, muscles and joints, together with impulses from the eyes and the ears. They are associated with the maintainance of balance and posture. These nerve impulses have two destinations.

    1. By a 3-neuron system, the impulse reaches the sensory area of opposite cerebral hemisphere.
    2. By a 2- neuron system, the nerve impulse reaches the cerebellar hemisphere on the same side or opposite side.

Motor tracts (descending tracts)

Neurons transmit nerve impulse away from the brain are motor (efferent) neurons. The efferent tracts descend from the brain and decussate in the brain stem and reach the spinal cord. When it reaches its appropriate level in the cord, it synapses with a cell in the anterior horn of the grey matter. Then these fibres pass through the spinal nerves and reach in the motor end plates of the skeletal muscles. The motor path ways from the brain to the muscles are made up of two neurons.

1. **Upper motor neurons:** They are situated in the precentral sulcus area of the cerebrum. The axons pass through the internal capsule, pons and decussate in the medulla and in the spinal cord form as lateral cortico spinal tracts. The fibres terminate with the cells of the lower motor neurons in the anterior grey matter. If the axons of upper motor neurons did not decussate in the medulla. They descend in the ventral cortico-spinal tract and cross over just before terminating in the anterior horn.

2. **Lower motor neurons:** The nerve cells are in the anterior grey matter in the spinal cord. Its axons comes out from the spinal cord by the anterior root, joins posterior root to form mixed spinal nerve, pass through the inter vertebral formen and terminates in the motor end plate. The motor end-plates of each nerve and the muscle fibres which form a motor unit. Here, the chemical transmitter is acetylcholine. The neurons from various sites in the brain stimulate the cells of the lower motor neuron, while others have an inhibiting effect. The outcome of these influences is smooth, co-ordinated muscle movement, some of which are voluntary and some are involuntary.

3. **Spinal reflexes:** These consist of 3 neurons, sensory neurons, connector neurons and lower motor neurons in the spinal cord. This is called reflex arc. A reflex action is defined as an immediate automatic motor response to a sensory stimu-

lus. Many connector and motor neurons are stimulated by afferent impulses from a small area of skin eg: pain impulses.

4. **Stretch reflexes (Somatic reflexes):** In these reflexes only two neurons are involved. The cells of the lower motor neuron are stimulated by the sensory neuron. Here, no connector neuron is involved. The knee jerk is one example. By tapping the tendon just below the knee joint when it is bent, the sensory nerve ending in the tendon and in the thigh muscles are stretched, stimulating lower motor neurons on the same side. As a result, thigh muscles suddenly contract and the foot kicks forwards.

5. **Autonomic (visceral) reflexes,** generally are not perceived. These reflexes occur in smooth muscle, cardiac muscle and glands. The autonomic nervous system controls the heart rate, respiration, digestion, urination and defaecation through autonomic reflexes.

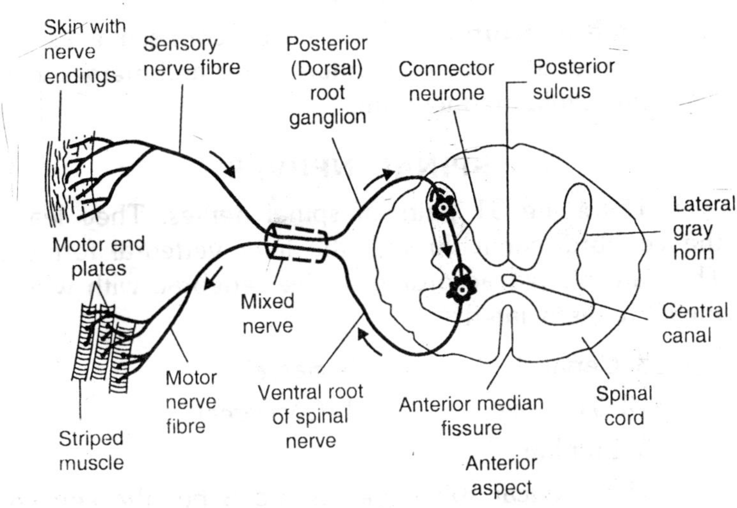

Figure 73. A single reflex arc

PERIPHERAL NERVOUS SYSTEM

This consists of

1. 31 pairs of spinal nerves.
2. 12 pairs of cranial nerves.

Most of the peripheral nerves are mixed nerves. They convey sensory impulses from sensory end organs to the brain and motor nerve impulses from the brain to effector organs through the spinal cord, eg: skeletal muscles and glands.

Structure

Each nerve consists of numerous nerve fibres and together called bundle. There is a connective tissue covering between fibres and nerve bundle.

1. **Epineurium:** It is a connective tissue which encloses groups of bundles of nerves in a big nerve. eg: sciatic nerve.
2. **Perineurium:** This connective tissue encloses each bundles of nerve fibres.
3. **Endoneurium:** It is a delicate connective tissue, surrounding each individual fibres and merges with the septa perineurium.

SPINAL NERVES

There are 31 pairs of spinal nerves. They leave the vertebral canal through the inter vertebral formen. They are named according to the vertebrae with which they are associated.

8 Cervical	5 Sacral
12 Thoracic	1 Coccygeal,
5 Lumbar	

The cervical spinal nerves are 8 but the cervical vertebrae are seven. The 1st cervical spinal nerve comes out between occipital bone and atlas, the 2nd cervical spinal nerve comes out between atlas and axis, the 8th cervical spinal nerve comes between 7th cervical and 1st thoracic vertebrae. There after, the nerves are given the name and number of the vertebrae immediately above. The lumbar, sacral and coccygeal nerves leave the spinal cord near its termination, and extend in the subarchnoid space, forming a sheath of nerves which resembles a horse's tail called the cauda equina. These nerves leave the vertebral canal at the appropriate lumbar, sacral or coccygeal level.

Nerve Roots

Each spinal nerve has two roots, the anterior (motor) root joins with the posterior (sensory) root having enlargement called spinal ganglia, to form spinal nerves. So spinal nerves are mixed nerves. The anterior roots from thoracic one to lumbar 2nd carry preganglionic fibres from the lateral grey horn of sympathetic nerve cells. The area of skin supplied by each nerve is called as dermatome. After emerging out from the intervertebral foramen, each spinal nerve divides into a ramus communicans, a posterior ramus and an anterior ramus. These rami communicans contain preganglionic sympathetic fibres.

The posterior ramus passes backwards to supply deep muscles and skin over the back of the neck and trunk.

The anterior rami, supply the muscles and structures of the anterior and lateral aspects of neck, trunk and the upper and lower limbs. In the cervical, lumbar and sacral regions, the anterior rami unite to form masses of nerves or plexuses. In addition to posterior and anterior rami, a meningeal branch comes out from the spinal nerves. This branch reenters the spinal canal through the intervertebral foramen and supplies the vertebrae, vertebral ligaments, blood vessels of the spinal cord and meninges. In the thoracic region the anterior rami supply the trunk musculature. There are five nerve plexuses on each side of the vertebral column.

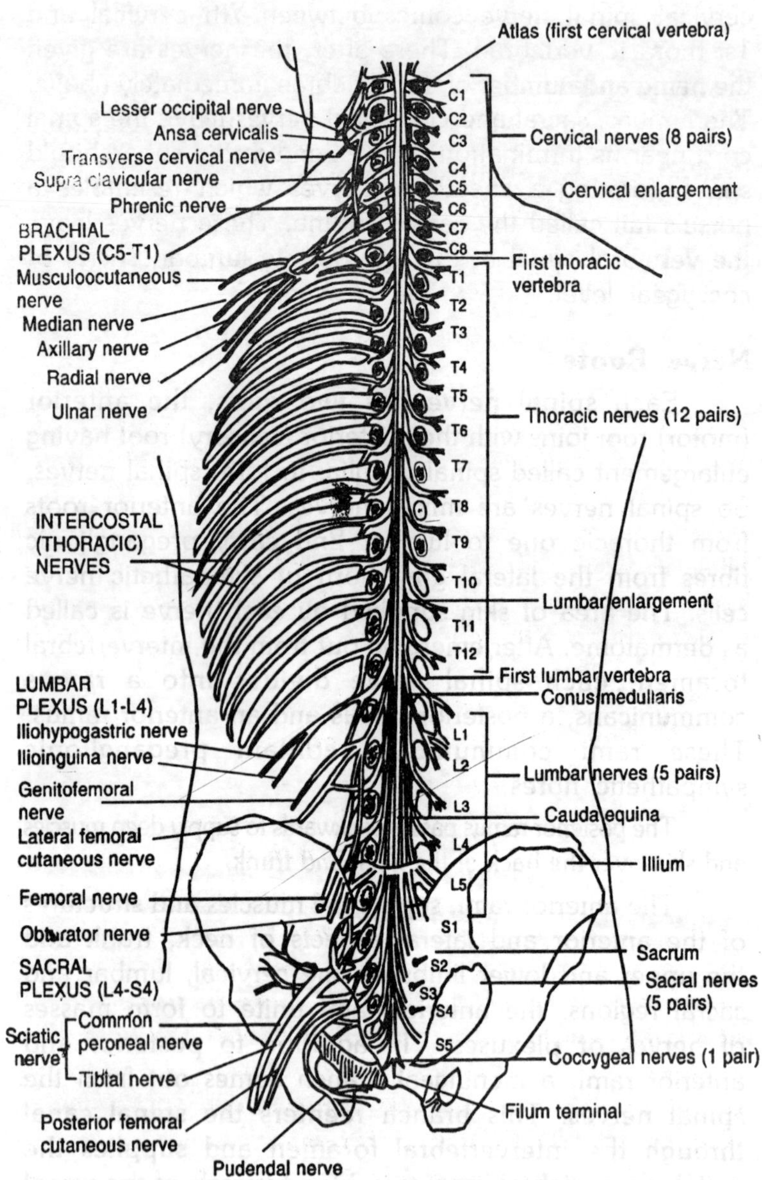

Figure 74. Spinal cord and Spinal nerves

Cervical plexuses, Brachial plexuses, Lumbar plexuses, Sacral plexuses, Coccygeal plexuses.

Cervical plexus

It is formed by the anterior rami of the first four cervical nerves and lies opposite to 1st, 2nd, 3rd and 4th cervical vertebrae. Branches from cervical plexuses supply back and side of the muscles of the neck. The phrenic nerve from cervical plexus of 3,4 and 5 passes downwards through the thoracic cavity in front of the roots of lungs to supply the Diaphragm.

The anterior rami of the lower 4 cervical nerves and 1st thoracic nerve form the brachial plexus situated in the axilla, and supply the skin and muscles of upper limb, and some chest muscles. Each branches with contribution from more than one nerve root, containing sensory, motor and autonomic fibres.

1. Axillary Nerve $C_{5,6}$
2. Radial Nerve $C_{5,6,7,8}$ T_1
3. Musculo Cutaneous Nerve $C_{5,6,7}$
4. Median Nerve $C_{5,6,7,8}$ T_1
5. Medial Cutaneous Nerve C_8 T_1
6. Ulnar Nerve $C_{7,8}$ T_1

The axillary or circumflex nerve encircles the surgical neck of the humerus and supplies the deltoid muscle, skin over the shoulder region and the shoulder joint.

The radial nerve supplies posterior compartment muscles of upper limb.

The musculo-cutaneous nerve supplies the anterior compartment muscles of the upper arm and cutaneous supply of lateral side of fore arm.

The median nerve supplies flexor muscles of fore arm and thenar muscles of the hand.

The Musculo-cutaneous nerve supplies cutaneous areas of the arm and forearm.

The ulnar nerve supplies flexor muscles of fore arm hypothenar and small muscles of the hand.

Lumbar plexus is formed by the anterior rami of the first four lumbar nerves situated in front of the transverse processes of lumbar vertebrae and behind the psoas muscle. The main branches are,

Ilio hypogastric nerve L_1

Ilio inguinal nerve L_1

Genitò femoral $L_{1,2}$

Later cutaneous nerve of thigh $L_{2,3,4}$

Femoral nerve $L_{2,3,4}$

Obturator nerve $L_{2,3,4}$

Lumbo sacral trunk $L_{4,5}$

The femoral nerve is the largest branch enters the thigh under the inguinal ligament and supplies the skin and quadriceps muscle of the thigh.

The obturator nerve supplies the adductor compartment muscles and skin on the medial side of the thigh.

The lumbo sacral trunk descends into the pelvis and gives contribution to the sacral plexus.

Sacral plexus is formed by the anterior rami of the lumbo sacral trunk and the 1st, 2nd and 3rd sacral nerves. The plexus divides into a number of branches supplying the muscles and skin of the pelvic floor and muscles around the hip joint. The sciatic nerve is the largest branch contains fibres from $L_{4,5}$ $S_{1,2,3}$.

The sciatic nerve is the largest nerve in the body passes through the greater sciatic foramen into the gluteal region. It descends through the posterior aspect of thigh supplying the hamstring muscles, then divides into tibial and the common peroneal nerves.

The Tibial nerve supplies muscles of the posterior compartment of the leg and continues into the sole of the foot to supply muscles of the foot. The common peroneal nerve descends obliquely along the lateral aspect of the popliteal fossa, winds round the neck of the fibula and divides into the deep peroneal (anterior tibial) and the superficial peroneal (Musculo-cutaneous) nerves. These nerves supply the skin and muscles of the anterior and lateral aspect of the leg, and the dorsum of the foot,

Coccygeal plexus: It is a very small plexus formed by part of the 4th and 5th sacral and the coccygeal nerves. Nerves from this plexus supply the skin in the area of coccyx and levator ani and coccygeal muscles of the pelvic floor.

Thoracic nerves: The ventral (anterior) rami of spinal nerves T_2-$T_{12.}$ do not form plexuses. They supply skin and trunk muscles. They are known as intercostal (thoracic) nerves.The dorsal (posterior) rami of the intercosal nerves supply the deep back muscles and skin of the dorsal aspect of the thorax.

Cranial nerves

There are 12 pairs of cranial nerves originating from nuclei in the brain and brain stem. Some are sensory, some are motor and some are mixed nerves.

1. Olfactory nerve (sensory)
2. Optic nerve (sensory)
3. Oculomotor nerve (motor)
4. Trochlear nerve (motor)
5. Trigeminal nerve (mixed)
6. Abducent nerve (motor)
7. Facial nerve (mixed)
8. Vestibulo cochlear (auditory or acoustic) nerve (sensory)
9. Glossopharyngeal nerve (mixed)
10. Vagus nerve (mixed)
11. Accessory nerve (motor)
12. Hypoglossal nerve (motor)

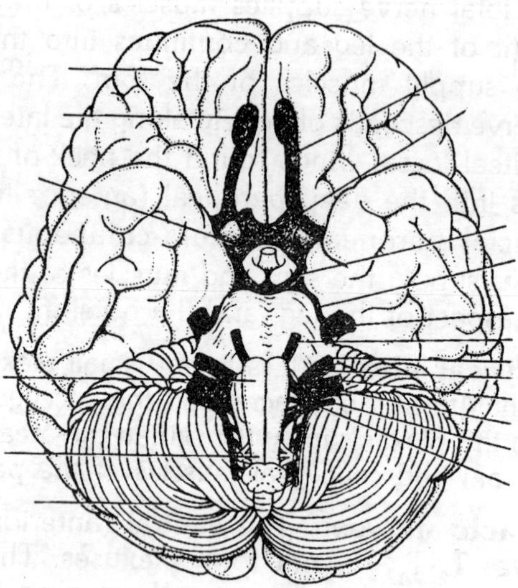

Figure 75. Base of the brain showing the origins of cranial nerves

1. **Olfactory nerve or nerve of smell:** It starts from nasal mucosa, passes upwards through cibriform plate of the ethmoid bone and ends in olfactory bulb.

2. **Optic nerve or nerve of the sense of sight:** The nerve fibres originate from retina of the eyes and form optic nerve, passes backwards through optic formen and each joins other optic nerve to form optic chiasma, then the nerves proceed backwards as the optic tracts to the lateral geniculate body. The impulses pass from these areas to the centre for the sight in the occipital lobes of the cerebrum and to the cerebellum.

3. **Oculomotor nerve :** This nerve arises from nerve cells near the cerebral aqueduct of the mid brain. It supplies

   1 Levator palpebrae muscle which raises the upper eye lid.

2 Four extra ocular muscles

3 Intra ocular muscles

   a) Ciliary muscles

   b) Circular muscles of the iris.

4. **Trochlear nerve:** This nerve arises from the mid brain and supplies extra-ocular muscle i,e superior oblique muscle.

5. **Trigeminal nerve:** It is a mixed nerve and largest among the cranial nerves. It is the chief sensory nerve for the face and head receiving impulses of pain, temperature and touch. The motor fibres supply the muscles of mastication. There are 3 main branches of the trigeminal nerve.

   a) The ophthalmic nerves are sensory and supply the lacrimal glands, conjunctiva of the eyes, fore head, eye lids, anterior surface of scalp and mucous membrane of the nose.

   b) The maxillary nerves are sensory and supply the checks, upper gums, upper teeth and lower eyelids.

   c) The mandibular nerve is mixed nerve, sensory fibres supply to teeth and gums of lower jaw, pinna of the ears and tongue. The motor fibres supply to muscles of mastication.

6. **Abducent nerve:** It arises from the neurons situated in the floor of 4th ventricle and supplies the lateral rectus muscle of the eyeball.

7. **Facial nerve:** It is a mixed nerve arises from pons. The motor fibres supply the muscles of facial expression. The sensory fibres convey impulses from the taste buds in the anterior two-thirds of the tongue.

8. **Vestibulo cochlear (Auditory or Acoustic) nerve:** The vestibular part the nerve arises from

the semicircular canals of the inner ear and conveys impulses to the cerebellum. The semicircular canals are associated with the maintenance of posture and balance. The cochlear part originates in the organ of corti (spiral organ) in the inner ear and conveys impulses to the hearing area in the cerebral cortex where sound is perceived.

9. **Glossopharyngeal nerve:** It arises from the nerve cells in medulla oblongata. The motor fibres supply the muscles of the pharynx and the secretory fibres supply the parotid glands. The sensory impulses are conveyed to the cerebral cortex from the posterior third of the tongue, the tonsils, and pharynx, also from taste buds in the tongue and pharynx.
10. **Vagus nerve:** It is a mixed nerve. It has extensive distribution than any other cranial nerves. It arises from nerve cells in the medulla oblongata, passes down through the neck into the trunk. It is a parasympathetic nerve. The motor fibres supply the smooth muscles and secretory fibres to G.I.system, respiratory system, cardio vascular system and urogenital system.
11. **Accessory nerve:** It arises from neurons in medulla oblongata and cervical spinal cord. The motor fibres supply the sternocleido matoid and trapezius muscles.
12. **Hypoglossal nerve:** It arises from the nerve cells in the medulla oblongata. The motor fibres supply the muscles of the tongue.

AUTONOMIC NERVOUS SYSTEM

The autonomic or involuntary part of the nervous system controls the functions of the body automatically. It is divided into 2 parts.

1. Sympathetic (thoraco-lumbar out flow)
2. Parasympathetic (cranio-sacral out flow)

The effects of autonomic control are mainly stimulation or depression of glandular secretion and control on heart rate and smooth muscles.

Sympathetic nervous system

This system consists of 3 neurons, conveying impulses from their origin in the hypothalamus, reticular formation and medulla oblongata to effector organs and tissues.

1. Neuron situated in the hypothalamus and its fibres extend into the spinal cord.
2. Neuron situated in the lateral grey column of spinal cord of thoracic region. The preganglaic fibres relays in lateral chain of sympathetic ganglia.
3. Neuron in a ganglion and terminates in the organ or tissue supplied.

Sympathetic chain

A pair of sympathetic chains situated on either side of vertebral column extending from the base of the skull to anterior surface of coccyx. In the chain, there are accumulations of nerve cells to form ganglia. There may be 22-24 sympathetic ganglia. The preganglonic fibres from the spinal cord relay in these ganglia. Then the post-ganglionic fibres come out from these chain to supply effector organs. The sweat glands, the skin and blood vessels of skeletal muscles are supplied by only sympathetic fibres.

Prevertebral ganglia

There are 3 prevertebral ganglia situated in the abdominal cavity close to the origin of arteries of the same names:

1. The coeliac ganglion.
2. The superior mesentric ganglion.
3. The inferior mesentric ganglion.

Second neuron: Sympathetic fibres pass through the lateral chain to reach these ganglion.

Parasympathetic nervous system

Two Neurons are involved in the transmission of impulses from their source to the effector organ. The first neuron is situated in the brain or spinal cord. The cranial out flow through the cranial nerves of 3,7,9 and 10. Their nerve fibres terminate outside the brain. The cells of the sacral outflow for lateral grey column of sacral spinal segments 2,3, and 4. Their nerve fibres terminate outside the brain. The cells of the sacral outflow for lateral grey column of sacral spinal segments 2,3 and 4. Their fibres leave through 2,3 and 4 sacro spinal nerves and relay with 2nd neuron cells in the walls of pelvic organs.

The second neuron is situated either in a ganglion or in the wall of the organ supplied.

Functions of the autonomic nervous system

This system is involved in a complex of reflex activities depending on sensory input to the brain or spinal cord and/or motor out put. The reflex action is contraction or inhibition of involuntary, smooth and cardiac or glandular secretion. These reflexes are co-ordinated in the brain below the level of consciousness i.e., below the level of the cerebrum. The majority of the organs of the body are supplied by sympathetic and parasympathetic nerves which have opposite effects to ensure the optimum functioning of the organs.

Sympathetic stimulation: It prepares the body to deal with exciting and stressful situation. The nerve ends and adrenal medulla produce adrenaline and noradrenaline.

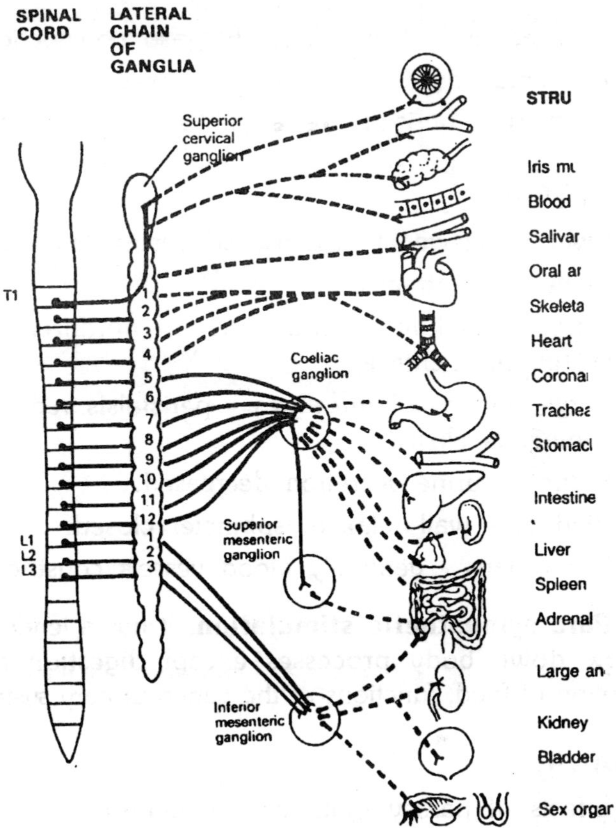

Figure 76. Effects of sympathetic stimulation

Structural effects of sympathetic stimulation

1. Iris muscle - pupil dilated
2. Blood vessels in head - constricted
3. Salivary glands - secretion is inhibited
4. Oral and Nasal mucosa - mucus secretion is inhibited.
5. Skeletal blood vessels - dilated
6. Heart rate and force of contraction increased.
7. Coronary arteries - dilated

8. Trachea and bronchi - slight vaso constriction.
9. Bronchial muscle (Asthma) - relaxed.
10. Stomach - peristalsis reduced, sphincters closed.
11. Intestine - peristalsis and tone decreased, vaso constriction.
12. Liver - glycogen to glucose conversion increased.
13. Spleen - contracted
14. Adrenal medulla - adrenalin and noradrenaline secretions increased.
15. Large and small intestines - peristalsis reduced, sphincters closed.
16. Kidney - urine secretion decreased.
17. Bladder - wall relaxed, sphincter closed.
18. Sex organs - generally blood vessels constricted.

Para sympathetic stimulation: It has a tendency to slow down body processes except digestion and absorption of food, functions of the genito urinary system.

ORGANS

Effects of parasympathetic stimulation

1. Iris muscle - pupils constricted.
2. Lacrimal gland - tear secretion increased
3. Salivary glands - increased secretion
4. Heart - rate and force of contraction decreased.
5. Coronary arteries - constricted
6. Trachea and bronchi - constricted
7. Stomach - increased gastric secretion and motility.
8. Small intestine - digestion and increased absorption.
9. Liver and gall bladder - blood vessels dilated, secretion of bile increased.
10. Pancreas - increased secretion of pancreatic juice.
11. Small Intestine - increased secretion of intestinal juice and motility increased.

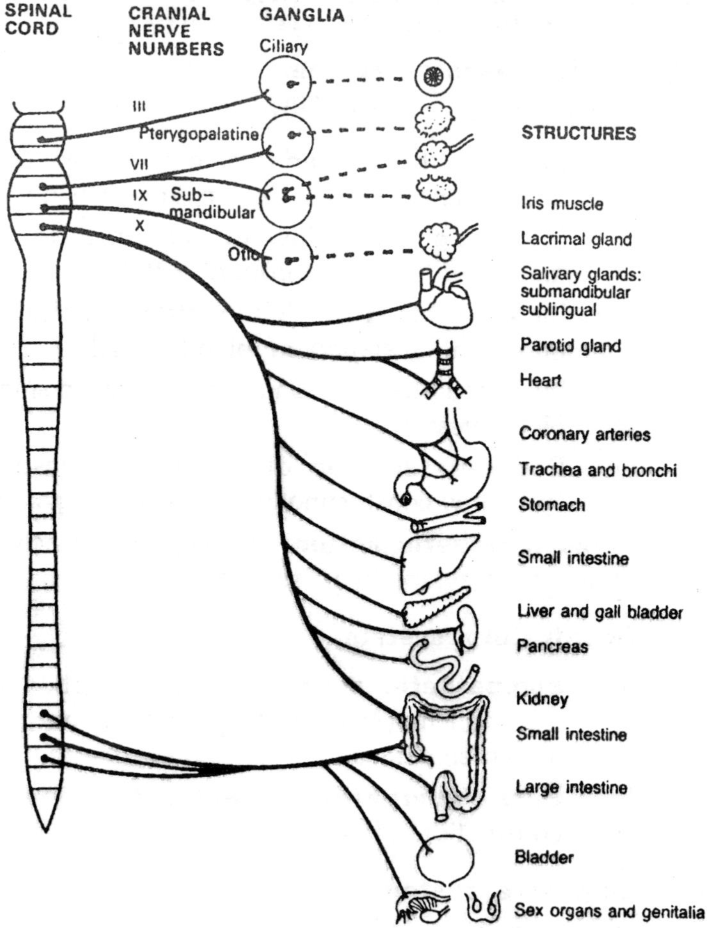

Figure 77. Effects of parasympathetic stimulation

12. Large intestine - secretion and motility increased, sphincter relaxed.

13. Sphincter relaxed

14. Sex organs – male – vasodilation and erection of genitalia.
 – female – vasodilation and erection.

AUTONOMIC STIMULATION ON VARIOUS SYSTEMS OF THE BODY

1. Cardio-vascular system

Sympathetic stimulation

a) Increased the rate and force of heart beat and accelerating effect upon the sinoatrial node.

b) Increasing blood flow to heart muscle by means of dilating coronary arteries.

c) Increased blood supply to skeletal muscles by means of dilatation of blood vessels.

d) Increased blood pressure by constricting small blood vessels.

e) Reduced secretion of glands in digestive system by constricting blood vessels of glands.

Parasympathetic action: It has opposite action of those of sympathetic stimulation.

2. Respiratory system

a) **Sympathetic action:** Causes dilatation of the bronchi (Asthma) so greater amount of air enters at each inspiration.

b) **Para sympathetic action:** produces constriction of the bronchi.

3. Digestive system

Sympathetic stimulation

a) Liver converts glycogen to glucose to provide energy.

b) Stomach and small intestine - reduced secretion of digestive juice, delayed movement and absorption of food, the tone of sphincter is increased.

c) Adrenal medulla is stimulated to secrete adrenalin and nor-adrenaline.

d) Increased metabolic rate.

Parasympathetic stimulation

a) Stomach and small intestine: The rate and motility are increased and rate of digestion and absorption are increased.

b) Pancreas: Increased secretion of pancreatic juice and hormone insulin.

4. **Urinary system**

Sympathetic action

a) Urethral Sphincters: The muscle tone of the spincters are increased inhibiting micturition.

b) Bladder wall relaxes.

Parasympathetic action: Relaxation of the internal sphincter with contraction of the urinary bladder and micturition occurs.

5. **Skin**

Sympathetic stimulation

a) Increased secretion of sweat, so increased heat loss of the body.

b) Contraction of the arrectores pilorum muscles produces appearance of goose flesh.

c) Constriction of the blood vessels preventing heat loss.

No parasympathetic supply of the skin

6. **Eye**

Sympathetic action: Retraction of the levator palpbral muscles occur, giving wide opening of the eyes. The pupil is dilated, the ciliary muscle adjusts the thickness of the lens.

Parasympathetic action: The eye lids tends to close, appearance of sleepiness, the pupil is constricted.

7. **Sex organs**

Sympathetic stimulation

In female - uterus - Inhibits contraction in nonpregnant woman,
Promotes contraction in pregnant woman.

Parasympathetic stimulation

In female - uterus - Minimal effect

Sympathetic action in male causes ejaculation.

Parasympathetic action causes vasodilatation, and erection of penis in the male.

in female - vasodilation and erection.

Questions

1. What are the main parts of the brain?
2. Describe the cerebellum.
3. Describe the coverings of the brain.
4. Where is cerebrospinal fluid secreted? Where does it flow?
5. Describe lumbar puncture and how a nurse can assist during and after the procedure.
6. List the cranial nerves. State their functions.
7. Describe the spinal cord with its cross section.
8. Write short notes on
   a) Reflex action
   b) Neuroglia
   c) Autonomic nervous system
   d) Reticular formation
   e) Basal ganglia
   f) Limbic system

Study the following:

1. Membrane potential
2. Resting membrane potential
3. Graded potentials
4. Action potential
5. Neurotransmitters
6. Neuropeptides

Learn the following procedures:

1. Lumbar Puncture
2. Electro-encephalogram.

UNIT 6

The Cardiovascular System

The life of all cells of the body is dependent on constant supply of food materials and oxygen and the removal of waste products formed in them. These functions are carried out by the cardio vascular system. The blood, heart and blood vessels together make up the cardio-vascular system.

Blood is a specialised form of connective tissue and is composed of transparent fluid plasma in which different types of cells are suspended. Plasma forms about 55% and cells constitute about 45% of blood volume.

Blood is thicker, heavier and more viscous than water. The temperature of blood is about 38^0 C (100.4^0 F). Blood is slightly alkaline having a pH of about 7.4(normal range is 7.35 to 7.5). The total blood volume in the average adult is 5 to 6 litres in males and 4 to 5 litres in females. Blood makes up about 8% of total body weight.

The study of blood, blood forming tissues and their associated disorders is called haematology.

Composition of blood: Blood plasma is made up of a straw coloured fluid and is slightly alkaline. Plasma contains

1. Water - 91%

Dissolved substances

2. Proteins - 8%
3. Salts - 0.9%

1. Plasma proteins : albumin, globulin and fibrinogen.
2. Nutrient materials (from G.I. tract)

   Mono saccharides from carbohydrates, amino acids from proteins, fatty acids and glycerol from fats, vitamins from foods.
3. Inorganic salts (Minerals)

   Sodium chloride, Sodium bicarbonate, Magnesium, iron, calcium, phosphorus copper, iodine, potassium.
4. Organic materials - urea, uric acid, creatinine, ammonium salts, bilirubin and cholesterol
5. Enzymes
6. Hormones
7. Antibodies.
8. Gases - oxygen, carbon dioxide, nitrogen

Functions of plasma

1. Transporting oxygen from lungs to tissues and carbon dioxide from tissues to lungs.
2. Transporting nutrient materials from G.I. tract to tissues and waste materials to excretory organs, eg : kidneys.
3. Transporting hormones from glands to their target organs.
4. Protective substances. Eg; transporting antibodies (gamma globulins) or antigens to infected area.
5. Factors containing clotting mechanism, so preventing blood loss from ruptured blood vessels.

1. **Plasma proteins**

a) **Albumins** are formed in the liver and their function is to maintain the plasma osmotic pressure and they provide protein to tissues. Albumins may be 3 to 5 gms per 100ml of blood. (54%of plasma proteins)

b) **Globulins:** They may be 2 to 3 gms per 100ml of blood (38%), formed in the liver and lympoid tissue. Their activities are :

   i) Immune response in the presence of antigens.

   ii) Transportation of some hormones, for ex : thyroid hormone and

   iii) Inhibition of some proteolytic enzymes. Eg : trypsin, chymotrypsin.

c) Fibrinogen may be 0.32 to 0.49 gm per 100ml of blood (7%) is synthesised in the liver and is essential for blood coagulation.

Fibrinogen can be removed from the plasma by various methods. Then the remaining fluid is called serum.

Plasma - fibrinogen = serum.

Clotting factors : These substances are essential for coagulation of blood.

2. **Nutrient materials**

Absorbed food materials from gastro-intestinal tract i.e. monosaccharides, amino acids, fatty acids and glycerol and vitamins, are required for body cells to provide energy, repair and replacement.

3. **Mineral salts**

Minerals (sodium bicarbonate) play an important role to maintain pH 7.4. Blood is slightly alkaline in reaction. Alkalinity and acidity are expressed in terms of pH. The usefulness of minerals are for cell formation, contraction of muscles, transmission of nerve impulses, and maintenance of the balance between acids and alkalies.

4. Waste products

They are urea, uric acid, creatinine, ammonia, bilirubin and carbon dioxide.

Urea and uric acid are waste products of protein metabolism, formed in the liver and excreted by the kidneys. Carbon dioxide is conveyed to the lungs for excretion. Excretion of acids and CO_2 also helps in the maintenance of normal pH of plasma.

5. Antibodies (Immunoglobulins)

Produced in lymphoid tissue, eg : lymph nodes and spleen. They are protective substances, fight against foreign materials eg : microbes, antigens.

6. Hormones

Hormones are secreted by endocrine glands and poured into blood which transports them to their target organs.

7. Gases

Oxygen and carbon dioxide are transported in blood in combination with haemoglobin in red blood cells.

CELLULAR CONTENT (FORMED ELEMENTS) OF BLOOD

1. Leukocytes or white blood cells.
2. Erythrocytes or red blood cells.
3. Thrombocytes or platelets.

Erythocytes account for 95% of the volume of formed elements. Leucocytes and thrombocytes account for the remaining 5% of the volume of formed elements.

Leukocytes or white blood cells

There are about 6000 to 10000 (average 8000) white blood cells per cubic millimeter of blood of an adult. The cytoplasm of the cells contains nuclei and some have granules in their cytoplasm. They are classified into,

a) Granulocytes or polymorphonuclear leukocytes
   1. Neutrophils 2. Eosinophils 3. Basophils.

b) Agranular leukocytes
   1. Monocytes
   2. Lymphocytes.

Leukopoiesis is the term used for the formation and development of the various types of white blood cells.

Granulocytes: They develop from stem cells (Haemocytoblast) in red bone marrow and pass through different stages of development before entering into circulation. This process is called as granulopoiesis. The stage from myeloblast or myelocyte, they are named according to the stain they take up. During staining, eosinophils take up red acid dye-eosin, basophils take up alkaline methylene blue, and neutrophils are purple because they take up both dyes.

Neutrophils: They number about 60 to 70 percent. They form largest percentage of white blood cells, and their function is defence mechanism against microbes. The phagocytes are attracted in large numbers to infected or inflammed area by chemical substances released by microbes and inflammed tissues. This phenomenon is called chemotaxis.

Neutrophils go to infected area by amoeboid movement, then they ingest and kill the microbes. This process is called phagocytosis. The pus is formed in the affected area by dead tissue cells, dead and live microbes. Neutrophils may increase in allergy, and in parasitic infections. Neutrophils also contain defensins which act against bacteria, fungi and viruses.

Eosinophils: They number about 1 to 4 percent. The number of eosinophils is increased in allergic conditions, such as, asthma, food and drug sensitivities and skin conditions. They migrate into mucous membranes of the respiratory and digestive systems to protect the body against foreign materials, especially, invasion by parasites. They neutralise histamine.

Basophils are difficult to find in human blood because they constitute only about 0.5 to 1.0 percent of total number of leukocytes. They are fewer in number and more irregular in size and shape than any other granulocytes. Morphologically, there are two types of basophilic cells, the basophil leukocytes of the blood and basophil cells of tissues called Mast cells. Both have granules that contain heparin and histamine.

Agranular leukocytes: The leukocytes with no granules in their cytoplasm are monocytes and lymphocytes. They form about 25% to 35% of all leukocytes.

Monocytes: They number about 3 to 8 percent. They are large mononuclear cells developed from monoblasts in red bone marrow. They circulate in blood and are actively motile and phagocytic. They migrate out into the tissues, enlarge and develop into macrophages. The Macrophage system : It consists of fixed phagocytic cells which multiply in situ, and has wide distribution in the body.

For example, Microglia in the brain, Histiocytes in connective tissue, Kupffer's cells in liver sinusoids, alveolar macrophages in the lungs, tissue macrophages in the spleen, lymph nodes and bone marrow. The function of macrophages is phagocytic with monocytes and lymphocytes. Their number may increase in microbial infection and collagen disease.

Lymphocytes: They number about 20 to 25 percent. They are associated with defence mechanism of the body. They develop from haemocytoblasts (stem cells) in red bone marrow, then circulate in blood stream. Immunologically, they are competent to respond to antigen or foreign materials . They are of three types- T - lymphocytes, B-lymphocytes and natural killer cells. The T - lymphocytes are activated in thymus gland, and B - lymphocytes are activated in lymphoid tissue and in the walls of intestine. Both types circulate in the blood, and settle in lymph nodes, spleen and aggregated lymphatic nodules in intestine. Each type divides into 2 groups, the effector cells that promote destruction of their specific antigen, the other memory cells that remain in lymphoid tissue and multiply, passing on their specific antibody forming character to subsequent generation cells.

T - Lymphocytes: They are sensitised when they encounter with an antigen for the first time. The effector cells act directly against antigens with phagocytes. The memory cells confer cell-mediated immunity. These lymphocytes produce lymphokinase that attract macrophages to the site. The lympho-toxin kills foreign cells for (ex:- organ transplants) and interferons prevent virus reproduction inside the cells. T-cells also attack cancer cells. They are unable to divide and they cannot carry on extensive metabolic activities. Each R.B.C. measures about 7.7 X 2.2 micrometers (mm) . Each R.B.C consists of an outer coat inside of which contains haemoglobin. The haemoglobin accounts for about one third of cells volume and gives whole blood its red colour.

B - lymphocytes are stimulated by both microbes and their toxins. They grow into plasma cells which secrete antibodies (immunoglobulins). The antibodies promote phagocytosis of foreign particles and neutralise toxins. The immune system works by a clonal selection process whereby T or B cells are grouped into different clones or sets. Each set consists of cells committed before being exposed to a particular antigen, for making a particular antibody.

Natural Killer Cells attack mocrobes and certain spontaneously arising tumour cells.

Erythrocytes or Red Blood Cells

The red corpuscles are flattened nonnucleated biconcave discs. They are the most numerous of the formed elements of the blood. In the normal adult male, they number about 5 million per cubic millimeter. In the adult female, they number about 4½ million per cubic millimeter.

Development: RBC's are formed in red bone marrow present in long bones, flat and irregular bones. They pass several stages of development before they enter into circulation. About 2 million mature R.B.C's per second enter the circulation. Their life span is about 120 days. The process of development of RBC's is called Erythropoiesis. They are derived from Haemocytoblasts during maturation of cell, then the haemoglobin formation takes place inside the cell. Maturation of the cell depends on a number of factors, the one is presence of vitamin B_{12} and folic acid. They are present in normal diet i.e., meat, liver and green vegetables. If the diet contains more than the body requirement, they will be stored in the liver. Absorption of vitamin B_{12} depends on a glycoprotein, called intrinsic factor, secreted by parietal cells in the gastric glands. Both together form vitamin B_{12} complex. It is absorbed by cells in the distal part of the ileum. The normal daily requirement of vitamin B_{12} is about 1-2 /ug.

Folic acid is absorbed by cells in the walls of the duodenum and jejunum. The normal daily requirement of folic acid is 100 to 200 /mg.

Haemoglobin: It consists of a complex protein called globin and iron containing red pigment haem. Each haemoglobin molecule consist of four globin proteins and four nonprotein red pigments called haems. A normal adult male contains 14 to 16 gm of haemoglobin/

100 ml of blood. and a normal adult female contains 12 to 16 gm/100ml of blood. Infants contain 14 to 20 gm/100ml of blood. Each haem contains one iron atom which is necessary for normal functioning of haemoglobin. A normal diet containing meat, eggs, bread and green leafy vegetables contains more iron. Women lose blood during menstruation and need more iron throughout the reproductive years and during pregnancy. Haemoglobin in RBC combines with oxygen to form oxyhaemoglobin. Each RBC contains about 280 million molecules of haemoglobin. Each haem containing an iron atom combines with one oxygen molecule. One gram of haemoglobin carries about 1.34 ml of oxygen. Haemoglobin carries 97% of oxygen in blood. The remaining 3% is carried in dissolved plasma. So oxygen is carried from lungs to tissues and carbon dioxide form tissues to lungs. Hypoxia is a stimulus to erythropoiesis. Hypoxia stimulates the production of hormone erythropoietin, mainly, by kidneys. This hormone stimulates an increase in the production of pro-erythroblasts and RBCs. The erythroprotein regulates normal red blood cells replacement.

Haemolysis: The life span of RBC is about 120 days and their break down is carried out by phagocytic reticulo endothelial cells. This process is called haemolysis. About 2 million R.B.C's per second are haemolysed.This occurs in spleen, liver and bone marrow. The iron released by haemolysis is retained in the body and reused in the bone marrow to form haemoglobin. Biliverdin is formed from the protein part of the erythrocytes. It is reduced to the yellow pigment bilirubin in the liver. It is excreted as part of bile and enters into small intestine. Bilirubin is converted into urobilinogen by bacteria present in large intestine. Some urobilinogen is absorbed back into the blood, converted to urobilin, a yellow pigment and excreted in urine. Urobilinogen is converted into stercobilin which is a brown pigment and excreted in the faeces.

Blood groups

Karl Landsteiner discovered human blood groups. ABO blood group system is used to categorize blood of human beings. The surface of erythrocytes contains ABO antigens (agglutinogens). A person with A group blood has type A antigens, type B group has type B antigens, type AB blood has both A and B antigens. In addition, the plasma of type A blood contains Type B antibodies (agglutinins), which act against type B antigens. Plasma of type B blood contains type A antibodies (agglutinins), which act against type A antigens. Type AB blood has neither type of antibody and type O blood contains both type A and B antibodies (agglutinins).

A donor is a person who donates blood. A recipeint is a person who receives blood. If donors blood does not match with that of the recipient, the incompatibility results in agglutination and lysis of donated red blood cells occurs after transfusion, This may lead to serious condition and may cause death.

ABO System

	Blood group	RBC antigens	Antibodies serum	Can donate to groups	Can receive in from groups
1.	AB	A & B	None	AB	All groups
2.	A	A	Anti – B	A and AB	A and O
3.	B	B	Anti – A	B and AB	B and O
4.	O	None	Anti A and Anti B	All groups	' O '

Rhesus system: The rhesus factor is present on red blood cell membrances that is, Rhesus positive (Rh +ve) and those who lack Rh antigens are designated as Rhesus negative (Rh -ve). The Rhesus factor has a number of antigens of which 'D' is the most common. The individuals with 'D' antigen are classified as Rhesus positive. Administration of Rh +ve blood to Rh –ve recepients stimulates an immune response with the production of antibodies that cause haemolysis of RBCs.

Thrombocytes or platelets

They are very small nonnucleated discs derived from megakaryocytes in red bone marrow. They are about 2 to 4 μm in diameter. The normal platelet couunt is between 250000 to 400000 per cu. mm of blood. They adhere to injured regions of blood vessels, producing a white thrombus, which covers injured surfaces and plugs deficiencies within the vessel walls. They are presumed to produce an enzyme, thrombo plastin, which is of importance in the clotting mechanism. Thromboplastin aids in the transformation of prothrombin into thrombin. Thrombin, in turn, transforms fibrinogen into fibrin. Serotonin, an agent that causes contraction of smooth muscle in small blood vessels, is also present in platelets. A decrease in the number of circulating platelets is seen clinically in a condition, known as thrombocytopenia.

Blood clotting (coagulation)

When a blood vessel is damaged bleeding occurs. Loss of blood is stopped by a formation of blood clot. The formation of a blood clot depends upon twelve clotting factors. Normally the clotting factors are inactive and do not cause clotting. Injury activates the clotting factors to produce a clot. Blood clotting is a complex process involving a number of chemical reactions. Three main stages are explained here

1. Injured tissues release chemicals which cause activation of clotting factors. Each clotting factor activates the next clotting factor in the series until the clotting factor prothrombinase is formed.

2. Prothrombinase and calcium act on inactive prothrombin and convert it into active thrombin.

3. Thrombin converts fibrinogen (inactive form) into fibrin (active form). The fibrin is a thread like protein. A network is formed from the fibrin threads which traps blood cells and platelets to form the clot. Condensaton and consolidation of the clot help to stop the flow of blood. In this way infection is reduced and healing is enhanced.

Leukocyte disorders

1. Leukopenia is the condition in which WBCs are reduced below normal i.e., less than 4000/cu.mm. of blood.

2. Agranulocytosis is an acute condition in which there is a great reduction in the number of polymorphonuclear leukocytes (frequently less than 500 granulocytes per cu. mm of blood)

3. Lymphopenia is a condition in which there is decrease in the number of lymphocytes in the blood.

4. Leukocytosis : An abnormal increase of circulating leukocytes in pathological condition.

5. Leukaemia is a malignant myeloproliferative disease of the bone marrow that results in the abnormal increase in the production of leukocytes and their precursors.

Disease of RBC's and haemoglobin

Anaemia : In this condition there is decrease in the amount of haemoglobin or a number of R.B.C's or both. So less amount of haemoglobin is available to carry sufficient oxygen from the lungs to the tissues.

THE CIRCULATORY SYSTEM

It consists of the heart which acts as a pump to expel the blood, and the blood vessels through which the blood circulates.

Blood Vessels: They are small tubes of different diameters ranging from 0.5 mm to 3 cms. They include the arteries, arterioles, veins, venules, and capillaries.

Arteries and arterioles: These blood vessels transport blood away from the heart. They vary in size.

Structure of blood vessels: Tunica adventitia or outer coat made up of loose areolar tissue containing blood capillaries and fibrous tissue.

Tunica media or middle coat consists of smooth muscle and elastic tissue.

Tunica intima or inner coat made up of inner lining of squamous epithelium called endothelium.

The proportion of smooth myocytes and elastic fibres varies according to its function, eg : elastic arteries i.e., aorta has more elastic tissue than smooth muscle in tunica media.

Anastomoses and end arteries: Anastomosis means two arterial branches joining or two veins joining called arterial anostomosis and venous anastomosis to have collateral circulation. If, by chance, one branch is obstructed, the tissue can get blood from another branch to prevent damage to tissues or organs. Eg : anastomosis channel at the base of the brain.

End arteries: These are distal branches of artery and there is no anastomoses with any branches, that is, only arterie supply blood to organs. By chance, if these arteries are obstructed death of the tissue or organs will occur. Eg : branches from circle of willis, central artery of retina of the eye.

Veins and Venules: These are blood vessels that transport blood to the heart. The structure of the veins are same, having 3 layers but thinner and the lumen is collapsed because of less elastic tissue. Some veins possess valves, that ensure the blood flow towards the heart and prevents back flow. Any damage to these valves occurs then the concerned vein gets dilated and tortuous course occurs. Then they are called varicose veins, eg: veins of the lower limb. The valves are reduplication of the endothelium. The smallest veins are called venules.

Capillaries: The smallest arterioles break up into a number of minute vessels called capillaries. The walls of which are made up of single layer of endothelium. Through these, fenestration of water and other small molecule substances can pass. The Capillaries of arterioles anastomose with smallest venules to form capillary anastomoses. Their diameter may be about 5 to 7 µm.

Sinusoids: They are wider in diameter than capillaries. They have very thin walls which separates blood from the neighbouring cells. The sinusoid wall is having phagocytic macrophages, eg : Kupffer's cells in the liver sinusoids, sinusoids present in endocrine glands and spleen. Because of the wider calibre, the blood pressure in sinusoids is lower than in capillaries and there is slower rate of blood flow.

Control of blood vessels: The blood flow in muscular arteries are under the control of the autonomic nervous system. The vaso motor centre is situated in the medulla oblongata. This centre controls the calibre of muscular and small arteries. The nerves that reduce the lumen of the blood vessels are vasoconstrictors, and those nerves which increase the lumen are called vasodilators.

Blood supply: The blood vessels get nutrition by means of diffusion. The inner two third gets nutrition by diffusion, the outer one third by small arterioles. These small arterioles are called vasa vasorum.

Capillary Exchange: In the capillaries at the arterial end the blood pressure is about 35 mm of Hg. It is the hydrostatic pressure of blood. The osmotic pressure in the capillaries is 25 mm of Hg. The difference of pressure between the two is 10 mm of Hg. This difference of pressure (10 mm of Hg) forces fluid from the capillaries into tissue spaces. Blood flows slowly through the large network of capillaries from the arterial end to the venous end. At the venous end the hydrostatic pressure of blood is 15 mm of Hg and the osmotic pressure is 25 mm of Hg. The difference of pressure between the two is 10 mm of Hg. The effect of osmotic pressure is to suck fluid from tissue spaces into capillaries. About nine-tenth of tissue fluid is sucked into the capillaries. About one tenth of tissue fluid does not return to the blood capillaries. They are drained from tissue spaces into minute lymph capillaries which originate as blind end tubes with similar walls, but more permeable than that of blood capillaries. From the lymph capillaries, they enter into lymph vessels and from there to the blood stream.

HEART

Cardiology is the study of the normal heart and its diseases. The heart is a hollow muscular organ. It weighs about 200 – 250 gms. It weighs less in women. The size is about one's own hand fist.

Position: The heart is situated in the mediastinum between the lungs, in the thoracic cavity, more inclined to the left than the right. Its base is directing posterio-superiorly and apex directing anterio inferiorly to wards the left. The apical beat can be felt in 5th intercostal space about 5 cms from the median plane, a little below the left nipple.

Relations : Anteriorly: The sternum, ribs and intercostal muscles.

Posteriorly: The oesophagus, trachea, left and right bronchus,descending aorta, inferior vena cava, and thoracic vertebrae.

Laterally : The lungs - The left lung overlaps the left side of the heart.

Superiorly : The great blood vessels, the aorta, pulmonary artery, superior vena cava and inferior vena cava.

Inferiorly : The apex rests on the central tendon of the diaphragm.

Structure: The heart has 3 layers, pericardium, myocardium and endocardium.

Pericardium: It consists of a touch, fibrous outer layer called the fibrous pericardium. Inside the fibrous sac, there is a double layer of serous membrane. The fibrous sac is continuous and merges with tunica adventitia of the blood vessels. Below, it is adherent to the diaphragm. So, it keeps the heart in position during contraction.

Serous pericardium: This has 2 layers. The outer parietal layer lines the inner surface of fibrous pericardium. The inner viceral layer lines the heart. Between the parietal and visceral pericardium is the pericardial sac which contains a thin film of serous fluid. This fluid helps reduce friction as the heart moves within the pericardial sac.

Myocardium: It is a specialised cardiac muscle tissue found only in the heart. Microscopically, the cardiac myocytes branch and their ends are in close contact with adjacent myocytes. These joints are called intercalated discs. The nucleus is situated centrally, and there are tranvere striations. They are the thick connections between two myocytes. The impulse of contraction spreads from cell to cell over the whole of cardiac muscle.

Endocardium: It lines the myocardium and is a thin, smooth, glistening membrane made up of flattened epithelial cells.

Interior of the heart: The heart is divided into right and left side by interatrial and interventricular septum. The septum is made up of myocardium and covered by endocardium. After birth, formen ovale, an opening in the interatrial septum closes. This is seen as a remnant (depression) named as fossa ovalis in this septum. Each side is divided by an atrio ventricular valve into an upper chamber, the atrium and a lower chamber, the ventricle. The atrio ventricular valves are formed by double folds of endocardium supported by fibrous tissue.

Valves of the heart

The right atrioventricular valve (tricuspid) has 3 valves or 3 cusps, and the left atrioventricular valve (mitral valve) has two cusps. The valves between the atria and ventricles open and close according to changes in pressure in the chambers. During ventricular systole the pressure in the ventricles rise higher than that in atria, closing the valves and preventing backward flow of blood. To the margin of valves, is the attachment of chordae tendinae. These tendinae help tight closure of valves. There are 3 papillary muscles in the right ventricle and there are two papillary muscles in the left ventricle. The base of muscles is attached inside the ventricle. The apices of papillary muscle are attached to the chordae tendinae. The trabeculae carneae are the irregular surface of folds and ridges of ventricular myocardium covered by endocardium.

Blood flow through the heart: The superior and inferior vena cava bring blood from all over the body and empty into the right atrium. The blood passes via atrioventricular valve into the right ventricle and from there it is pumped to the lungs through the pulmonary artery (deoxygenated blood). The opening of pulmonary

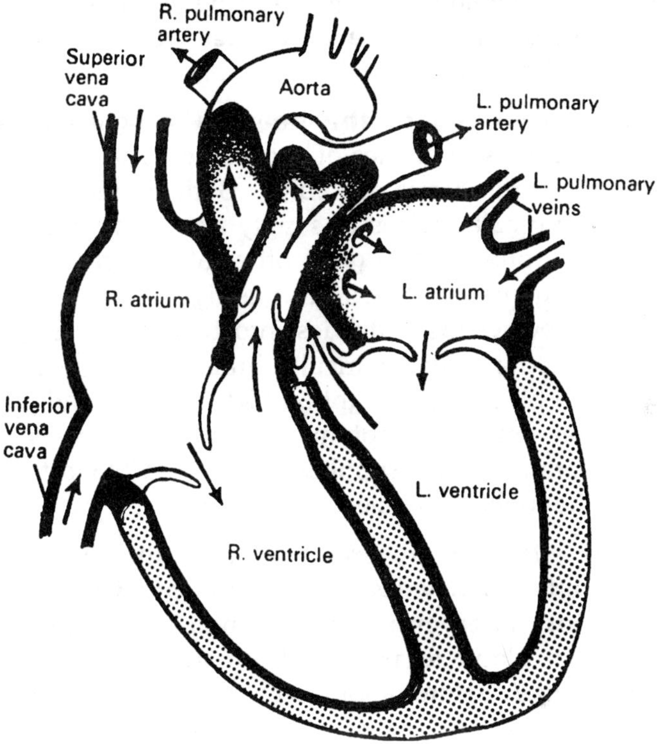

Figure 78. The Heart

artery is guarded by pulmonary semi lunar valves (3 valves). These valves prevent back flow of blood. The pulmonary artery divides into two branches and carry blood to the corresponding right and left lungs for the purification of blood.

Two pulmonary veins from each lung carries oxygenated blood and opens into the left atrium. Then the blood passes through the left atrio ventricular valve to the left ventricle, from there it is pumped into the aorta. The ascending aorta is guarded by 3 aortic semilunar valves. These valves prevent back flow of blood. It can be seen that the blood passes from the right to the left side of the heart via the lungs. Both atria contract at the same time and this is followed by the simultaneous contraction of\lungs where as the left ventricle pumps blood to whole of the body.

Blood supply to the heart: The right and left coronary arteries, branches of ascending aorta, arise just above the aortic semilunar valve. Both arteries run in the atrioventricular sulcus to supply atria and ventricles. The right coronary artery gives off small branches which supply oxygenrated blood to the right atrium. As it descends downwards it divides into two branches. One is the posterior inter ventricular branch which supplies oxygenated blood to the right and left ventricle and parts of the interventricular septum. The other branch is the marginal branch which supplies oxygenated blood to the wall of the right ventricle.

The left coronary artery is larger than the right coronary artery. It devides into two branches. One branch is anterior interventricular branch and supplies oxygentated blood to right and left ventricles and the interventricular septum. It joins with the terminal branches of circumflex artery of the right coronary artery and forms anastamosis. The other branch is the circumflex branch which supplies oxygenated blood to the walls of the left atrium and left ventricle. These arteries are end arteries. Stenosis (narrowing) of one or more branches of coronary arteries by atheroma restricts the flow of blood through it (them). The symptom which may result from this stenosis of one or more vessels is angina pectoris. Any blockage of these branches causes myocardial infarction. Most of the venous blood is collected into small veins which join to form coronary sinus which opens into the right atrium. Some small veins (thebesian veins) directly open into the right atrium.

The main veins carrying blood into the coronary sinus are the great cardiac vein which drains blood from the anterior aspect of the heart and the middle cardiac vein which drains blood from the posterior aspect of the heart.

The coronary sinus is a venous space consisting of a thin wall without a smooth muscle to alter its diameter.

Conducting system of the heart

There are some specialised neuro muscular cells (autorhythmic cells) in the myocardium, which initiate and conduct impulses of contraction throughout the muscle of the heart.

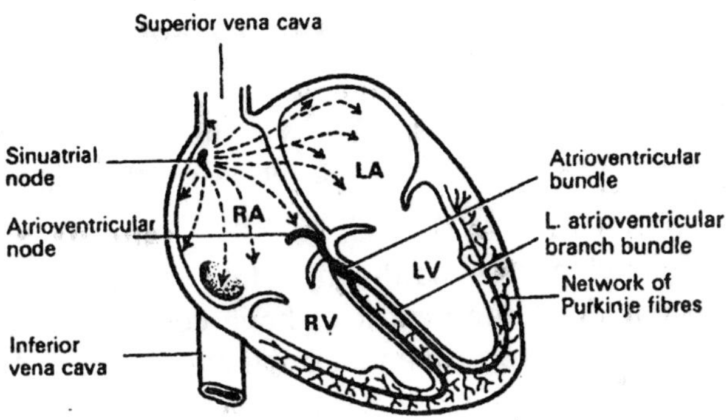

Figure 79. Conducting system of the heart.

a) **Sinoatrial node (SA node)** : It is the specialised cells in the wall of the right atrium near the opening of superior vena cava. The SA node is often called 'pacemaker' because it initiates impulse of contractions of the heart. From this cardiac action potentials spread over the right and left atria, causing them to contract and the blood enters into the ventricles.

b) **Atrio ventricular node** (AV node) It is also the specialised cells situated in the wall of the atrial septum near the atrioventricular opening.

Normally, the AV node is stimulated by the impulse of contraction that sweeps from the SA node.

c) **Atrio ventricular bundle** (AV bundle or bundle of His.) It is a specialised mass fibres that originate from AV node. The AV bundle crosses the fibrous ring at the upper end of the ventricular septum. It divides into right and left branch bundles, dessends on either side of ventricular septum, then the branches break up into fine fibres called purkinje fibres. These fibres spread in the myocardium and also in the papillary muscles. These fibres convey impulse of contraction from the AV node to the ventricles.

Action potentials spread over the ventricles causing them to contract and the blood is pumped out into the aorta and pulmonary artery.

Following their contraction the ventricles begin to relax. After the ventricles have completely relaxed, another action potential originates in the S.A. node and the next cycle of contractions begins.

Autonomic nerve supply

The heart is influenced by nerves originating from the cardiac centre in the medulla oblongata. The nerves reach the heart through the autonomic nervous system. These have sympathetic and parasympathetic nerves. They are antagonistic to one another.

Sympathetic nerves supply the SA and AV nodes and the myocardium of atria and ventricles. This stimulation increases the rate and force of the heart beat.

Parasympathetic nerves (vagus nerve) supply mainly SA and AV nodes and atrial muscle. This stimulation decreases the rate and force of the heart beat.

Cardiac activity usually decreases during rest and increases during excitement and exercise.

Cardiac cycle: The heart acts as a pump and its action consists of a series of contractions and relaxations. These events are known as the cardiac cycle. The number of cardiac cycles per minute varies from 60 to 80, the average is 72 per minute. Each cycle lasts about 0.8 of a second.

Atrial systole – Contraction of the atria.

Ventricular systole– Contraction of the ven tricle.

Cardiac diastole – relaxation of the atria and ventricles.

The superior and inferior vena cava pour deoxygenated blood into the right atrium. At the same time the four pulmonary veins pour oxygenated blood into the left atrium. The atrioventricular valves open and blood flows through the openings to the ventricles. During ventricular systole the AV valves close and the semilunar valves of aorta and pulmonary artery open. The blood from the ventricles goes to aorta for circulation into the body and to the lungs through the pulmonary arteries. The contraction of impulse from SA node spreads over the myocardium of both atria and the atria contracts and ventricular filling takes place (aterial sysole 0.1 sec). The wave of contraction reaches the AV node and spreads through AV bundles, branch bundles and purkinje fibres. This results in contraction of ventricles (systole 0.3 sec). and empty the contents. After ventricular contraction, there is complete cardiac diastole (0.4 sec); both atria and ventricles are relaxed.

Heart sounds: If a stethoscope is placed on the chest wall a little below the left nipple and on left side of chest wall, two heart sounds can be heard. The two sounds are separated by a pause, can be clearly distinguished. They are described in words as "Lub and dub"

The first sound "Lub" is fairly loud and is due to the closure of atrioventricular valves, soon after ventricular systole begins.

The second sound "dub" is softer and is due to the closure of aortic and pulmonary semilunar valves at the beginning of the ventricular diastole.

Normally the third and fourth heart sounds (S_3 and S_4) are not heard. The third heart sound (S_3) occurs in early diastole, is associated with rapid ventricular filling and the fourth heart sound (S_4) occurs in late diastole and is associated with atrial contraction.

Abnormal heart sounds are called murmurs. They are named as systolic murmur and diastolic murmur.

Other abnormal heart sounds are crescendo, decresendo, ejection click and thrill. `Fremitus' is another term used in relation to thrill.

Cardiac output

The volume of blood pumped out of the left ventricle (or right ventricle) into the aorta (or pulmonary trunk) each minute is called cardiac output.

It is measured by multiplying the stroke volume into the heart rate. If the stroke volume is 70 ml and the heart rate is 70 per minute the cardiac output is as follows

SV X HR = CO
70 ml/beat X 70 beat/min
= 4900 ml, rounded off to 5000 ml or 5litres.

This volume is close to the blood volume which is about 5 litres in an adult male. Exercise increases the stroke volume and heart rate thus increasing the cardiac output. During exercise it may increase upto 20 litres per minute.

The Normal Electro Cardio Gram (ECG)

As the cardiac impulses pass through the heart, electrical currents spread into the tissues surrounding the heart, and a small proportion of these spreads all the ways to the surface of the body. If the electrodes are placed on the skin on opposite side of the heart, electrical potentials generated by these currents can be recorded. The recording is known as Electrocardiogram. A normal electro-cardio-gram of the heart is as follows.

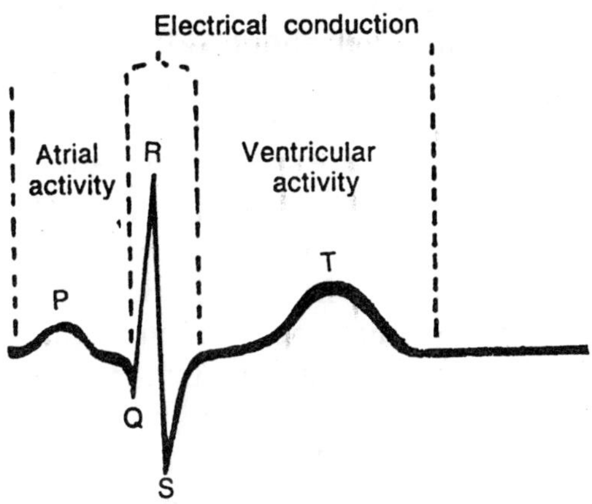

Figure 80. Normal E.C.G.

Normal ECG is composed of a P wave, a 'QRS' complex, and a 'T' wave. The QRS complex has often three separate waves, the Q wave, the R wave, and the S wave.

The P wave is caused by electrical potentials generated in the atria prior to contraction (atrial depolarization).

The QRS complex is caused by potentials generated in the ventricle prior to contraction (onset of ventricular depolarization).

The T wave is caused by potentials generated as the ventricular relaxation (ventricular repolarization). By examining the pattern, the waves and the time interval between cycle, the physician obtains valuable information regarding the condition of myocardium and conducting system.

Blood Pressure: It may be defined as the force or pressure which the blood exerts on the walls of blood vessels in which it is contained. Arterial blood pressure is more than the venous pressure. When the left ventricle contracts and pushes blood into the aorta, the pressure produced is called the systolic blood pressure. In adults, it is about 120 mm of Hg. When cardiac diastole occurs and the heart is resting following ejection of blood, the pressure within arteries is called diastolic blood pressure. In adult, it is about 80 mm of Hg. It increases with age and is usually higher in women than in men. Blood pressure is expressed as following, Bp = 120/80 mm of Hg. The blood pressure is maintained within normal limits by involving a number of factors i.e., cardiac out put, venous return, blood volume, peripleral resistance and elasticity of the aterial wall.

Pulse pressure : The difference between the systolic and diastotic pressure is called the pulse pressure. If a person has a systolic pressure of 120 mm Hg and a diastolic pressure of 80 mm Hg. The pusle pressure is 40 mm Hg. Pulse pressure inceases in a person suffering from arteriosclerosis.

Blood pressure above 140/90 mm Hg is considered high blood pressure.

Measurement of blood pressure

A sphygmonometer is used to measure the blood pressure. In clinical conditions, the auscultatory method is used to determine blood pressure. A sphygmo-monometer consists of a blood pressure cuff which s placed around the patient's arm and a stethoscope is placed

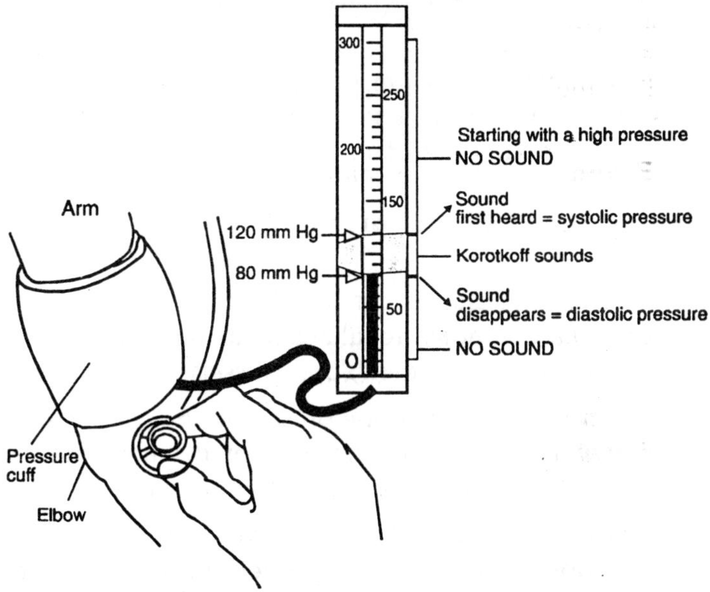

Figure 81. Blood pressure measurement

over the brachial artery. Inflating the blood pressure cuff blocks the brachial artery completely. Then the blood does not flow through the constricted area, so no sounds can be heard through the stethoscope at this point. The pressure in the cuff is then gradually lowered. Gradually deflating the blood pressure cuff allows the column of mercury to fall. As soon as the pressure in the cuff declines below the systolic pressure, blood flows through the constricted area. This produces vibrations in the blood and surrounding tissues that can be heard through the stethoscope. These sounds are named as KOROTKOFF sounds. The pressure at which the KOROTKOFF sound is heard is the systolic pressure.

As the pressure in the blood pressure cuff is lowered stil more, the pressure drops and at a point the sound disappears completely. Then continuous blood flow is reestablished. The pressure at which the KOROTKOFF sound disappears is the diastolic pressure

The blood pressure varies with rest, activity, emotion and age.

A low blood pressure or hypotension is present in shock due to blood loss, septicaemia, myocardial infarction and in other conditions.

Regulation of blood pressure and blood flow :

1. The cardiovascular centre which is present in the medulla oblongata regulates heart rate, contractility and diameter of the blood vessels.
2. Baroreceptors which are present in the carotid sinus (carotid bodies) and the arch of the aorta and in the right atrium monitor blood pressure
3. Chaemoreceptors of the carotid sinus and arch of the aorta monitor blood levels of O_2, CO_2 and hydrogen ions.
4. Hormones that help regulate blood pressure are epinephrine, norepinephrine, ADH (vasapressin), angiotensin II and atrial natriuretic peptide (ANP).

Pulse: It is described as a wave of distension and elongation felt in an artery wall due to the contraction of the left ventricle. The lefft ventricle pumps about 60 to 80 ml of blood into aorta. When the aorta is distended, a wave passes along the walls of the arteries and can be felt at any point where an artery can be compressed against a bone. The radial artery at the wrist is most commonly used to feel the pulse. Pulse is felt in the following arteries namely temporal artery, facicial artery, common carotid artery, brachial artery, fernoral artery, popliteal artery, posterior tibial artery and dorsalis pedis artery. The number of pulse beats per minute varies in different people and in the same person at different times and ages. An average pulse rate is 60 - 80/minute. During exercise and emotion of a person,the pulse rate is increased. The pulse gives certain information

3. The rate at which the heart is beating
2. The rhythm gives regularity of heart beats.
3. The volume or strength of the beat, compression of the artery moderately, gives some indication of the blood pressure and the state of the wall of the blood vessel.

Circulation of Blood

William Harvey first explained the circulation of blood. The blood circulation of the body is continuous around the body. It may be divided into

1. Pulmonary circulation
2. Systemic circulation
3. Hepatic Portal circulation
4. Coronary circulation

Pulmonary Circulation

It consists of circulation of blood from the right ventricle of the heart to the lungs and back to the left atrium. In the lungs, carbon dioxide is excreted and oxygen is absorbed. The pulmonary artery, carrying deoxygenated blood, leaves the right ventricle of the heart. It passes upwards and divides into left and right pulmonary arteries.

The right pulmonary artery passes to the root of the right lung and divides into branches that enter the right lung.

The left pulmonary artery passes to the left root of the lung, where it divides into branches and enter the left lung.

Within the lungs, these arteries divide and sub divide into smaller arteries, arterioles and capillaries. The capillaries are in contact with alveoli of lungs for exchange of gases. In each lung, the venules containing oxygenated blood join up and form two pulmonary veins.

The two pulmonary veins leave each lung, carrying oxygenated blood to left atrium. During atrial systole, this blood passes into left ventricle and during ventricular systole, it is forced into the aorta for systemic circulation.

Systemic Circulation

The blood from the left ventricle is carried by ascending aorta, branches of the arch of aorta and descending aorta to circulate around the body and is returned to the right atrium by the superior and inferior vena cava. This is called systemic or general circulation, In the systemic circulation, the blood passes through arteries and veins of body.

Arteries carry oxygenated blood to supply the body tissues.

The Aorta begins at the upper part of the left ventricle, passing upwards for a short way, then arches backwards and to the left, descends behind the heart through the thoracic cavity to a little left of the thoracic vertebrae at 12th thoracic vertebra. This part in the thoracic cavity is called thoracic aorta. It enters the abdominal cavity through the opening in the diaphragm. In abdominal cavity, it is called abdominal aorta. At the level of 4th lumbar vertebra, it divides into right and left common iliac arteries.

Thoracic aorta

1. Ascending aorta
2. Arch of the aorta.
3. Descending aorta.

Ascending aorta starts from the left ventricle. It is about 5 cms long, passes behind the sternum. At its origin there are three dilations called aortic sinuses, two of these, the right and left sinuses - give rise to the right and left coronary arteries respectively. Arch of the aorta, is

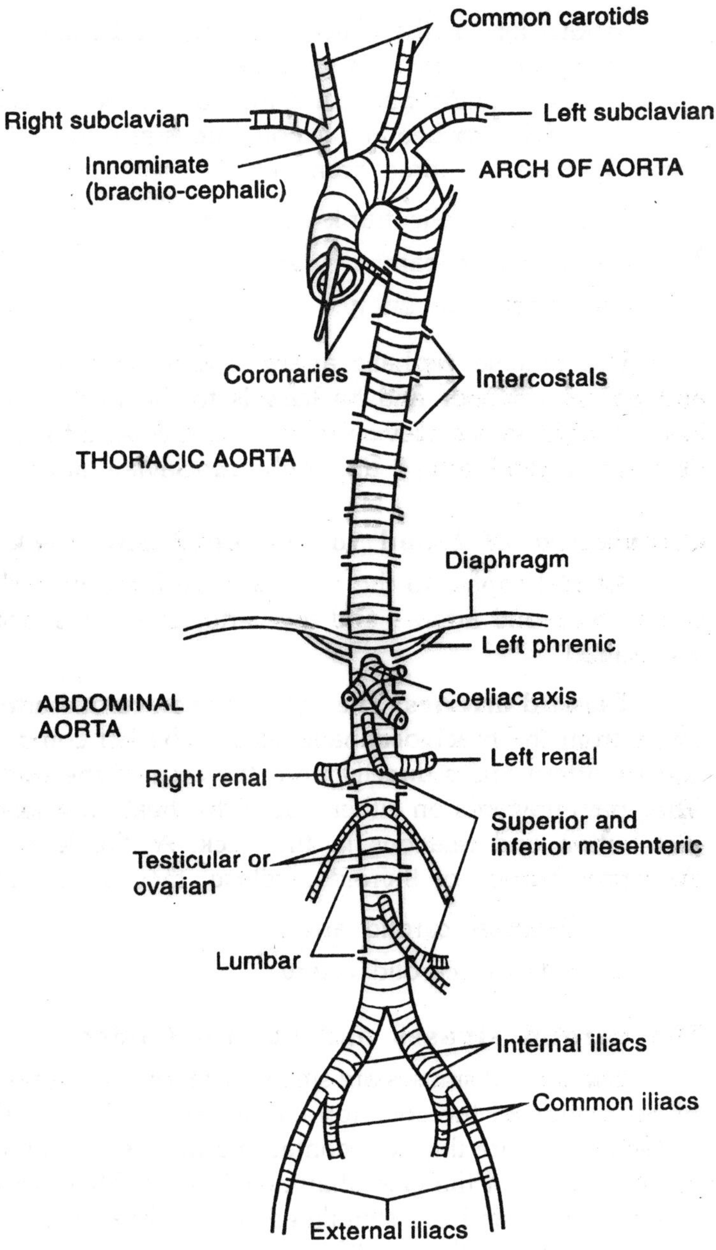

Figure 82. The aorta and its main branches

the continuation of the ascending aorta is behind the manubrium sterni and runs upwards, backwards and to the left in front of the trachea. It then passes downwards to the left of the trachea and is continuous as descending aorta. It gives off three branches.

Brachio cephalic trunk or artery.

Left common carotic artery.

Left subclavian artery.

The brachio cephalic artery is about 5 cms long and passes upwards and backwards to the right at the level of right sterno clavicular joint. It divides into right common acrotid artery and right subclavian artery.

Circulation of blood to the head and neck

Arterial supply to the head and neck are from the common carotid arteries and the vertebral arteries, both are paired.

Carotid arteries: The right common carotid artery arises from the brachiocephalic artery. The left common carotid artery arises directly from the arch of the aorta. They pass upwards on either side of trachea, have same distribution and relations in the neck. At the level of the upper border of thyroid cartilage, they divide into

1. External carotid artery.
2. Internal carotid artery.

The carotid sinuses and carotid bodies

The carotid sinuses are small dilatations at the point of bifurcation of the common carotid arteries. The walls of the sinuses are thin and contain numerous specialised nerve endings of the glosspharyngeal nerve. They act as 'Barorecptors' and are stimulated by any change in the blood pressure in the carotid sinuses. The carotid bodies are small groups of specialised cells, lying in close association at the bifurcation of common carotid artery.

They are supplied by branches of glossopharyngeal nerve. These specialised cells are stimulated by any change in concentration of carbon dioxide and oxygen. These cells have connection to respiratory centre in the medulla oblongata to adjust the respiratory movements. They are also called chemo receptors.

External carotid artery: This artery supplies the structures in the head and neck through these branches.

1. The superior thyroid artery supplies the thyroid gland.
2. The lingual artey supplies the tongue and tonsil.
3. The facial artery supplies, face, muscles of the face and sub mandibular gland. One can feel the facial artery at the base of the mandibule.
4. The occipital aretry supplies the posterior part of the scalp.
5. The ascending pharyngeal aretry supplies the pharynx and prevertebral muscles.
6. The posterior auricular artery supplies the auricle and auricular muscles of the ear.
7. The maxillary artery supplies the muscles of mastication. The important branch is a middle meningeal artery which enters the head and supplies the covering of the brain and skull.
8. The superficial temporal artery passes over the zygomatic arch in front of the ear, and supplies the frontal, temporal and parietal parts of the scalp. The pulse may be felt on this artery in front of the ear.

The internal carotid artery: It is the major contributor to the circle of willis which supplies the greater part of the brain. It ascends to the base of the brain through the carotid foramen. It also supplies the eyes, forehead and nose.

The circulus arteriosus (circle of willis)

It is the arterial anastomoses channel situated at the base of the brain in subarchnoid space to supply the brain. It is formed by four arteries. The vertebral arteries unite to form basilar aretry. This artery runs on the anterior surface of the pons to its upper margin, where it divides into the posterior cerebral arteries. The internal carotid artery enters into the cranial cavity through the carotid formen. At the base of the brain, the internal carotid artery divides into the anterior and middle cerebral arteries. Both the right and left anterior cerebral arteries are connected by anterior communicating artey. In between posterior and middle cerebral arteries they are connected by posterior communicating arteries to complete the circle of willis. Its branches are

2 Anterior cerebral arteries
1 Anterior communicating artery
2 Middle cerebral arteries
2 Posterior communicating arteries
2 Posterior cerebral arteries.

Branches of circle of willis namely the basilar artery and vertebral arteires supply the brain and spinal cord.

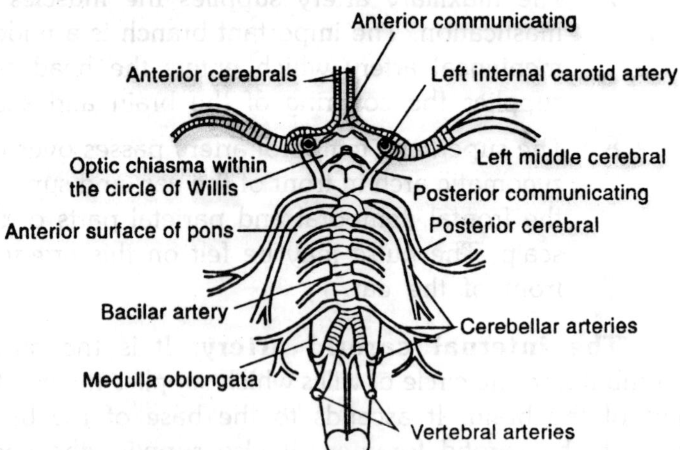

Figure 83. The circulus arteriosus

Venous return from the head and neck

The venous blood from the head and neck is returned by deep and superficial veins. The superficial veins have the same name as the branches of external carotid artery. They drain venous blood from the superficial structures of the face and scalp, and unite to form the external jugular vein at the angle of the mandible. It passes downwards on the anterior surface of sterno mastoid muscle and joins the subclavian vein behind the clavicle. The venous blood which returns from the brain is collected into sinuses. These venous sinuses are formed by layers of durameter lined by endothelium.

The main venous sinuses are

1 Superior sagittal sinus

1 Inferior sagittal sinus

1 Straight sinus

2 Transverse sinuses

2 Sigmoid sinuses.

The straight sinus continues as right and left sigmoid sinuses on either side of tentorium cerebelli. These sinuses pass through the jugular foramen as internal jugular veins out side the cranial cavity. They run downwards in the neck behind the sterno - mastoid muscle and join the subclavian veins carrying blood from the upper limbs to form the brachio cephalic veins. The brachio cephalic veins are situated one on either side in the root of the neck. The left brachio cephalic vein is longer than the right and passes obliquely behind the manubrium sterni, where it joins the right brachio cephalic vein to form the superior vena cava.

The superior vena cava drains all the venous blood from the head, neck and upper limbs. It passes downwards along the right border of the sternum and opens into the right atrium of the heart.

Circulation of blood to the upper limb

Arterial blood supply: The right subclavin artery arises from the brachio cephalic artery where as the left branch arises from the arch of the aorta. They pass behind the clavicle and over the first rib and at lower margins of 1st rib continue as axillary artery. The artery before entering the axilla gives off two branches. The vertebral artery which passes upwards to cranial cavity to supply the brain. Another artery is the internal mammary artery which descends in the anterior thoracic wall to supply the breast and the thoracic and anterior abdominal wall.

The axillary artery is the continuation of sub clavian artery and supplies the breast and the thoracic wall and axilla.

The brachial artery is the continuation of axillary artery in the arm and supplies blood to the humerus and muscles of the arm.

The radial artery is the terminal branch of the brachial artery which descends down to supply the forearm muscles and hand. This artery can be palpated against radius just above the wrist joint on the anterior surface. The ulnar artery is the terminal branch of the brachial artery to supply the forearm muscles and hand.

The superficial and deep palmar arches: These are the anastomatic channels between the radial and ulnar arteries to supply the digits.

Venous blood return from the upper limb

The venous blood is drained by two sets of veins. They are superficial veins and deep veins. The deep veins accompanying arteries take the same names. The superficial veins are

1. Cephalic vein
2. Basilic vein
3. Median cubital vein.

The cephalic vein: It starts on the dorsum of the hand as laternal continuation of dorsal venous arch. It winds round the radial side to the anterior aspect of the forearm. After crossing the elbow joint, it passes up the lateral aspect of the arm and in front of the shoulder joint to end in the axillary vein.

The basilic vein is the continuation of dorsal venous arch on the medial side. It ascends on the medial side of the fore arm, then crosses the elbow on medial side, passes upwards to the arm. In the middle of the arm it pierces the deep fascia to join the brachial vein.

The median cubital vein: It is a connecting channel between the cephalic and basilic veins in front of the elbow joint. Most of the blood from the cephalic veins drains to the basilic vein. This vein is commonly used for drawing blood samples and also for intra venous drips.

Descending aorta in the thorax: The arch of the aorta continues downwards at the level of the 4th thoracic vertebra as descending aorta on the left and anterior surface of bodies of vertebrae up to the level of 12th thoracic vertebra where it passes through an opening in the diaphragm and becomes abdominal aorta. The branches of the descending aorta in the thorax are-

1. Bronchial arteries that supply the lung tissue and structures at the root of the lungs.
2. Oesophageal arteries supply the oesophagus.
3. Intercostal arteries : There are 11 pairs of intercostal arteries. Each lie in the sub-costal groove of rib to supply the thoracic and abdominal walls.

Venous blood return from the thoracic cavity: The venous blood from the thoracic cavity is drained into the azygos vein and the hemiazygos vein. Tributaries to the azygos and hemiazygos veins are,

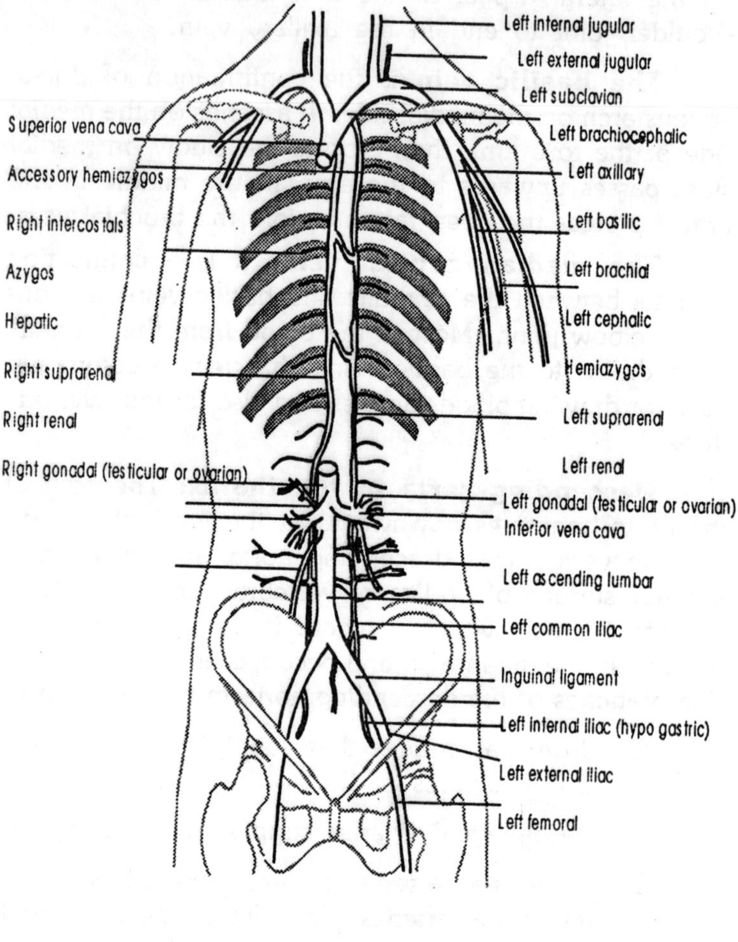

Figure 84. New figure

bronchial, oesophageal and intercostal veins. The azygos vein joins the superior vena cava and the hemiazygos vein joins the left brachio cephalic vein. At the distal end of the oesophagus, some oesophageal veins join the azygos vein and others, the left gastric vein to form venous plexus. This is the anastomatic channel between portal and systemic circulation.

Abdominal aorta: It is the continuation of thoracic aorta in the abdominal cavity. It descends in front of the bodies of the thoracic vertebrae to the level of 4th lumbar vertebra where it divides into right and left common iliac arteries.

The branches of abdominal aorta are paired and unpaired.

a) Unpaired arteries

1. Coeliac trunk have three branches

   Common hepatic aretery - supplies liver, gall bladder, parts of stomach, duodenum and pancreas.

   Left gastric artery - supplies most of the stomach and part of oesophagus.

   Splenic artery - supplies the speen, part of pancreas and part of stomach.

2. Superior mesentric artery - supplies the whole of small intestine, ascending colon and part of the transverse colon and part of the pancrease..
3. Inferior mesentric artery - supplies part of the transverse colon and descending colon, sigmoid colon including the rectum.
4. Medial sacral artery supplies the sacrum,coccyx and rectum.

b) Paired arteries

1. Inferior phrenic arteries - supplies the inner surface of the diaphragm and part of suprarenal glands.

2. Renal arteries - supplies blood to the kidneys and part of supra renal glands.
3. Supra renal arteries - supply suprarenal glands.
4. Gonadal arteries.

   Male - testicular arteries - supply testes and scrotum.

   Female - Ovarian arteries - supply overies
5. Lumbar arteries - supply the spinal cord and its menenzes and the muscles and skin of the lumbar region of the back.

So the branches of the abdominal aorta supplies all the viscera in the abdominal cavity and also the abdominal wall.

Venous blood returns from the abdominal organs to join the inferior vena cava. The inferior vena cava is formed by the left and right common iliac veins at the level of 5th lumbar vertebra. This is the largest vein in the body. It receives blood from all the viscera in the abdominal cavity and passes through the diaphragm to the right atrium of the heart. It enters the central tendon of the diaphragm at the level of 8th thoracic vertebra. The blood from the digestive system enters the liver through the portal circulation. The blood from the liver drains into the inferior vena cava by two hepatic veins.

HEPATIC PORTAL CIRCULATION

Portal circulation carries blood between two capillary networks (beds), from one location in the body to another without passing through the heart.

In this case, the venous blood passes from the capillary bed of the abdominal part of the digestive system, the spleen, and pancreas to the liver. In the liver sinusoids the portal veins ends into capillary bed. The blood in the portal circulation contains high concentration of nutrient materials absorbed from the stomach and intestine and goes to the liver for metabolism. Then it enters the systemic circulation to distribute nutrient materials to the body.

The portal vein is formed by the union of the splenic and the superior mesentric veins posterior to the neck of the pancreas.

The splenic vein drains blood from the spleen, the pancreas and part of the stomach.

The inferior mesentric vein returns blood from the rectum, pelvic and descending colon. This vein joins the splenic vein.

The superior mesentric vein returns venous blood from the small intestine and the proximal parts of large intestine i.e. the caecum, ascending and transverse colon. It unites with the splenic vein to form the portal vein.

The gastric vein drains the blood from the stomach and distal end of the oesophagus to portal vein.

The cystic vein drains venous blood from the gall bladder and joins the portal vein.

The hepatic veins are short veins. They leave the liver and join the inferior vena cava.

Circulation of blood to the pelvis and lower limb:

Arterial blood supply

Common iliac arteries : The right and left common iliac arteries are terminal branches of abdominal aorta. In front of the sacro iliac joint, each artery divides into

1. Internal iliac artery
2. External iliac artery

The Internal iliac artery runs medially to supply the organs within the pelvic cavity. In the female, the uterine arteries branches of the interal iliac arteries (hypogastric) supply the female reproductive organs namely the uterus and vagina.

In the male,branches of the internal iliac arteries supply the prostate gland and vas deferens.

In both males and femles, branches of the internal iliac artries supply psoas major, gluteal muscles, quadratus lumborum, medial side of each thigh, urinary bladder and rectum.

The external iliac artery runs obliquely downwards, passes behind the inguinal ligament into the thigh where it becomes the femoral artery.

The femoral artery begins at the mid point of inguinal ligament where one can feel the pulse of femoral artery. It passes downwards, then turns medialy and passes into the medial aspect of the femur to enter the popliteal space where it continues as popliteal artery. The femoral artery and its branches supply blood to complete thigh muscles and femur. The popliteal artery passes behind the knee joint and at the lower border of popliteal area, it divides into anterior and posterior tibial arteries. The popliteal artery supplies the knee joint. The anterior tibial artery passes forwards between the tibia and fibula and enters the anterior compartment of leg and descends down upto the ankle joint where it continues as the dorsalis pedis artery on the dorsum of the foot. The anterior tibial artery supplies blood to the anterior compartment of the leg.

The dorsalis pedis artery is in continuation of the anterior tibial artery, runs forwards and enters into 1st interosseous space and supplies blood to plantar surface of the foot. It can be palpated between the great toe and 2nd toe.

The posterior tibial artery is the branch of popliteal artery. It descends in the posterior compartment of the leg upto the ankle joint. It gives peroneal branch and supplies lateral compartment muscles. The posterior tibial artery supplies contents of the posterior compartment. It enters the sole of the foot where it continues as the plantar artery.

The planter artery supplies the structures in the sole of the foot and it joins the dorsalis pedis artery to complete the plantar arch. From the arch, the digital branches supply blood to the toes.

Venous blood return from lower limbs and pelvis:

The venous blood from the lower limb is drained by superficial and deep veins, and from pelvis by internal iliac veins. The deep veins of the lower limb accompanies the arteries, where as, the superficial veins run in superficial fascia. Both veins are connected by perforating veins. All the veins have valves. These valves allow the blood flow to the deep veins and the blood ascends upwards by contraction of the muscles of lower limb. The valves help the blood to pass against gravity. Any damage to the valves, accumulation of blood occurs, that leads to dilatation of veins resulting in varicosity of the veins.

The deep veins accompany the arteries and having the same names as arteries.

The femoral vein continues upwards under the inguinal ligament as external iliac vein. This vein joins with internal iliac vein from pelvic cavity to form the common iliac vein.

The two common iliac veins begin at the sacroiliac joint. They ascend obliquely and a little to the right of 5th lumbar vertebra and join the inferior vena cava.

The superficial veins

Short saphenous vein is in continuation of the dorsal venous arch on the lateral side of the dorsum of the foot. This vein ascends to the lateral side and posterior surface of leg to end in popliteal vein.

The long saphenous veins: It is the longest superficial vein in the body. It is the continuation of dorsal venous arch on medial side on dorsum of the foot. It ascends to the medial side of the ankle and anterior to the medial malleoulus. Here, doctors do venesection to put the venous catheter in conditions of shock when other veins are collapsed. It ascends to the medial aspect of the knee joint, then in the anterior surface of the thigh it ascends and ends in the femoral vein passing through the saphenous opening. Commonest clinical problem is varicosity of the long saphenous vein.

The perforating veins: These are communicating veins from superficial to deep veins. In these veins, blood flow is superficial to deep, having valves.

Questions

1. Write the composition of blood.
2. Name the plasma proteins and list their functions.
3. Give a brief account of Leucocytes (WBC).
4. What are the common disorders of leukocytes?
5. Locate exact position of the heart with a neat diagram.
6. Name the three layers of the heart and explain briefly the structure and function of each of the layers.
7. Define the blood pressure with a brief account.
8. What information can be gained of the pulse?
9. Name the types of circulation of blood.
10. What do you understand by "Systemic circulation" and "Pulmonary circulation"?

11. Write short notes on the following:

    a) Blood groups
    b) Coagulation of blood
    c) Interior structure of the heart

12. a) What is meant by portal circualtion?
    b) Name the three portal circulations in the body.
    c) Describe the hepatic portal circulation.

The Lymphatic system

Approximately nine tenths of the fluid that leaves the capillaries returns to the venous capillaries and the remaining one tenth of the fluid diffuse through the more permeable walls of the lymph capillaries. The tissue fluid after entering into the lymph capillaries is called lymph. The composition of lymph is similar to that of plasma but the constituents have some additional substances that are too large to pass through blood capillary walls, eg : macroparticles from damaged area, and cells damaged by disease and bacteria. Lymph passes through different size of vessels and a varying number of lymph nodes before returning to the blood.

The lymphatic system consists of

Lymph vessels

Lymph nodes

Lymphatic tissue eg: tonsils

Spleen, ed bone marrow and

Thymus gland.

The primary lymphatic organs of the body are the red bone marrow and the thymus gland because they produce B and T cells.

LYMPH VESSELS

These originate as blind end tubes in the interstitial spaces. Structurely, they are same as blood capillaries having a single layer of endothelial cells. Their walls are more permeable to all interstitial fluid including proteins and cell debris. The capillaries join to form larger lymph vessels. The walls of lymph vessels are about the same thickness as those of small veins and have the same layers of tissue. Lymph vessels have numerous cup shaped valves that prevent back flow of movement of lymph in vessels. Certain factors are believed to assist, include

1. Tissue fluid pressure
2. Contraction of surrounding muscles
3. Pressure caused by the pulsation of adjacent vessels
4. Negative pressure in the thorax during inspiration.

Lymph vessels join together to form two larger ducts, the thoracic duct and the right lymphatic duct, that empty lymph into the subclavian veins.

The thoracic duct

This duct begins at the upper end of cisterna chyli, which is a dilatation of lymph vessel in front of the bodies of 1-2 lumbar vertebrae. It is about 40 cms long ascends through the diaphragm and passes upwards in the thoracic cavity, enters into the root of the neck, and opens at the junction of internal jugular and left sub clavian veins. It drains lymph from both legs, the pelvic and abdominal cavities, the left half of the thorax, head and neck and the left upper limb.

The right lymphatic duct

It lies in the root of the neck and opens into the right subclavian vein. It drains lymph from right half of the thorax, head and neck and right upper limb.

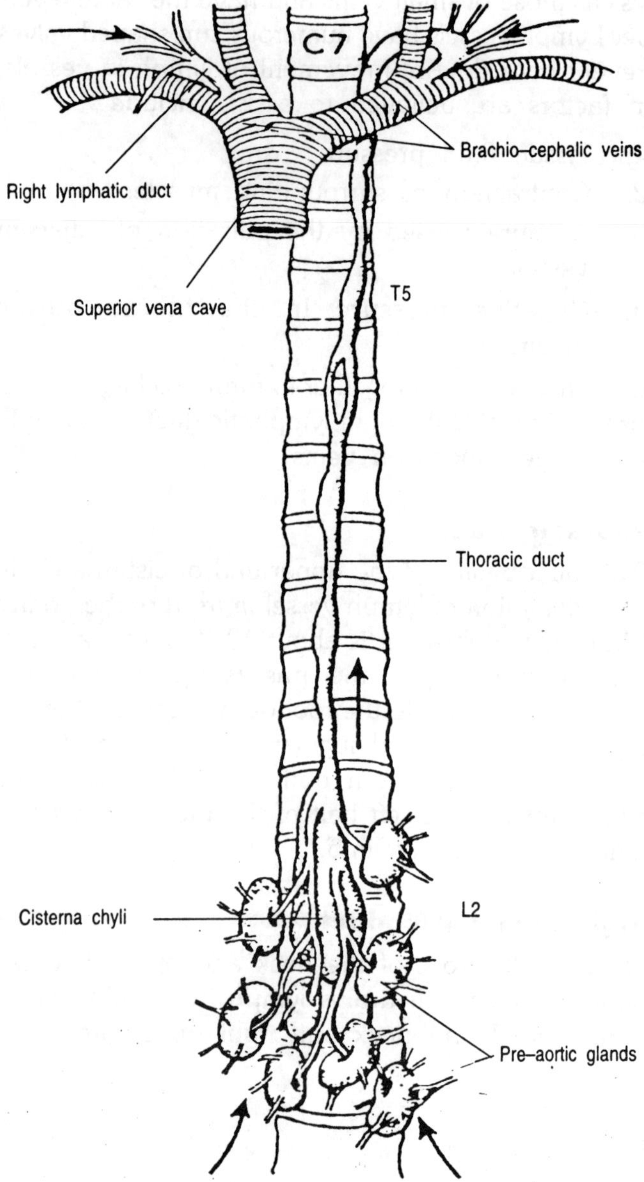

Figure 85. The thoracic duct

LYMPH NODES

All the small and medium size lymph vessels open into lymph nodes which are situated in the area where the bacteria enter or the tissues are exposed or more prone for infection. Throughout the body, the lymph drains through a number of nodes, usually, 5 to 10 before returning to the blood. The size of a node varies from pin head to the largest is about the size of an almond.

Structure: A lymph node has a fibrous capsule, which dips down into the node forming trabeculae that divide the node into compartments. Below the capsule is sub capsular substance. The frame work of the node is made up of the capsule, trabeculae, reticular fibres and fibroblats. The outer portion is called cortex.

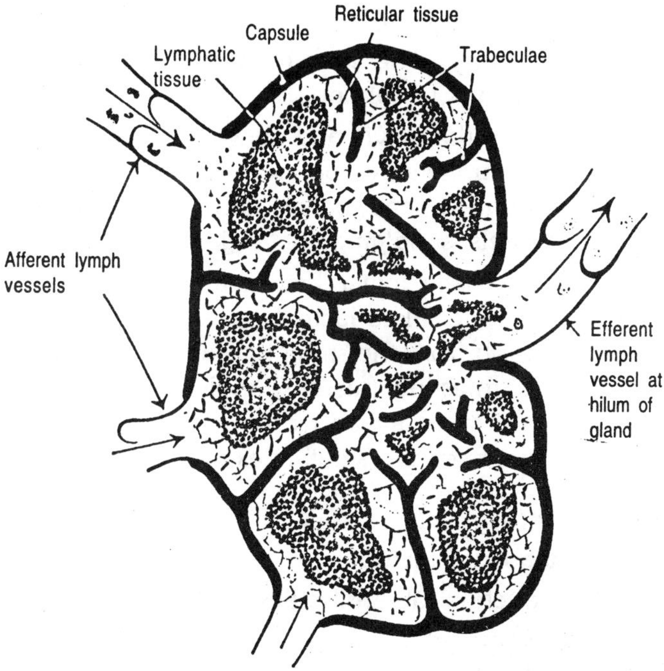

Figure 86. Section of a lymph node.

It has more aggregation of lymphocytes which are called lymphatic nodules and also present macrophages. The inner portion is called medulla. It has tightly packed lymphocytes, macrophages and plasma cells. The hilum of the node is in direct contact with the medulla, where there are no lymphatic nodules. In the hilus, the blood vessels and only one efferent lymph vessel leaves, where as, 4-6 afferent lymph vessels are present around the cortex, which enter the lymph node. Lymph flows through a node in one direction

Lymph is drained from the head and neck through deep superficial cervical nodes.

Lymph is drained from the upper limb and anterior chest wall through the axillary lymph nodes.

Lymphatic drainage occurs from the thoracic cavity through the groups of nodes. They are, parasternal intercostal, brachiocephalic, mediastinal, tracheobrachial, broncho pulmonary. The lymph of the breast passes through the axillary lymph nodes.

Lymph from the pelvic and abdominal cavities pass through many lymph nodes before entering the cisterna chyli. The abdominal and pelvic nodes are associated with blood vessels supplying the organs.

Lymph from the lower limb drains through deep and superficial nodes. The lacteals are lymph capillaries which drain lymph from the small intestine. Fat absorbed from the small intestine passes into lymph capillaries. This lymph gives a milky appearance. Lymph entering the thoracic duct from the small intestine is called Chyle.

Functions of lymph nodes

1. Phagocytic action
2. Production of antibodies
3. Enlargement of lymph nodes, when the area of drainage is infected or has malignancy.
4. Activated T- and B-lymphocytes multiply.
5. Filtration of lymph.

Lymphatic tissue

The lymphatic tissue is found in a number of situations in the body in addition to the lymph nodes.

1. Palatine tonsils - They lie between the mouth and oral part of the pharynx.
2. Pharyngeal tonsil - lie between the pillars of the fauces on the wall of the nasal part of the pharynx. Hypertrophy of the pharyngeal tonsil (Luschka's tonsil) is known as adenoids. (Meyer's disease).
3. Lingual tonsils : They are paired and lie at the base of the tongue.
4. Solitary lymphatic follicles - They are found in the duodenum and jejunum.
5. Aggregated lymphatic folliceles (peyer's patches) - They are found in the ileum. Typhoid is the disease of the peyer's patches.
6. Vermiform appendix : It consists of aggregation of lymphatic modules.

Spleen

The spleen is formed partly by lymphatic system. It lies in the left hypochondriac region of the abdominal

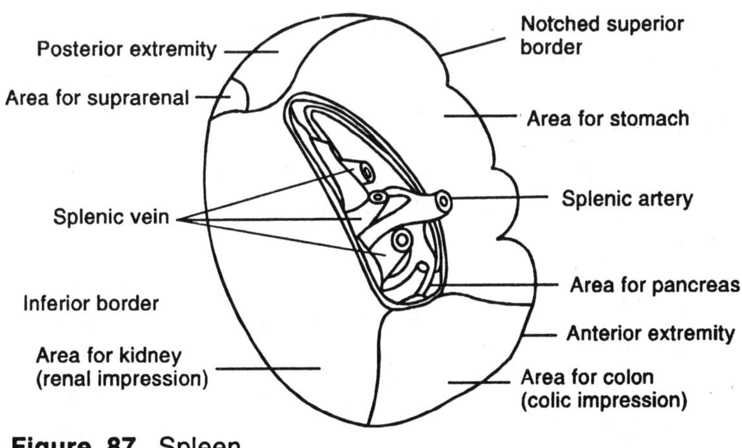

Figure 87. Spleen

cavity between the fundus of the stomach and diaphragm. It varies in size in different individuals, usually, about 12 cms long, 7 cms wide and 2.5 cms thick.

Relations

1. Posteriorly and Superiorlly - diaphragm

Inferiorly	:	left colic flexure of the large intestine
Anteriorly	:	fundus of the stomach
Medially	:	pancreas and left kidney.
Laterally	:	9th, 10th and 11th ribs and intercostal muscles, separated by diaphragm

Structure: It is oval in shape with the hilum on medial surface and enclosed in peritoneum. It is covered by a capsule. The capsule dips into the organ to form trabeculae. The trabaculae subdivides the structure into lobules. The spleen is composed of white pulp consisting of lymphatic nodules and diffuse lymphatic tissue and of red pulp consisting of venous sinuses between which are splenic cords. The stroma of both red and white pulp is composed of reticular fibres and cells. The spleen has no afferent lymphatic vessels. So it does not filter lymph. The structures at the hilum are splenic artery, splenic vein, lymphatic vessels and nerves.

Functions

The spleen is a blood forming organ in early life. It is a storage organ for red corpuscles. Other functions are:

1. Phagocytosis of bacteria
2. Break down of worn out of erythrocytes

} By red pulp

3. Immune reactions of lymphocytes to produce antibodies.
4. B-lymphocytes grow into plasma cells.

} By white pulp

Splenectomy

Spleen is often ruptured in abdominal trauma. A damaged spleen can cause severe harmorrhage, shock and possibly death. Removal of the spleen is performed to stop the bleeding. Other structures like the lymphatic organs, red bone marrow and the liver take over the functions of the spleen.

THYMUS GLAND

The thymus gland lies in the upper part of mediastinum behind the sternum and extends upwards into the root of the neck. It weighs about 15 gms at birth and grows upto puberty, then atrophies. Its weight may be same as at birth.

Relations:

Anteriorly	:	Sternum and upper 4 costal cartilages.
Posteriorly	:	Aortic arch and its branches.
Laterally	:	Lungs
Superiorly	:	Structures in the root of the neck.
Inferiorly	:	Heart

Structure: The thymus gland consists of two lobes. These lobes are divided into lobules. Each lobule has aggregation of lymphocytes. Outer thick aggregation is called cortex. The cortex is composed of aggregation of lymphocytes, epithelial cells and macrophages. The thymus gland develops pre - T cells into mature T cells. Inner portion is the medulla which contains less lymphocytes. There are Hassal's corpuscles in the centre of the lobules. The frame work is made up of epithelio-reticular cells.

Blood supply: By inferior thyroid and internal thoracic arteries. Its nerves are derived from sympathetic and vagus.

Functions

1. Activated T-lymphocytes
2. Producing thymosin, a hormone.
3. Production of antibodies.

   Thymectomy is done in selected cases of myasthenia gravis. It is a chronic disease in which there is weakness of certain skeletal muscles. It is attributed to an auto-immune process in which the receptor proteins of neuromuscular junctions are affected and antibodies are produced against these receptors.

   In some cases of myasthenia gravis a tumour thymoma is present.

Immunity

The ability of the body to resist imfectious disease toxins and foreign tissues.

The person is said to be immune if his body destroys bacteria and/or other microorganisms before any symptoms develop.

Immunology is the brach of science that deals with the various phenomena of immunity, induced sensitivity and allergy.

Antigen : Any substance (for Ex: Bacteria) which provoke (produce antibodies) is called an antigen.

Immunity differs from non-specific defences by having the property of specificity and memory. Immunity is named as innate immunity and adaptive immunity.

T cells and B cells

T cells and B cells are lymphocytes that they have developed the ability to carry out immune responses. T cells come out of thymus gland as T4 and T8 cells. They have different functions.

Antibody

It is a protein found in the plasma (or formed) that is responsible for antibody-mediated (humoral) immunity.

Immunoglobulins (Igs)

They are antibodies produced in the body in response to the introduction of antigens. There are five kinds of immunoglobulins

There are two kinds of immunity

1. Cell-mediated immunity and
2. Antibody-mediated (humoral) immunity.

Functions of antibodies

1. They neutralize antigens.
2. They cause motile bacteria to lose their motility.
3. They agglutinate (clump) the bacteria.
4. They activate complement. Complement is an enzyme like substance which is always present in normal blood and completes the work of lysis.
5. They enhance phagocytosis.
6. They provide foetal, and newborn immunity.

Questions

1. What is "Lymph"?
2. List the structures of lymphatic system.
3. Explain the structure and function of "Lymph nodes".

4. Give a brief account of structure and function of spleen.
5. Write short notes on
   a) Thymus gland
   b) Tonsils

Study the following

1. Interferon
2. Monoclonal antibodies

Define the following

1. Macrophages
2. Interlukins

UNIT 7

The Respiratory System

The respiratory system provides the route by which the supply of oxygen present in the atmospheric air gains entry to the body and the route of excretion of carbon dioxide. As the air breathed in, moves through the air passages to reach the lungs. It is warmed up or cooled down to body temperature, cleaned and filtered by cilia in nasal cavities. Dust stick to the mucus, which is secreted in the lining of nasal cavity. Blood provides the transport system for these gases between the lungs and the cells of the body. The organs of the respiratory system are,

Nose and nasal cavities Pharynx	Upper respiratory system
Larynx Trachea Two bronchi Two lungs and their coverings - the pleura.	Lower respiratory system

Muscles of respiration - the intercostal muscles and diaphragm.

Nose and nasal cavities

The nose opens anteriorly in the face and posteriorly to the pharynx. It is the beginning organ of the respiratory

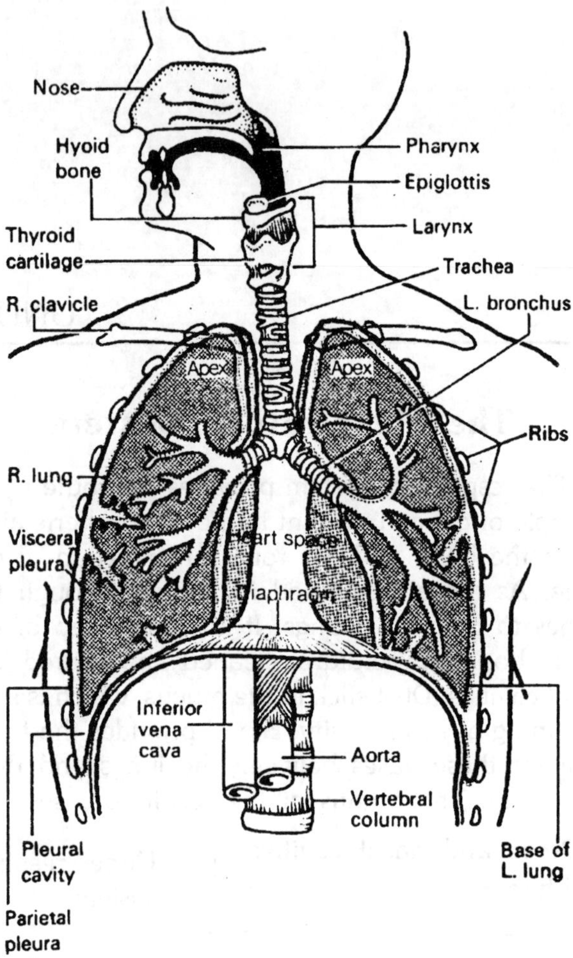

Figure 88. Organ of the respiration system

system. The nasal cavity consists of a large irregular cavity divided into two equal parts by a septum. The septum is formed by the vomer, the perpendicular plate of ethmoid bone and anteriorly the hyaline cartilage.

The roof is formed by the body of sphenoid, ethmoid, frontal and nasal bones.

The floor is formed by the hard and soft palate. The hard palate is formed by the maxilla and palatine bones. The soft palate is formed by involuntary muscles.

The medial wall is formed by the septum.

The later wall has irregular surface by elevation and depression, the former is called conchae by ethmoid and inferior concha. The latter is called meatus to that there is an opening of the para nasal air sinuses.

The lining of the nose is made of ciliated columnar epithelium which contains mucus secreting goblet cells. At the anterior nares the epithelium blends with the skin and at the posterior nares it extends as mucous membrane of the nasopharynx.

Openings of the nasal cavities: The anterior nares open to the exterior, the posterior nares open into the nasopharynx. Around the nose, there are bony spaces called as para nasal air sinuses. They are situated in the respective names of the bone, i.e. frontal, sphenoid, ethmoid and maxillary air sinuses. They contain air. The mucosa of the nasal cavities continues with these sinuses.

Functions of the Nose

The nose is the beginning organ of the respiratory system. As the air enters, it is warmed up or moistered and filtered. The cilia of the nose filters the air; the dust particles stick to the wet mucous membrane. The air is moistened by the large uneven surface of mucous membrane.

Olfactory function: The nose is the organ of the sense of smell. There are nerve endings in the mucosa at the roof of the nasal cavity. A dozen of olfactory nerve fibres passes on each side through the cribriform plate of the ethmoid bone. These fibres end in olfactory bulb, from the bulb it continues as olfactory nerve. The olfactory nerve conveys the sense of smell to the brain.

Pharynx: The pharynx is a fibro muscular tube of about 12 to 14 cms long. It extends from the base of the skull to the level of 6th cervical vertebra. It lies behind the nose, mouth and larynx and is wider at its upper end.

Relations

Superiorly	:	Inferior surface of the base of the skull.
Inferiorly	:	Continuous with the oesophagus.
Anteriorly	:	It communicates with nose, mouth and larynx.
Posteriorly	:	Loose areolar tissue, pre vertebral muscles and bodies of 1st to 6th cervical vertebrae.

For descriptive purpose, the pharynx is divided into nasal, oral and laryngeal parts.

The naso-pharynx: It extends from the internal nares of the nasal cavity to the level of the uvula a soft process that extends from the posterior edge of the soft palate. On its lateral wall, the opening of the auditory tube or pharyngo - tympanic tube or Eustachian tube communicates with the middle ear or tympanic cavity. On the posterior wall, there is a collection of lymphatic tissue called pharyngeal tonsil. In children, it may be enlarged (Adenoid) and cause respiratory obstruction and children breath through the mouth. There after, it gradually atrophies.

The oro-pharynx: It lies behind the oral cavity extending from the soft palate to the upper part of the body of the 3rd cervical vertebra. On each side, it has two folds i.e., one with soft palate, the palato pharyngeal fold and another with the tongue, the glossopharyngeal fold. In between the folds, the palatine tonsils are situated. In the middle of the inferior surface of the soft palate, the muscular uvula is present. This structure is important to stimulate vomiting sensation by touching.

The laryngeal-pharnyx lies behind the larynx. It extends from the oral part above and continues below as oesophagus, i.e., from level 3rd to 6th cervical vertebrae.

Structure: It has 3 layers.

1. **Mucous membrane lines** the entire pharynx but there are different types at different regions. The nasopharynx is lined by ciliated columnar epithelium. The oro-pharynx and laryngeal-pharynx are lined by stratified squamous epithelium which continues to oesophagus.
2. **Fibrous tissue:** It is the middle layer. It is thicker in the nasal part and becomes thinner towards the lower end.
3. **Muscle tissue:** It consists of 3 pairs of constrictor muscles. They are involuntary muscles and play an important role in the mechanism of deglutition.

Blood and nerve supply: Blood supply is from the branches of facial artery. The venous blood drains into facial and internal jugular veins. The nerve supply is by autonomic nerve plexus formed by the sympathetic and para sympathetic nerves.

Functions: The pharynx is an organ of respiratory and digestive systems. The nerve endings in the oral part carry sense of taste through cranial nerves. The auditory tube equalise the tympanic pressure with external atmospheric pressure to stabilise tympanic membrane. The lymphatic tissue in pharynx acts as phagocytic and production of antibodies.

Larynx

The larynx or voice box extends from the root of the tongue and hyoid bone to the trachea. It lies in front of the laryngeal part of the pharynx at the level of 3rd to 6th cervical vertebrae. The thyroid cartilage of the voice box is very prominent in adult males than in females. This prominence is called the "Adam's apple" Generally, there is deeper voice in males.

Relations

Superiorly	:	The root of the tongue and the hyoid bone.
Inferiorlay	:	It is continuous with the trachea.
Anteriorly	:	The muscles are attached to the hyoid bone.
Posteriorly	:	The laryngeal part of the pharynx.
Laterally	:	The lobes of the thyroid gland.

Structure : The larynx is made up of irregularly shaped cartilages (3 single and 3 paired) attached to each other by ligaments and membrane.

1.	Thyroid cartilage	Hyaline cartilage.
1.	Cricoid cartilage	
2.	Arytenoid cartilages	
2.	Cuneiform cartilages	Elastic cartilage
2.	Corniculated cartilages	
1.	Epiglottis	

The thyroid cartilage is the most prominent in the neck and consists of two flat pieces of cartilage or laminae fused anteriorly, forming an angle superior to the laryngeal prominence (Adam's apple). On the angle there is thyroid notch. The laminae are free on the posterior border. On the superior and inferior ends of the posterior border form processes called superior and inferior cornu. The upper part of the cartilage is lined by stratified squamous epithelium.

The cricoid cartilage is situated below the thyroid cartilage. It is shaped like a signet ring, completely encircling the larynx with the narrow part anteriorly and the broad part posteriorly. Tracheostomy is done in the cricoid cartilage.

The arytenoid cartilages are two, roughly, pyramid shaped cartilages situated on top of the cricoid cartilage forming the posterior wall of the larynx. They attach to the vocal cords and intrincic pharyngeal muscles.

Cuneiform cartilages Corniculate cartilages	They are paired elastic cartileges

The epiglottis is a leaf-shaped cartilage attached to the inner surface of the anterior wall of the thyroid cartilage, just below the thyroid notch. It rises as a free flap upwards behind the tongue and the body of the hyoid bone. The apiglottis (along with the false vocal cords) prevents food and liquids from entering the larynx.

Blood and nerve supply: Blood supply is by superior and inferior laryngeal arteries and the venous blood is drained by thyroid veins which join the internal jugular vein.

Nerve supply: Autonomic plexus formed by the branches of ganglion (sympathetic).

Voice box: It is formed by two vocal-folds or two folds of mucous membrane extending from inner wall of the thyroid prominence anteriorly, to the arytenoid cartilages posteriorly. The superior pair forms the false vocal cords and the inferior pair composes the true vocal cords. The true vocal cords are involved in voice production. When the muscles of arytenoid cartilages contract the cartilage adduct and rotate medially, pulling the true vocal cords together and narrowing the gap between them, forming the chink of the glottis. If air is forced through this chink, it causes vibration of the cords and sound is produced. When muscles relax, cartilages rotate laterally and abduct, separating the cords. Sound has the properties of pitch, loudness and quality. The pitch of the voice depends on the length and lightness of the cord. In adults, the vocal cords are longer in the male than in the female, thus male voice has lower pitch.

The loudness of the voice depends upon the force with which the cords vibrate. The greater the force of expired air, the more the cords vibrate and the louder the sound.

The quality and resonance of the voice depend upon the shape of the mouth, the position of the tongue and the lips, the facial muscles and the air sinuses in the bones of the face and skull.

Speech consists of the combination of the sound produced by the true vocal cords, by the tongue and cheeks.

Functions:

1. Air passage.
2. Production of sounds.
3. Helps during swallowing.

Trachea

The trachea or wind pipe is a continuation of the larynx and extends upto the level of 5th thoracic vertebra where it divides into right and left bronchi. The point of bifurcation has an internal ridge called carina. This is formed by the last tracheal cartilage. The mucous membrane of the carina is very sensitive which triggers a cough reflex. Its length is about 10 to 12 cms. The adult trachea is about 1.4 to 1.6 cm in diameter. It is situated in the median plane in front of the oesophagus.

Relations

Superiorly : The larynx.

Inferiorly : The right and left bronchi.

Anteriorly : Upper part - the isthmus of the thyroid gland, Lower part - the arch of the aorta and sternum.

Posteriorly : The oesophagus.

Laterally : The lungs and the lobes of the thyroid gland.

Structure: It is made up of 16-20 C-shaped rings (incomplete) of hyaline cartilage situated one above the other. The connective tissue and involuntary muscle join both ends of the cartilage. The posterior wall is related with the oesophagus.

Layers: The inner layer consists of pseudo stratified columnar epithelium of cilia, containing mucus-secreting goblet cells. The cilia propel mucus produced by goblet cells as well as foreign particles, towards the larynx. There are serous and mucous glands below the epithelium.

The middle layer consists of C-shaped hyaline cartilage and trachealis smooth muscle. Some areolar tissue is present having blood and lymph vessels and nerves.

The outer layer is a fibro-elastic layer which encloses the cartilages. The absence of cartilages posteriorly allow the trachea to dilate. The cartilage prevents collapse of the tube when the internal pressure decreases.

Blood and nerve supply

Blood supply is by the inferior thyroid and bronchial arteries; the venous drainage is by inferior thyroid veins into the brachio-cephalic veins; nerve supply is by the autonomic nerve plexus.

BRONCHI

The trachea divides into 2 bronchi at the level of the 5th thoracic vertebra.

The right bronchus is wider and shorter tube than the left bronchus. It lies in more vertical position. Its length is about 2.5 cms. After entering the right lung at hilum, it divides into 3 branches and enters into 3 lobes. Each branch is then subdivides into numerous smaller branches.

The left bronchus is about 5 cms long and narrower than the right, then it divides into two branches and enters into two lobes. Within the lung tissue, it subdivides into smaller branches.

Foreign body commonly enters into the right lung because the right bronchus is wide, short and straight than the left bronchus.

Structure: Same as trachea. The bronchi subdivide progressively into Brochioles, terminal bronchioles, respiratory bronchioles, alveolar ducts, and finally alveoli. The cartilage is absent at the bronchiole level, the epithelium changes, ciliated columnar epithelium becomes cuboidal, and in alveolus, it becomes the simple squamous epithelium. The alveolar epithelium is called alveolar I and modified alveolar II cells. The alveolus II, secretes surfactant substance that reduces the surface tension between the collapsed walls of the distal air passages and alveoli in newborn infants. The outer surface of alveolus closely invested with the network of capillaries. The exchange of gases takes place across two membranes, the alveolar and capillary membranes during respiration.

Blood supply and nerve supply

The alveoli are supported by a loose network of elastic connective tissue in which macrophages, fibroblasts, blood, nerves and lymph vessels are embedded.

Blood supply is by right and left bronchial arteries, venous drainage is by bronchial veins. Nerve supply is by autonomic nerve plexus. Lymphatic drainage is from the walls of the air passages into a network of lymph vessels.

Functions of air passages

1. The hyaline cartilage keeps the potency of the tube.

2. The dust particles adhere to sticky mucus secreted by goblet cells.
3. The wave of contraction of cilia of the epithelium moves the dust particles toward the larynx.
4. The diameter of air passage is altered by contraction of smooth (trachealis) muscle.
5. The macrophages and lymphocytes in connective tissue produce antibodies and act as phagocytes.
6. Inspired air is warmed upto body temperature by contact with mucus membrane of air passage.

LUNGS AND PLEURA

There are two lungs, the right and left situated on each side of the mid line in the thoracic cavity. They are cone-shaped, having base, apex, costal and medial surface.

The apex is rounded and rises into the root of the neck about 2.5 cms above the level of the middle third of the clavicle. It is related with blood vessels and nerves.

The base is concave and closely related with the upper surface of the diaphragm.

The costal surface is convex and related with the costal cartilages, ribs and intercostal muscles.

The medial surface is concave having the hilum. The structures which leave and enter from the root of each lung are :

1. Bronchus
1. Pulmonary artery
2. Pulmonary veins
1. Bronchial artery and bronchial veins

   Lymphatic vessels

   Nerves that enter and leave

MEDIASTINUM

The area between the lungs in the median plane is called mediastinum. The contents are the pericardium and heart, great blood vessels of the heart, trachea, right and left bronchus, oesophagus, lymph nodes, lymph vessels, thoracic duct, thymus gland, the phrenic and vagus nerves, azygos and hemiazygos veins.

The right lung

The right ling is thicker and broader than the left. It is also shorter than the left lung because the diaphragm is higher on the right side inorder to accommadate the liver that lies inferior to it.

The left lung

There is a concavity on the medial side of the left lung called cardiac notch in which the heart lies.

Pleura: It is a closed serous sac which encloses the lungs. It has two layers - The parietal pleura is lining the inner surface of chest wall and the thoracic surface of the diaphragm and is reflected at the hilum to become the visceral pleura. The visceral pleura lines the outer surface of lungs and its fissures.

The pleural cavity: It is a potential space between the two pleurae. They are separated by a thin film of serous fluid, sufficient to prevent friction between them during breathing.

The lobes of the lung: The right lung is divided into 3 lobes i.e. superior, middle and inferior lobes. They are separated by oblique and horizontal fissures.

The left lung is divided into 2 lobes i.e., superior and inferior lobes. They are separated by oblique fissure.

Lobules : Each lobe is subdevided into a number of lobules. Each lobule is composed of terminal bronchioles, respiratory bronchioles, alveolar ducts, atrium and alveoli. The cartilage becomes irregular in size and shape, eventually disappear, the walls become thinner until muscles and connective tissue are replaced by a single layer of flattened epithelial cells. Each alveolar duct contains a number of alveoli. The alveolar walls consist of type I and type II alveolar cells. Type I alvelar cells are the main site where gas exchange takes place. Type II alveolar cells secrete a phospholipid surfactant. This surfactant helps to prevent the movement of water from capillary blood into alveoli and keeps the potency of alveoli. The production of surfactant occurs by viable foetus i.e., by 7th month. The Pulmonary artery divides into right and left to carry deoxygenated blood to the lungs. The artery divides into many branches, and at the end, a capillary network surrounds the walls of the alveoli. The walls of the alveoli and that of capillaries consist of only one layer of squamous epithelial cells. The exchange of gases between air in the alveoli and blood in capillaries takes place by diffusion across these two very fine membranes. These layers are collectively known as alveolar capillary (respiratory) membrane. It consists of the following

1. A layer of type I and type II alveolar cells with wandering alveolar macrophages that constitute the alveolar (epithelial) wall.
2. An epithelial basement membrane beneath the alveolar wall.
3. A capillary basement membrane that is often fused to the epithelial basement membrane
4. The endothelial cells of the capillary.

The thickness of the alveolar capillary membrane is about 1/2 Um, the diameter is 1/16 of a red blood cell. This permits rapid diffusion of respiratory gases. There are about 300 million alveoli in the lungs. This provides vast surface about the size of a hand ball court for the exchange of gases. The pulmonary capillaries join up to form two pulmonary veins in each lung. They leave the lungs at hilum, convey oxygenated blood to the left atrium of the heart.

RESPIRATION

Expansion and contraction of lungs makes a regular exchange of gases between the alveoli and the external air. This is dependent upon the arrangement of the contraction and relaxation of the muscles of respiration.

Physiology of respiration: The process of contraction and relaxation of lungs to take and expel air is called the cycle of respiration. This process occurs about 15-18 times per minute and it consists of 3 phases

1. Inspiration
2. Expiration
3. Pause

The expansion of the chest during inspiration occurs as a result of muscular activity, by voluntary and partly involuntary. The muscles of respiration in normal breathing are the intercostal muscles and the diaphragm. During deep breathing, they are assisted by the muscles of the neck and abdomen.

Intercostal muscles: They are 11 pairs. They occupy between the 12 pairs of ribs. They are arranged in two layers, the external and internal inter costal muscles.

The external intercostal muscle fibres extend downwards, forwards from the lower border of the rib above, to the upper border of the rib below. The internal intercostal muscle fibres extend downwards and backwards from the lower border of the rib to the upper border of the rib below, crossing the external muscles fibres at right angles. The first rib is fixed. When the intercostal muscles contract, they pull the other ribs towards the first rib. The ribs move outwards when pulled upwards. In this way the thoracic cavity is enlarged anterioposteriorly and laterally.

Nerve supply By intercostal nerves.

DIAPHRAGM

Is a dome-shaped muscuulo-tendinous structure separating the thoracic cavity from the abdominal cavity. It forms the floor of the thoracic cavity and the roof of the abdominal cavity. The origin of the diaphragm is from sternum, lower 6 ribs and attached to the lumbar vertebrae by two crura. The muscle fibres radiate inwards and are inserted into the central tendon. When it contracts, its muscle fibres are shortened and the central tendon

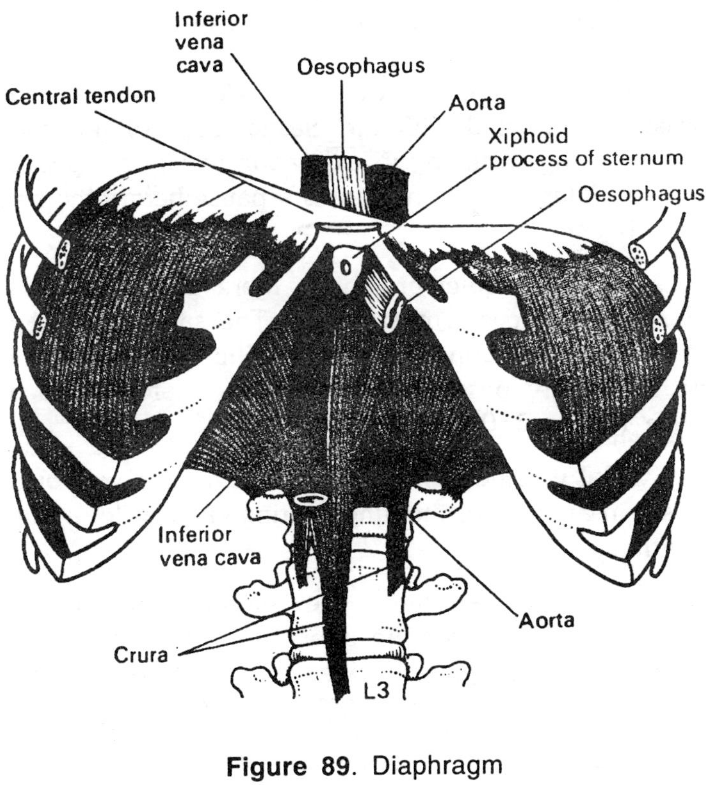

Figure 89. Diaphragm

is pulled downwards enlarging the vertical diameter of the thoracic cavity. It decreases the pressure in the thoracic cavity, and the lungs expand and air enters into the lungs.

Nerve supply: Motor & Sensory supply by phrenic nerve.

Respiratory cycle: There is a potential space between these two layers of serous membrane called the pleural cavity, containing a thin film of fluid. When the capacity of the thoracic cavity is increased by contraction of the intercostal muscles and diaphragm, the parietal pleura moves with walls of the thorax and the diaphragm. This reduces the pressure in the pleural cavity, causes negative pressure. The visceral pleura follows the parietal pleura. So the lungs are stretched and the pressure within the lungs is reduced, drawing air into the lungs to equalise the atmospheric and alveolar air pressure. This is the inspiration and it is described as active. When the diaphragm and intercostal muscles relax, the inspiratory process is reversed with the elastic recoil of the chest wall and lungs resulting in expiration which is a passive process. After expiration there is a pause before the next cycle begins.

In normal quiet breathing, there are about 15 to 18 respiratory cycles per minute. The same amount of air is left over during each cycle. The air remaining in the respiratory passages is called the anatomical dead space (about 150 ml).

Tidal volume (about 500 ml) is the amount of air passes in and out of the lungs during each cycle of quiet breathing.

Inspiratory capacity is the amount of air that can be inspired with maximum effort. It consists of the tidal volume (500 ml) plus the inspiratory reserve volume.

Functional residual volume is the amount of air remaining in the air passages and alveoli at the end of quiet expiration. Tidal air mixes with this air. The functional residual volume prevents collapse of the alveoli on expiration.

Vital capacity is the tidal volume plus the inspiratory and expiratory reserve volumes.

Alveolar ventilation is the amount of air which moves into and out of the alveoli in each minute.

Alveolar ventilation = Respiratory rate - (tidal volume - dead space volume)

= 15 (500 - 150) ml

= 5.25 litres per minute

Interchange of gases in the lungs occurs between the blood in the capillary network surrounding the alveoli and the air in the alveoli. Some properties of gases,

1. The gas molecules are always in motion.
2. The gases always tend to diffuse from an area of higher concentration to the area of lower concentration.
3. The gases exert pressure upon all the walls.

The total pressure exerted on the walls of the alveoli by the mixture of gases is the same as atmospheric pressure 101.3 k pa (760 mm Hg). Each gas in the mixture exerts a part of the total pressure proportional to its concentration, i.e., the partial pressure.

The partial pressure of nitrogen (PN2) is the same in the alveoli as it is in the blood. This stable state is maintained because nitrogen, as a gas, is not used up by the body but it can diffuse across the walls of the alveoli and the capillaries. The partial pressure of oxygen (PO_2) in the alveoli is higher than that of capillaries of the pulmonary arteries, as gases diffuse from an area of higher concentration to the area of lower concentration. So, the movement of oxygen is from alveoli to the blood. the reverse is true of CO_2. The PCO_2 is higher in deoxygenated blood than in alveolar air. So, CO_2 passes across the walls of the capillaries and the alveoli into the alveolar air. The partial pressure of each gas in the blood in the pulmonary veins and in the alveolar air is same. The slow movement of blood through the capillaries surrounding the alveoli allows time for the inter change of gases to take place and for the uptake of oxygen by the erythrocytes in the blood with haemoglobin in the erythrocytes. The amounts of O_2 and CO_2 in inspired (atmospheric) air, alveolar air and expired air are as follows

Composition of inspired air, alveolar air and expired air			
	Inspired air (Dry) %	Alveolar air %	Expired air %
Nitrogen	78.98	74.9	74.5
Oxygen	20.98	13.6	15.7
Carbon Dioxide	0.04	5.3	3.6
Water Vapour	0.0	6.2	6.2

Internal respiration

The exchange of O_2 and CO_2 between tissue blood capillaries and tissue cells is called internal (tissue) respiration. In this process oxygenated blood is converted into deoxygenated blood. Oxygen diffuses from the tissue blood capillaries into tissue cells and CO_2 diffuses from the tissue cells into tissue blood capillaries. The deoxygenated blood returns to the heart. The heart pumps this deoxygenated blood to the lungs for another cycle of external respiration.

Control of respiration

Nervous control : Respiration is partly but mainly involuntary. Voluntary control is exerted during physical activities and controlled by a centre in cerebral cortex for a very short time. Involuntary respiration needed to maintain life is controlled by the respiratory centre in medulla oblongata and pneumotaxic centre in the pons. The inhibition of inspiration results in expiration. Nerve impulse from respiratory centre passes to the phrenic nerve of the diaphragm and to the intercostal muscles in the intercostal nerves to contract these muscles and inspiration occurs.

Chemical control : When the alveoli of lungs are inflated the stretch sensory impulses are passed to the pneumotaxic centre through the afferent fibres of the vagus nerves and expiration occurs.

There are chaemoreceptors in the aortic and corotid bodies consisting of cells that are sensitive to changes in PCO_2 and PO_2 in the blood. The nerve impulses are transmitted to respiratory centre through the glosso-pharyngeal and vagus nerves. The chaemoreceptors and the respiratory centre are stimulated by increase in PCO_2 in the blood which results in increased ventilation of the lungs. A small reduction in the PO_2 has the same effect. Normally, quiet breathing is sufficient to maintain a balance between the blood PCO_2 and PO_2. During exercise, breathing becomes deeper because the muscles need more oxygen.

In normal quiet breathing, the inter costal muscles and the diaphragm are involved, but in deep or forced breathing, other muscles come into play. They are the accessory muscles of respiration. They are the sternomastoid muscles. The contraction of these muscles causes maximum increase in the capacity of the thoracic cavity.

The following factors take part in the regulation of respiration.

1. Blood pressure
2. Limbic system

3. Temperature
4. Pain
5. Stretching the anal canal sphincter muscle.
6. Irritation of airways

Effect of exercise on respiration

Exercise accelerates the function of the respiratory and cardiovascular systems. During exercise increased cardiac output increases the blood flow to the lungs. This is called as pulmonary perfusion which rises about five times. The O_2 diffusion capacity increases three times during maximal exercise.

Muscles consume large amounts of O_2 when they contract during exercise and produce large amounts of CO_2. Pulmonary ventilation increases upto 30 fold from the resting state.

Neural changes that bring excitatory impulses into the inspiratory area in the medulla oblangata cause the abrupt increase in ventilation at the start of exercise.

At the end of exercise, pulmonary ventilation abruptly decreases. This is followed by a gradual decline to the resting level.

Words used in relation to exchange and transport of oxygen and carbon dioxide

1. Eupnoea means normal quite breathing.
2. Pulmonary ventilation means the movement of air in and out of the lungs. It is also called breathing.
3. Hyperventilation means rapid and deep breathing.
4. Hypoventilation means slow and shallow breathing.
5. Hypoxia means decreased amount of oxygen in the tissues.

Classification of hypoxia according to the cause.

a) Hypoxic hypoxia - This condition is due to decreased oxygen content in arterial blood as a result of obstruction in air ways or high altitude.

b) Anaemic hypoxia - In this condition there is dificiency of haemoglobin in the blood as in case of anaemia or harmorrhage or defeciency of functioning haemoglobin as in carbon monoxide poisoning.

c)) Stagnant hypoxia - In this condition tissues receive less blood supply and receive inadequate oxygen though the amount of haemoglobin is normal.

d) Histotoxic hypoxia - In this condition the cells are unable to use adequate oxygen though the blood delivers adequate oxygen. For ex: cyanide poisoning.

6. Hypoxaemia means decreased amount of oxygen in the blood.
7. Hypercapnia means increased amount of CO_2 in the blood.
8. Dyspnoea means difficulty in breathing.
9. Orthopnea means difficulty in breathing except in the upright position.
10. Apnoea means cessation of breathing for a short period.
11. Hyperpnoea means deeper and more rapid respiration than normal.
12. Polypnoea or Tachypnoea means very rapid breathing

Breathing accompanied with sound

1. Wheezing is a type of noisy breathing in which the air passes through narrow bronchial airways as seen in Asthma.

2. Stertorous breathing is a noisy inspiration occuring in coma or deep sleep (snoring)
3. Stridor is a high pitched noisy respiration, like the blowing of the wind, a sign of respiratory obstruction, especially in the trachea or larynx.

Abnormal respiratory sounds

1. Rale - is a bubbling or rattling sound of varied character,heard on auscultation of the chest in the diseases of the lung or bronchi (a small rhonchus)
2. Rhonchus - (Pl. Rhonchi) means a loud rale, especially a whistling or sonorous (snoring) rale produced in the larger bronchi or the trachea.

Questions

1. a) Define respiration
   b) Name the organs of the respiratory sytem.
   c) Describe the structure of the nasal cavity.
2. Name the parts of the pharynx. With what structures does each part communicate?
3. Describe the structure of the larynx. How do the vocal cords produce sound?
4. Describe the structure of the lungs with diagram.
5. Describe the mechanism of respiration.
6. Describe the regulation of respiration.
7. Write short notes on
   a) Pleura
   b) Effect of exercise on respiration
   c) Pulmonary volumes.
   d) Breathing pattens.

UNIT 8

The digestive system

The alimentary canal begins at the mouth, passes through the thorax, abdomen and pelvis and ends at the anus. It is associated with accessory organs. They secrete secretions which contain enzymes necessary for digestion. These enzymes modify the food so as to be absorbed by the digestive system. After they are absorbed, the nutrient materials are used in the synthesis of the constituents of the body and provide energy for the body. The activities in the digestive system can be grouped as

1. **Ingestion:** Taking food into the alimentary canal.
2. **Digestion:** It is the breakdown of food by mastication (chewing) and chemical breakdown by enzymes secreted by glands of the digestive system. The following secretions assist in digestion - saliva from the salivary glands, gastric juice from the stomach, intestinal juice from the small intestine, pancreatic juice from the pancreas and bile from the liver.
3. **Absorption:** Absorption of digested food substances takes place in the walls of alimentary canal, from there they are carried to the liver for metabolism.

4. **Elimination:** Food substances that cannot be digested and absorbed are excreted by the bowel as faecal matter.

The gastro-intestinal tract consists of a long tube through which food passes. It starts at mouth and ends at the anus. The different parts are

Mouth	Small intestine
Pharynx	Large intestine
Oesophagus	Rectum and anus
Stomach	

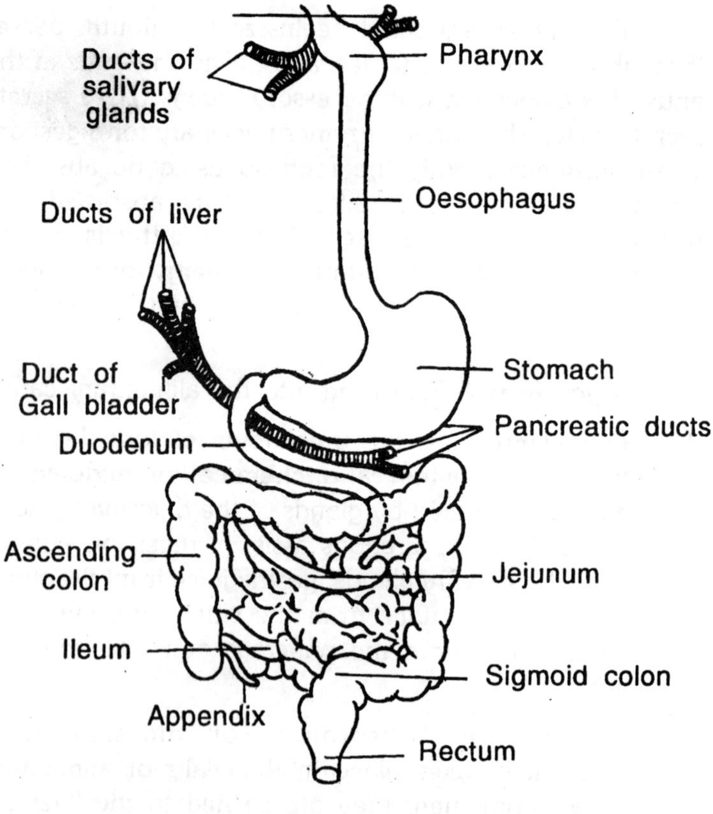

Figure 90. Organs of the digestive system.

Accessory organs secrete various secretions which are poured into the alimentary canal. The glands are situated outside the tract. Their secretions are passed through the ducts to enter the alimentary tract. They are

3 pairs of salivary glands

Pancreas and

Liver

General structure of the alimentary canal: The walls of the alimentary tract are formed by four layers of tissue from inside to outside of the tube.

1. Mucous membrane
2. Submucous layer
3. Muscular layer
3. Serous or peritoneal layer.

Mucous membrane : This layer has three main functions; protective, secretory and absorptive. This layer has three divisions, i.e., epithelium, lamina propria and muscularis mucosa. The epithelium of the alimentary system consists of simple columnar cells except in the mouth, oesophagus and terminal part of anus. The columnar cells are modified into secretory cells i.e., cells of small intestine. Some columnar cells are modified into absorptive cells. The lamina propria contains loose (areolar) connective tissue, with blood and lymphatic vessels and glands i.e., in the stomach. Large amount of simple tubular glands secrete gastric juice. The intestine contains glands of Lieberkuhn which secrete intestinal juice. In the terminal part of ileum, there are aggreation of lymphoid tissue called peyer's patches. They produce lymphocytes which act as phagocytes. The smooth muscle layer is called muscularis mucosa which separates the mucous membrane from the submucos layer.

2 **Submucous layer :** It consists of loose connective (areolar) tissue with some elastic fibres, blood capillaries, lymphatic vessels, nerve plexus of

Meissner's made up of autonomic nervous system. In the duodenum, there are glands and their secretion is poured into the lumen by ducts.

3. **Muscular layer:** It consists of smooth muscles arranged in layers, inner circular and outer longitudinal layers. Between these two layers of muscle, there are blood vessels, lymph vessels, and autonomic nerves of Mesenteric or Auerbach's plexus. A wave of alternate contraction and relaxation of the muscle is called peristalsis. Peristalsis assists in onward propel of the contents of the canal. Other movements of the intestine help to mix food with digestive juices. On certain points, the circular muscle is well developed into sphincters.

4. **Serous or peritoneal layer:** The alimentary canal in the abdomen is lined by serous coat i.e., visceral peritoneum.

Nerve supply: The G.I. tract is supplied by autonomic nerve plexus i.e., parasymphathetic and sympathetic nerves.

Peritoneum: It is the largest serous membrane of the body. It has two layers; the parietal and visceral layers. The parietal layer lines the inner surface of the abdominal cavity. The visceral layer covers most of the abdominal viscera contained therein. In between the two layers of the peritoneal cavity there is only a potential space contains sac, where as, in female, it is an open sac because the uterine tubes enter into the sac.

The peritoneum is divided into three parts:

1. Omentum
   i) Greater
   ii) Lesser
2. Mesentery
3. Peritoneal ligaments

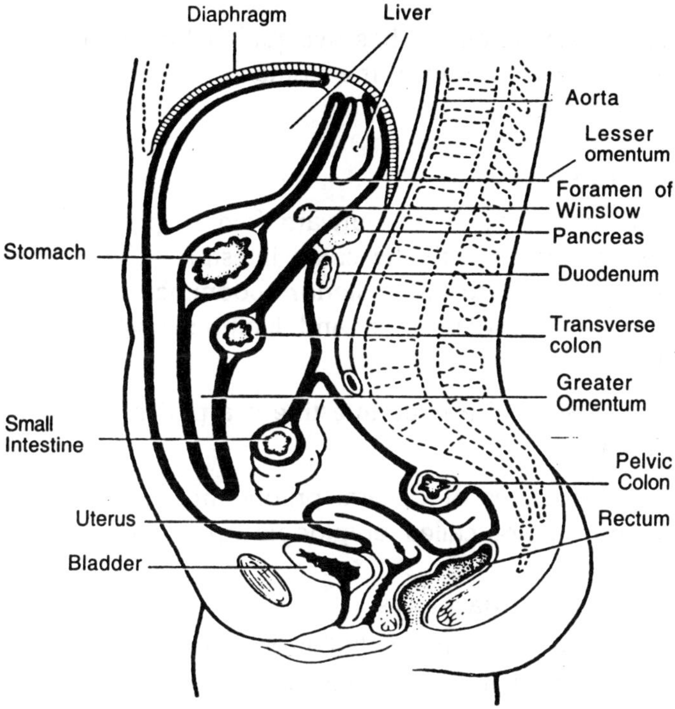

Figure 91. Peritoneum

Omentum

i) The greater omentum is long, double fold of connective tissue sheet that extends inferiorly from the stomach and drapes over the transverse colon and coils of the small intestine. Large quantities of adipose tissue accumulate in the greater omentum which appears like a "fatty apron". It creates the omental bursa. It covers the anterior surface of the abdominal viscera. It becomes a four layered structure as its double sheet folds upon itself. Many lymph nodes are contained in the greater omentum. These lymph nodes form plasma cells that may produce antibodies to combat the infection and help prevent it from spreading to the poritoneum.

ii) The lesser omentum has two folds which connects the lesser curvature of the stomach to the liver and diaphragm.

2. Mesentary

The mesentary is an outward fold of peritoneum which is associated with the small intestine. The tip of the fold is attached to the posterior abdominal wall. The mesentery also carries blood and lymphatic vessels to the intestine.

The sersosa of a large intestine is a part of visceral peritoneum.

Small pouches of visceral pritoneum are attached to taeniae coli are called epiploopic appendages.

3. Peritoneal ligaments

They are the folds in the peritoneum. There are several peritoneal ligaments, few are mentioned here.

a) The falciform ligament attaches the liver to the anterior abdominal wall

b) Mesocolon is a fold of peritoneum which binds the large intestine to the posterior abdominal wall. It also carries blood and lymphatic vessels to the intestines.

c) Pelvic Peritoneum : The broad and round ligaments of the uterus.

The lower part of the peritoneum forms the outer layer of uterus called perimetrium. A layer of peritoneum covers the superior surface of the urinary bladder is called the serosa.

The following organs lie behind the pritoneum (retro-peritoneal). They are the duodenum, pancreas, ascending colon, descending colon, rectum, kidneys, adrenal glands, and urinary bladder.

Functions of the peritoneum

1. Being a serous membrane it enables the abdominal organs to glide over each other without friction.
2. The abdominal organs are covered partly or completely.
3. The ligaments and mesenteris of the peritoneum help to keep the organs in position.
4. Adipose tissue is deposited in omenta and mesentary. They are the fat storage organs.
5. The omentum helps to prevent the spread of infection to the rest of the peritoneum.
6. It has the ability to absorb large amounts of fluids.

Peritoneal dialysis

The peritoneum acts as a selectively permeable membrane. This property is made use of in dialysis. Dialysis means the separation of smaller molecules from larger ones (crystalloid from colloid substances) through the use of a selectively permeable membrane. This procedure is used in the treatment of some cases of kidney failure.

Peritonitis is an inflammation of peritoneum.

Mouth

The mouth or oral cavity or buccal cavity is bounded by muscles and bones. The relations are:

Anteriorly : The lips.

Posteriorly : Opens into oropharynx.

Laterally : By the muscles of the cheeks.

Superiorly : By the bony hard palate and muscular soft palate.

Inferiorly : By the muscles of the floor of the oral cavity and root of the tongue.

The lips form the opening of the mouth. They are fleshy folds. They are covered externally by skin and internally by mucous membrane. Between the skin and mucous membrane is a zone called the vermillion. This is the nonkeratinized portion of the lip. Labial frenula (sing. frenulum) are the folds of mucous membrane which attach the inner surface of the lip to their corresponding gums.

The oral cavity is lined by stratified squamous epithelium. The part of the mouth between the gums and the cheeks is the vestibule and the remainder of the cavity is the mouth proper. The parotid ducts open into the vestibule of the mouth. The palate is divided into the anterior hard palate and posterior soft palate. The hard palate is formed by the maxilla and palatine bones. The soft palate is muscular, curves down wards to form the posterior end of the hard palate. The uvula is a curved fold of muscle covered with mucous membrane hanging down from the middle of the free posterior border of soft palate. On either side, there are two mucosal folds, the posterior folds, one on each side is the palato pharyngeal fold and the 2nd anterior fold is palatoglossal fold. One each side, between these folds, there is a collection of lymphoid tissue called the palatine tonsil.

Tongue: The tongue is a voluntary muscular organ covered with mucous membrane. It is situated in the floor of the mouth. It is attached by its root to the hyoid bone and by a fold of its mucous membrane covering called the frenulum. The upper surface and lateral surface of the mouth is lined by the stratified squamous epithelium with numerous papillae which contain taste buds.

Filiform papillae are pointed and thread like. They are ditributed over the entire surface of the tongue. They rarely contain taste buds.

Fungiform papillae are knob like elevations scattered over the entire surface of the tongue. Most of them contain taste buds.

Circumvallate papillae, the largest type and circular and are arranged on the posterior surface of the tongue in the form of an inverted V.

Function: It plays an important role in mastication, deglutition and speech. It is the main organ of taste. The nerve endings of the sense of taste are present in the papillae. They are widely distributed in the epithelium of tongue, soft palate, epiglottis and pharynx.

Teeth: They are embedded in the alveoli or sockets of the alveolar ridges of the mandible and maxilla. Each person has two sets of teeth, the temporary, deciduous teeth or milk teeth and the permanent teeth. At birth, the teeth of both dentitions are present in immature form in the mandible and maxilla. The temporary teeth are 20 in number, 10 in each jaw. They begin to erupt at 6 months old and should all present by the end of 24 months. Milk teeth in each jaw are,

Incisors,	Canine,	Molars
4	2	4

The permanent teeth begin to replace the deciduous teeth in the 6th year of age. The permanent set consists of 32 teeth. Eruption usually completes by the 24th year. On each jaw has 16 teeth

Incisors,	Canine,	Premolar,	Molar
4	2	4	6

The incisors are cutting teeth, canine teeth are for tearing, the premolars and molar teeth are for the grinding or chewing the food.

Structure of a tooth: Each tooth has a crown, a neck and a root. The crown consists of one or more cusps. It is the part that protrudes outsie the gum. The root is the part embedded in the bone. The neck is the slightly constricted part where the crown merges with the root. In the centre of the teeth, is the pulp cavity. It is filled with pulp, a connective tissue containing blood vessels, lymphatic vessels and nerves. Surrounding this, is a hard-ivory like substance called dentine. On the crown the dentine is covered by a thin and hard layer called enamel. Enamel is the hardest substance in the body which protects the tooth against abrasion and acids produced by bacteria in the mouth. The roots are fixed to the alveolar sockets by the cement like substance called cementum. The roots number from one to three. The teeth are held in place by periodontal ligaments that extend from the alveolar walls and are embedded into the cementum. The alveolar walls are lined with a periodontal membrane. The blood vessels and nerves enter at the root of the teeth.

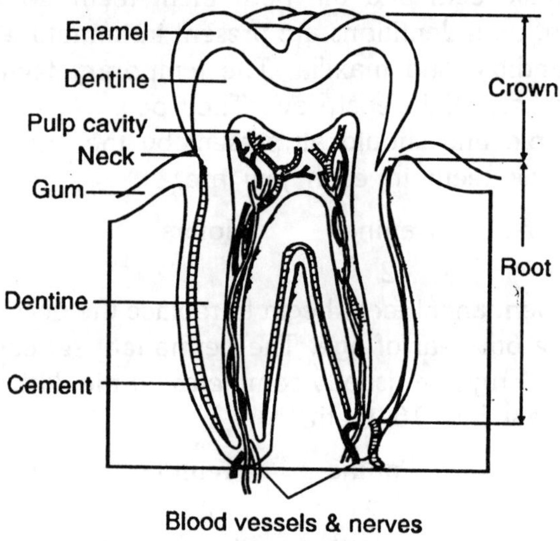

Figure 92. A section of a tooth

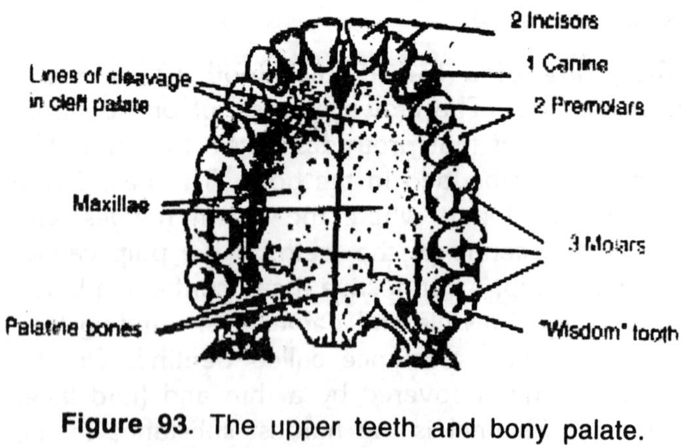

Figure 93. The upper teeth and bony palate.

Nerve supply: The upper teeth are supplied by maxillary nerves. The lower teeth are supplied by the branches of mandibular nerves. These two nerves are the branches of trigeminal nerve or 5th cranial nerve.

The Pharynx

It is divided into 3 parts for descriptive purpose-the naso-pharynx, oro-pharynx and laryngeal- pharynx. The oro-pharynx and laryngeal-pharynx are concerned with the alimentary canal. Food passes from the oral cavity to the pharynx, then it passes into the Oesophagus below. The details are already described.

Structure: The inner layer is composed of stratified squamous epithelium of oral cavity and continuous below with oesophagus.

The middle layer consists of fibrous tissue, containing blood, lymph vessels and nerves.

The outer layer is made up of a number of involuntary constrictor muscles which are involved in swallowing.

Blood supply is by several branches of the facial artery. The venous drainage is into the facial vein and into the internal jugular vein.

Nerve supply is from the pharyngeal nerve plexus.

Salivary glands

They are three pairs of salivary glands. They are compound racemose glands. They pour their secretion into the mouth.

2 Parotid glands

2 Submandibular glands

2 Sublingual glands.

Pam glands

They are serous glands are situated on each side of the face just below the external acoustic meatus. Their secretion is drained by parotid ducts (Stenson's ducts) which pierces the buccinator muscle and open into the vestibule of the mouth at the level of the second upper molar tooth.

Submandibular glands

These glands are situated below and posterior to the base of the mandible. The two sub mandibular ducts (Wharton's ducts) open on the floor of the mouth, one on each side of the frenulum of the tongue. They produce more serous than mucous secretions.

Sublingual glands

These glands are situated in the floor of the mouth under the mucous membrane. These glands have a number of ducts. They are named as duct of Bartholin and ducts of Rivinus. They produce primarily mucous secretions.

Structure: All the glands are surrounded by a fibrous capsule. They consist of a number of lobules. These are made up of small alveoli lined with secretory cells. The secretions are collected in smaller ducts. These ducts unit to form larger ducts leading into the mouth.

Nerve supply by autonomic nerves.

Parasympathetic - stimulates secretion.

Sympathetic - depresses secretion.

Blood supply: Branches of the external carotid arteries and venous drainage is into external jugular veins.

Saliva

Saliva is the secretions from the salivary glands mixed with mucus from the oral cavity. It consists of water, mineral salts, an enzyme ptyalin, mucus, lysozymes, immunoglobulins and blood clotting factors. Saliva also contains lingual lipase secreted by glands of the tongue.

Oesophagus

The oesophagus or gullet is about 25 cm long and about 2 cm in diameter. It lies in the median plane in the thorax in front of the vertebral column, behind the trachea and the heart. It continues with the pharynx above, passes below through an opening in the diaphragm, joins with the stomach. The upper and lower ends have sphincter muscles. Above, is the cricopharyngeal sphincter which prevents air passage into the oesophagus. Below, is the cardiac sphincter which prevents the reflux of acid gastric contents into the oesophagus.

Structure: It consists of four layers as in general pattern of alimentary tract, but the epithelium is the stratified squamous epithelium on the upper end. The distal end is lined by columnar epithelium. The middle third is lined by a mixture of the two.

Blood supply: By the oesophageal branches of the aorta. The abdominal part is supplied by branches of inferior phrenic arteries and the left gastric branch of the coeliac artery.

Venous drainage is into the azygos and hemiazygos veins. From the abdominal part of oesophagus, the venous blood is returned to left gastric vein. So, at the terminal end of oesophagus, the venous blood is drained into systemic and hepatic portal circulations.

Nerve supply: By autonomic nerve plexus.

Functions of the mouth, pharynx and oesophagus

Mouth: In the mouth food is masticated or chewed by the teeth and mixed with saliva by use of tongue and muscles of cheek. Then it is formed into a soft mass or bolus. It is ready for deglutition or swallowing.

Saliva: Saliva is a clear, tasteless, odourless, slightly acid (pH 6.8) viscid fluid, consisting of secretion from the parotid, suubligual and submaxillary salivary glands and the mucous glands of the oral cavity. Saliva contains water, mineral salts, enzyme Ptyalin (Salivary amylase), linguinal lipase mucus, lysozymes and immunoglobulins. Daily secretion is 1000 to 1500 ml.

Function: Its function is to keep the mucous membrane of the mouth moist and to lubricate the food during mastication. The enzyme ptyalin converts cooked starch into maltose.

Lingual lipase starts digestion of dietary triglycerides into fatty acids and monoglycerides.

Lysozymes and immunoglobulins prevent infection.

Taste: The tongue contains different kinds of taste buds. From this, sense of taste is carried to the brain.

Secretion of saliva: It is under the autonomic nervous control. The parasympathetic stimulation causes vaso dilatation and profuse secretion. Reflex secretion occurs when there is food in the mouth and the reflex secretion by the sight or smell. Even the thought of food stimulates the flow of saliva.

Mechanism of deglutition or swallowing

This mechanism occurs in three stages.

1. When mastication of food is over, bolus forms. Then the lips are closed, the voluntary muscles of the tongue and cheeks push the bolus backwards into the oro pharynx. This is the voluntary stage of swallowing.
2. Here the involuntary pharyngeal stage of swallowing begins. The bolus stimulates raceptors in the oropharynx. These receptors send afferent impulses to the swallowing centre in the medulla oblongata and lower pons of the brain. The efferent impulses cause the soft palate and uvula to move upward

to close off the nasopharynx. The larynx is lifted upward and forward. The epiglottis comes into contact with the base of the tongue to cover the glottis. Breathing is temporarily withheld. In this way food is prevented from entering the trachea.

3. The muscles of the pharynx propel the bolus down into the oesophagus through the upper oesophageal sphincter. The presence of the bolus in the oesophagus stimulates peristalsis, which propels the bolus downwards in the oesophagus. The cardiac sphincter relaxes and the bolus enters the stomach. This is the involuntary oesophageal stage of swallowing.

The walls of the oesophagus are always relaxed, when the bolus enters, then only the peristaltic waves of contraction and relaxation start. The walls of the oesophagus are lubricated by mucus secretion by submucosal glands.

STOMACH AND GASTRIC JUICE

The stomach is a J-shaped dilated portion of the alimentary tract, situated just below the diaphragm and liver. It is related to epigastric, umbilical and left hypochondriac regions of the anterior abdominal wall. The stomach is continuous with the oesophagus at the cardiac orifice with the duodenum at the pyloric orifice. It has two borders, shorter the lesser curvature and another longer, the greater curvature. Stomach has two surfaces, anterior and posterior. The part of the stomach above the level of cardiac orifice on left side is the fundus, the middle and main part is the body and the lower part is pyloric antrum. At the distal end of the pyloric antrum is the pyloric sphincter, guarding the opening between the stomach and the duodenum. When the stomach is inactive, the pyloric sphincter is relaxed and open. When it contains food, the sphincter is closed.

Relations

Anteriorly : Left lobe of liver and anterior abdominal wall.

Posteriorly : Stomach bed formed by left kidney, left adrenal gland, spleen, pancreas and abdominal aorta.

Superiorly : Diaphragm, oesophagus and left lobe of liver.

Inferiorly : Transverse colon and small intestine. To the left diaphragm and spleen. To the right liver and duodenum.

The peritoneum covers the anterior and posterior surfaces. The peritoneal folds at lesser curvature is lesser omentum. It extends from the lesser curvature to the liver and diaphragm. The peritoneal folds which connects the greater curvature of the stomach to the transverse colon and posterior abdominal wall is called greater omentum. It extends downwards in front of the abdominal organs like an apron. It contains large amount of fat, is richly supplied with blood and lymph vessels. It protects the abdominal viscera.

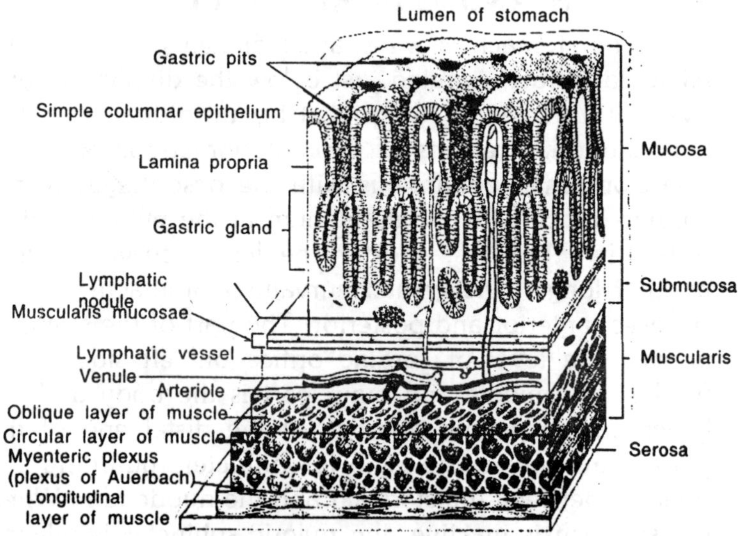

Figure 94. Layers of the stomach

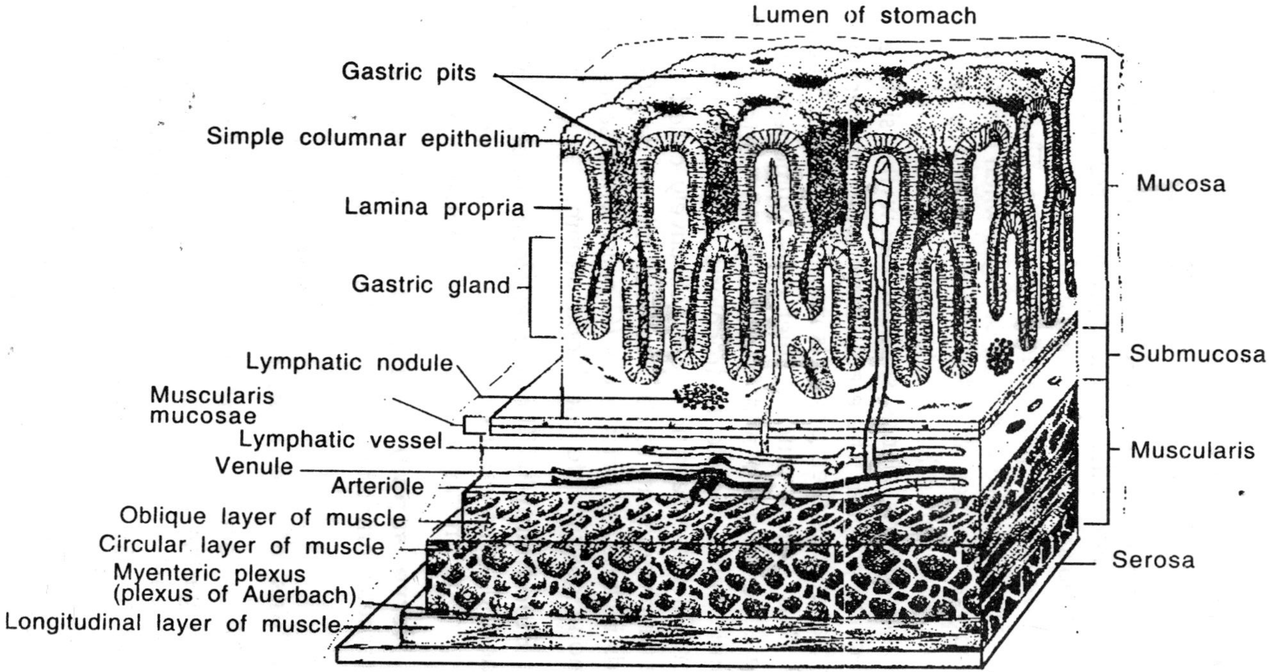

Figure 94. Layers of the stomach

Structure

As the general plan of alimentary canal with a little modification, the muscle has 3 layers, outer has longitudinal fibres, the middle layer has circular and inner layer has oblique fibres. This type of muscle arrangement has churning and peristaltic movement. The mucous membrane is thrown into folds or rugae when the stomach is empty and when it is full the rugae disappear. The surface has smooth velvety appearance. There are numerous gastric glands situated below the surface in the lamina propria. There are three types of specialised cells that secrete their products into the stomach. Mucous neck cells secrete mucus, chief cells (xymogenic cells) secrete pepsinogen and gastric lipase, parietal cells (oxyntic cells) secrete hydrochloric acid and intrinsic factor. All these secretions are collectively called gastric juice which amounts to 2000 to 3000 ml. per day. Gastric glands include endocrine cells (G cells) which secrete the hormone gastrin into the blood stream.

Blood supply: The arterial blood supply is by left gastric and branches of splenic arteries from coeliac trunk. The venous drainage is to hepatic portal vein.

Nerve supply: The right and left vagus, the sympathetic branches from coeliac plexus.

Functions of the stomach

When food is in the stomach, gradually it mixes up with gastric juice. The food is sufficiently acidified to stop the action of ptyalin. The gastric muscle contraction makes churning movement and it breaks down the bolus and further mixes it with gastric juice. The peristaltic waves propels the stomach contents towards the pyloric antrum after they are sufficiently liquefied. Through the pylorus the gastric contents are passed into the duodenum in small spurts.

Gastric juice: The gastric juice is secreted by secretory glands in the mucosa. It contains

Enzymes- Pepsinogen secreted by chief cells in the glands.

Water and Mineral salts- by gastric glands.

Mucus-mucous neck cells.

Hydrochloric acid (HCl) and intrinsic factor - by parietal cells.

Functions of gastric juice

1. Water: Liquefies the food swallowed.
2. Hydrochloric acid:
   a) Kills many bacteria that may be harmful to the body.
   b) Acidifies the food and stops the action of plyatin.
   c) Provides the acid needed for effective digestion by pepsin.
3. Pepsinogen is activated to pepsin by hydrochloric acid. It begins the digestion of proteins, breaking into smaller molecules. Pepsin acts most effectively at pH 1.5 to 3.5.
4. Intrinsic factor is necessary for the absorption of vitamin B_{12} (extrinsic factor).
5. Mucus prevents mechanical injury to the stomach wall by lubricating the contents, also prevents chemical injury by acting as a barrier between the stomach wall and the gastric juice.

Mechanism of gastric juice secretion

A small amount of gastric juice is present in the stomach even though it contains no food. This is known as Fasting Juice. The secretion reaches its maximum level about 1 hour after a meal then it declines to the fasting level after about 4 hours. There are 3 phases of secretion,

1. Cephalic phase: Secretion of gastric juice before food begins in the stomach and is due to reflex stimulation of the vagus nerve by the sight, smell or taste of food.

2. Gastric phase: When the food is in the stomach the cells in the pyloric antrum (a small amount of gastrin is also secreted by the endocrine cells of duodenum) secretes gastrin - a hormone which passes directly into the circulating blood, reaches the stomach and stimulates gastric glands to produce more gastric juice. Gastrin also causes contraction of cardiac sphincter and increases the motility of the stomach. In this way the secretion of digestive juuice is continued after the completion of the meal and till the end of the cephalic phase. Gastric phase-secretion is suppressed when the pH in the pyloric antrum falls to about 1.5.

3. Intestinal phase: When the partially digested food contents leave the stomach and reach the small intestine, a hormone called enterogastrone is secreted by intestinal cells. It acts to slow down the gastric juice secretion and reduces gastric motility. When the meal contains a high fat, it stimulates the gall bladder to empty the bile into the duodenum. The contents of the duodenum become more thoroughly mixed with bile and pancreatic juice.

Functions of the stomach

1. As a temporary reservoir for food, allowing the digestive enzymes to act.

2. Production of gastric juice. (Functions are explained in page No. 260)

3. The muscular action mixes the food with gastric juice. The rate at which the stomach empties, depends to a large extent on the type of food eaten.

A carbohydrate meal leaves the stomach in 2 to 3 hours, a protein meal remains longer and a fatty meal remains in the stomach longest. The stomach contents entering the duodenum are called CHYME.

4. Selective absorption takes place i.e., water, alcohol and some drugs.
5. Secretion of intrinsic factor which is needed for the absorption of extrinsic factor.

EMESIS

Vomiting : It is the forcible ejection of contents of the stomach (sometimes duodenum) through the mouth. It is a reflex action. Gastric irritation and distention act as stimuli for vomiting. Other stimuli are unpleasant sights, dizziness, certain drugs, irritation in the pharynx, oesophages and intestines, raised intracranial pressure etc. Nerve impulses are carried to the vomiting centre in the medulla oblongata which sends impulses to the organs of the gastrointestinal tract, diaphragm and abdominal muscles to bring about the vomiting act.

Nurses have to observe, record and report about vomiting of patients.

After the vomiting centre is stimulated and the reflex is initiated, the following events occur.

1. A deep breath is taken.
2. The hyoid bone and larynx are elevated, opening the upper oesophageal sphincter.
3. The opening of the larynx is closed.
4. The soft palate is elevated, closing the posterior opening into the nasal cavity.
5. The diaphragm and abdominal muscles are forcefully contracted, strongly compressing the stomach and increasing the intragastric pressure.
6. The lower oesophageal sphincter is relaxed and the gastric contents are forcefully expelled.

SMALL INTESTINE

The small intestine is continuous with the stomach at the pyloric sphincter and ends at ileo-caecal valve. It is about 5 metres long and lies in the abdominal cavity surrounded by large intestine. In small intestine, most of digestion and absorption of nutrient materials take place. It has 3 parts.

1. The duodenum is about 25 cms long having a C-shaped curved around the head of the pancreas. The pancreatic duct and common bile duct open into the duodenum at an orifice called Ampulla of Vator.
2. The jejunum is the middle part and is about 2 meters long.
3. The ileum or terminal part is about 3 metres long. It opens into caecum. The junction is guarded by ileocaecal valve.

Structure: The small intestine has 4 layers as described by general plan. Some modifications are present in mucous membrane and mesentry. The peritoneal cavity is freely movable. The mesentry is attached to the posterior abdominal wall. It contains blood vessels, lymphatic vessels and nodes, autonomic nerve plexus.

Mucous membrane: The surface of mucosal area is increased by circular folds and villi. The circular fold distends when bolus enters the intestine. The villi are tiny finger like projections into the intestinal lumen. They are about 0.5-1 mm in length. Their walls are made up of simple columnar cells with microvilli on the luminal border. The goblet cells secrete the mucus. Some cells are modified into enzyme secreting cells. These villi contain blood capillaries and lymphatic lacteals (for absorption of fat). The surface epithelium between the villi, dips into lamina propria to form simple tubular glands

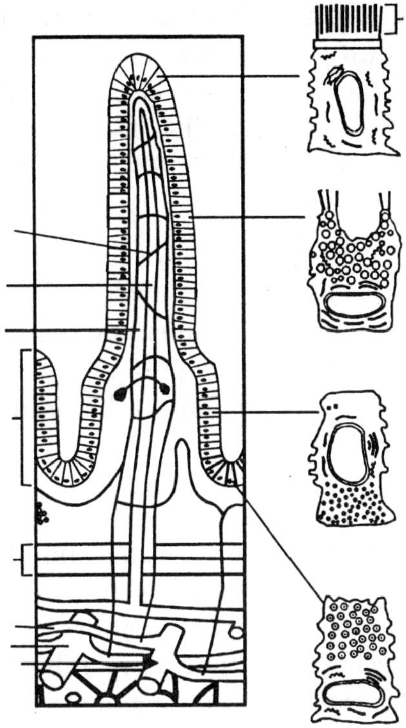

Figure 95. Digrams of villus

(Crypts of Lieberkuhn) throughout the small intestine. They are more concentrated in jejunum. They secrete intestinal juice that helps the digestion of carbohydrates, proteins and fats. The intestinal glands also contain paneth cells.

Lymphatic nodules: They are the accumulation of lymphocytes in the lamina propria. The smaller groups are known as solitary lymphatic follicles. Larger aggregation of these follicles are called peyer's patches. They are present in the ileum.

Blood supply: The arterial blood is supplied by branches from superior mesentric artery. The venous drainage is by the superior mesentric vein to the hepatic portal circulation.

Nerve supply: Autonomic nerve plexus.

Intestinal juice: The daily secretion is about 3 litres. It is alkaline in reaction with a pH 7.8 to 8.0. It is secreted by glands of the small intestine. It consists of, water, mucus, enzymes and mineral salts.

Functions

1. Onward movement of its contents by peristaltic, segmental and pendular movements.
2. Secretion of intestinal juice. (SUCCUS ENTERICUS)
3. The digestion of carbohydrates, proteins and fats.
4. Protection against infection, antimicrobial action by lysozyme, secreted by paneth cells of small intestine, by production of antibodies by lymphatic aggregations.
5. Secretion of the hormones, cholecystokinin, pancreozymin, and secretin by the duodenum.
6. Absorption of nutrient materials.

Digestion in the small intestine

When acid chyme passes into the small intestine it is mixed up with pancreatic juice, bile and intestinal juice. After digestion, it is absorbed by cells of mucous membrane. In the small intestine digestion of all the nutrients is completed i.e., carbohydrates to monosaccharides, proteins to amino acids, fats to fatty acids and glycerol. Pancreatic juice consists of water, mineral salts, enzymes i.e., amylase, lipase and peptidases including trypsinogen and chymo trypsinogen. Pancreatic juice is alkaline with a pH 8. When acid stomach contents enter the duodenum, they are mixed up with pancreatic juice and bile to raise the pH 6-8. The enzymes, trypsinogen and chymotrypsinogen are inactive enzymes. When they come in contact with enterokinase, an enzyme, secreted by the intestine, they are convertd into the active proteolytic enzymes trypsin and chymotrypsin. These enzymes convert some polypeptides to amino acids and some to smaller molecule polypeptides (dipeptides and tripeptides). Pancreatic amylase converts all polysaccharides (starches) to diasaccharides (sugars). Lipase converts emulsified fats into fatty acids and glycerol. Bile salts emulsify fats i.e., reduce the size of the fat globules. Presence of acid material in the duodenum stimulates the cells of the small intestine to produce the hormones, secretin, pancretozymin and cholecystokinin.

• **BILE:** It is secreted by the liver cells. When the sphincter of oddi is closed, bile cannot enter into the duodenum, so it enters into the gall bladder through the hepatic duct and the cystic duct. When a fatty meal enters the duodenum, the duodenal cells produce cholecystokinin (CCK). It stimulates the contraction of the gall bladder and relaxation of the sphincter of oddi. So, bile and pancreatic juice pass into the duodenum. The bile consists of water, mineral salts, mucus, bile salts and bile pigment bilirubin and cholesterol.

Functions

1. Bile pigment, bilirubin, is the waste product of the breakdown of erythrocytes. It colours and deodorises faeces. It has a laxative effect. It also colours the urine.
2. Bile helps the absorption of vitamin K and digested fats.
3. The bile salts, sodium taurocholate and sodium glycocholate emulsify fats, in the small intestine.

Intestinal juice (succus entericus): It is secreted by the glands of the small intestine. It consists of water, mucus and enzyme enteropeptidase (enterokinase). The digestive enzymes are secreted by the cells of the walls of villi. The digestion of carbohydrates, proteins and fats is completed by direct contact between these nutrients and the microvilli and within the enterocytes.

The enzymes involved in completing the digestion of food in the cells of the villi are - Peptidases, Lipase, Sucrase, maltase and lactase.

Functions

Alkaline intestinal juice raises the pH of the intestinal contents to between 6.5 and 7.5.

Enteropeptidase (Enterokinase) activates pancreatic peptidases which convert some polypeptides to amino acids and some to smaller molecule peptides. Lipase completes the digestion of fats to fatty acids and glycerol.

Sucrase, maltase and lactase complete the digestion of carbohydrates by converting diasaccharides to monosaccharides.

Secretion: Intestinal glands are stimulated by chyme to secrete intestinal juice.

Absorption of nutrient materials

1. Carbohydrates as monosaccharides, proteins as amino acids and fats as fatty acids and glycerol are slowly absorbed by diffusion but more rapidly by active transport.
2. Monosaccharides and amino acids pass into the capillaries in the villi and fatty acids and glyderol pass into the lacteals of the villi.
3. Some proteins are absorbed unchanged eg: antibodies present in mother's milk and oral vaccine, such as, poliomyelitis vaccine.
4. Other nutritional materials like vitamins, mineral salts and water are absorbed from the small intestine into blood capillaries.

SUMMARY OF CHEMICAL DIGESTION

Organ	Digestive fluid	Reaction pH	Enzymes/other substances	Chemical actions of Enzymes
Mouth	Saliva	Slightly acid pH. 6.8	Ptyalin (Salivary Amylase)	Converts cooked starches (polysaccharides) into maltose and dextrum. (only about 5% of carbohydrates are digested in the mouth)
			Lingual Lipase	Begins convertion of triglycerides into fatty acids and glycerol
Stomach	Gastric juice	Acid pH. 1.5 to 3.5	Pepsinogen	
			By HCl	
			Pepsin	Converts proteins into peptides.
			Renin (Present in small animal fats)	Converts caseinogen into casein (Curdle Milk), Pepsin converts casein into peptides
			Gastric lipase (very small amounts in stomach)	Begins digestion of fats
			Hydrochloric acid	Converts pepsinogen into pepsin. Kills microorganisms in food. Denatures Proteins.
			Intrinsic factor (glycoprotein)	Needed for absorption of Vitamin B_{12}
			Mucus	Forms a protective barrier which prevents digeston of stomach wall.

SUMMARY OF CHEMICAL DIGESTION (contd.)				
Organ	**Digestive Fluid**	**Reaction pH**	**Enzymes/other substances**	**Chemical Action of Enzymes**
Duodenum	Bile	Alkaline pH 7.6 to 8.6		Emulsifies fats. Enhances action of Pancreatic enzymes.
	Pancreatic Juice	Alkaline pH 7.1 to 8.2	Trypsin and chymotrypsin	Converts protein and peptides into di and tripeptides.
			Peptidases	Complete the conversion of peptides, di and tripeptides into amino acids.
			Nucleases	Converts DNA and RNA into nucleotides
			Pancreatic lipase	Converts emulsified fats into fatty acids and glycerol
Small Intestine			Enterokinase	Converts tripsinogen into trypsin
			Alpha dextrinase	Converts alpha dextrins into glucose
			Maltase	Converts maltose into glucose
			Sucrose	Converts sucrose into glucose and fructose
			Lactase	Converts lactose into glucose and galactose

5. The surface area of absorption is greatly increased by circular mucosal folds of mucous membrane and the very large number of villi present.

Large intestine, rectum and anal canal

The large intestine is about 1.5 metres long. It begins from the caecum at right iliac fossa and ends at the rectum in the pelvic cavity. Its lumen is bigger than the small intestine and forms an arch around the coils of small intestine. For descriptive purpose, it is divided into the caecum, ascending colon, transverse colon, descending colon, sigmoid or pelvic colon, rectum and anal canal.

The caecum is the first part of the colon. It is a blind dilated end lies inferiorly and is continuous with the ascending colon above. At the junction of the ileum and caecum there is a valve, called as ileo-caecal valve. The vermiform appendix is a tube closed at another end, which leads from the caecum. The appendix is about 1.8 cms long and structurally same as colon, and possesses more lymphoid tissue. Inflammation of this is called appendicitis. It is the commonest abdominal problem.

The ascending colon passes upwards from the caecum to the level of liver, where it bends to the left at the right colic or hepatic flexure to become transverse colon.

The transverse colon is a loop of colon extends from hepatic flexure to the spleen and bends downwards as descending colon. The bend at spleen is called left colic or splenic flexure.

The descending colon passes downwards on left side of the abdominal cavity to the pelvis to continue as pelvic colon.

The sigmoid or pelvic colon continues in pelvic cavity as S-shaped curve, then continues downwards to become the rectum.

The rectum is the slightly dilated part in the pelvic cavity. It terminates in the anal canal.

The anal canal is about 4 cms long, opens to the exterior and its opening is controlled by external and internal sphincters and is under voluntary nerve control.

Structure: It consists of 4 layers as in general plan of G-I tract. In muscular layer the longitudinal muscle fibres are modified and are collected in 3 bundles or bands called Taenia coli. They give a sacculated or puckering appearance of the colon. The anal sphicters are formed by thickness of the circular muscles. In the submucous layer, there is more lymphoid tissue. In the mucous membrane, the surface cells are modified into the goblet cells to secrete mucus to help lubrication of faecal matter. In the external opening, the anus is lined by stratified squamous epithelium. In the upper part of the anal canal, the mucous membrane is arranged in 6 to 12 vertical folds in the anal columns.

Blood supply is by the superior mesentric artery and inferior mesentric artery.

Venous drainage is by the same names of veins to hepatic portal circulation.

Functions of the large intestine

1. Absorption: The large intestine absorbs water. It continues until the familiar semisolid consistency of faeces is achieved. With water, some mineral salts and vitamins are absorbed. [This function of the large intestine is made use of in administering retention enema. For Ex: Rectal saline administration (Proctoclysis)].

2. Microbial activity: There are large numbers of bacteria or microbial flora to synthesise vitamin K and folic acid. They include, escherichia coli, streptococcus faecalis and clostridium welchii. These microbes are commensals in man. If they

enter the other system, they become pathogenic. Hydrogen, carbon di-oxide and methane gases are produced by bacterial fermentation of unabsorbed nutrients. These gases pass out of the bowel as flatus.

Defaecation: The large intestine, only at long intervals, has a wave of strong peristaltic movement along the transverse colon which forces its contents into the descending and pelvic colon. This is known as mass movement. The rectum is empty but when a mass movement forces the contents of the pelvic colon into the rectum, the nerve endings in its walls are stimulated by stretch. In the infant, defaecation occurs by reflex action which is not under voluntary control. The defaecation involves involuntary contraction of the muscle of the rectum and relaxation of the internal anal sphincter. The contraction of diaphragm and abdominal muscles increases intra abdominal pressure and so assists the process of defaecation.

Constituents of faeces consist of a semisolid brown mass. The brown colour is due to the presence of stercobilin. The water is about 60% of the weight of faeces. Other parts are indigestible food materials, dead and live bacteria, fatty acids, epithelial cells and mucus. The goblet cells secrete mucus that helps to lubricate faecal matter.

Enema is a liquid preparation injected into the lower bowel through the rectum. Left lateral position is suitable, to give enema as the sigmoid colon and descending colon are lower and the liquid flows easily because of gravity.

Pancreas: It is about 12-15 cms in length, situated transversely in the abdominal cavity. It extends from the C-shaped duodenum to the spleen.It lies in epigastric and left hypochondriac regions. It consists of a broad head, a body and a narrow tail. The head lies in the curve of duodenum. The body is behind the stomach and the tail is in front of the left kidney and reach the hilum of the spleen. The abdominal aorta and the inferior vena cava lie below the pancreas and it is intimately related to posterior abdominal wall. It lies behind the peritoneum.

Structure: It consists of exocrine and endocrine glands. The exocrine part consists of a large number of lobules made up of small alveoli. The alveolus wall is made up of secretary cells (acinar cells). Each lobule is drained by small ducts. These ducts unite to form the main pancreatic duct. It extends from the whole length of the gland and opens into the duodenum at its mid point. The pancreatic duct joins the common bile duct to form ampulla of the bile duct (ampulla of vator). The duodenal opening of the ampulla is controlled by the sphincter of oddi. The endocrine part is the islets of Langerhans. They consist of specialised groups of cells situated throughout the gland. They secrete the hormones insulin, glycogen, somatostatin and pancreatic polypeptide. The hormones pass directly into the blood stream.

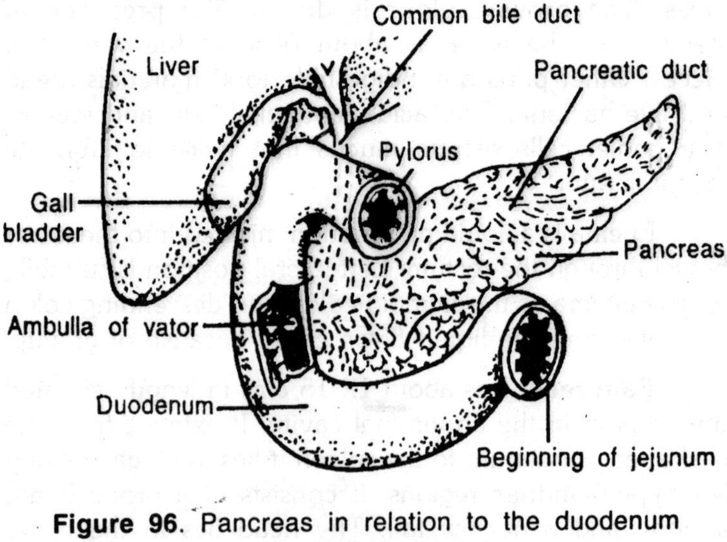

Figure 96. Pancreas in relation to the duodenum and biliary tract.

Blood supply: by splenic and superior mesentric arteries from coeliac artery. The venous drainage is to the hepatic portal vein.

Nerve supply: By autonomic nerve plexus, parasympathetic stimulation increases the secretion of pancreatic juice and sympathetic stimulation depresses it.

Functions: Pancreatic juice contains water, some salts, sodium bicarbonate and the enzymes that digest carbohydrates, proteins and fats namely pancreatic amylase, tripsinogen, chymotripsinogen, pancreatic lipase, elastase and nucleases (ribonuclease and deoxyriboneuclease).

Pancreatic juice is alkaline in reaction, the pH is 7.1 to 8.2. A slightly alkaline pH is due to sodium bicarbonate. Daily secretion is about 1200-1500 ml.

Liver

The liver is the largest gland in the body weighing about 1.5 to 2.5 kg. It is situated in the abdominal cavity occupying the right hypochondriac region, part of epigastric region and extending to the left hypochondriac region. Its superior and anterior surfaces are smooth to fit under the diaphragm.

Relations

Superiorly	:	Diaphragm
Anteriorly	:	Anterior abdominal wall.
Inferiorly	:	Stomach, bile ducts, duodenum, right colic flexure of the colon, right kidney and adrenal gland.
Posteriorly	:	Oesophagus, inferior vena cava, aorta, gall-bladder, vertebral column and diaphragm.
Laterally	:	Lower ribs and diaphragm.

The liver has a thin capsule and covered by a layer of peritoneum. The folds of peritoneum form supporting ligaments attaching the liver to the inferior surface of the diaphragm. It is held in position by hepatic veins and partly by peritoneal ligaments and partly by pressure of the organs in the abdominal cavity. The liver is having four lobes, the larger right lobe, and the smaller left lobe, the other two are the caudate and quadrate lobes.

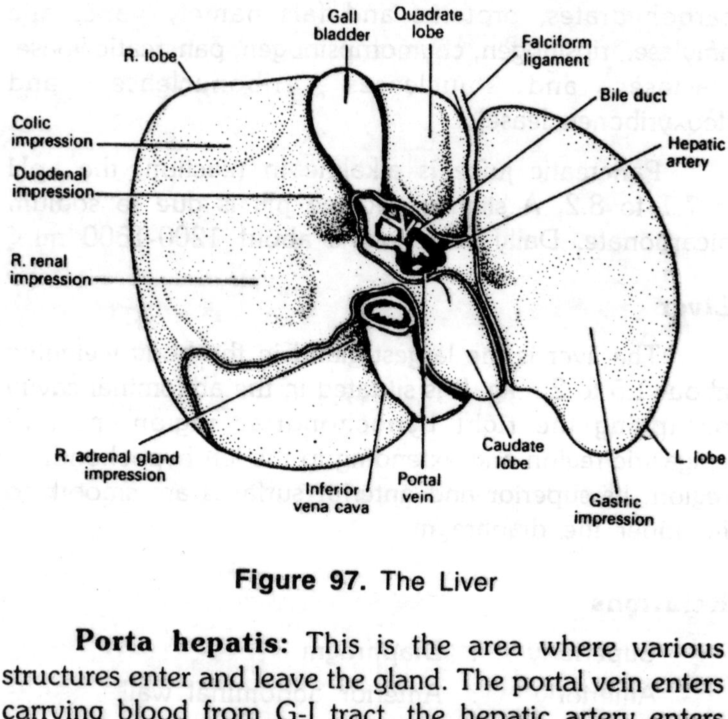

Figure 97. The Liver

Porta hepatis: This is the area where various structures enter and leave the gland. The portal vein enters carrying blood from G-I tract, the hepatic artery enters carrying arterial blood. It is a branch of coeliac trunk. The nerve supply is from the autonomic nerve plexus. The right and left hepatic ducts leave, carrying bile from the liver to the gall bladder. Lymph vessels leave the liver, draining to abdominal nodes.

Blood supply: By hepatic artery and protal vein. Venous drainage is by two hepatic veins situated on posterior surface of the liver which enpty into the inferior vena cava.

Structure: The lobes of the liver are subdivided into lobules. These lobules are hexagonal in outline,

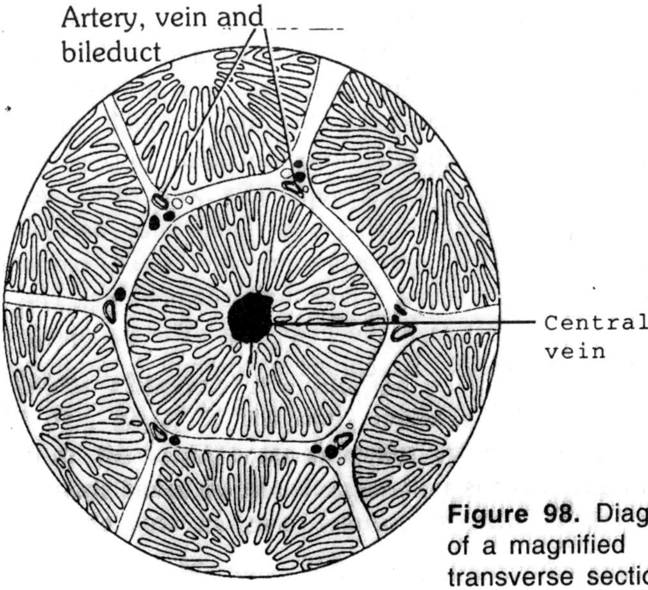

Figure 98. Diagram of a magnified transverse section of liver lobules

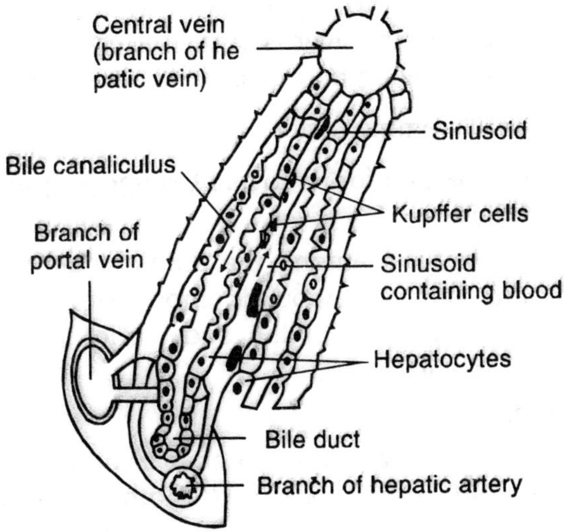

Figure 99. Microscopic structure of a lobule of the liver.

formed by polyhedral cells cailed hepatocytes. They are arranged in pairs radiating from a central vein. Between two pairs of column of cells there are sinusoids containing a mixture of oxygenated and deoxygenated blood from branches of portal vein and hepatic artery. These mixed blood will have contact with hepatocytes. The special cells lining the sinusoids are hepatic macrophages (Von kupffer's cells). These cells destroy worn out red and white blood cells and some bacteria in the blood which enters the sinusoids. Blood drains from sinusoids into central or centrilobular veins. These veins join with other veins of lobule to form larger veins and finally they become the hepatic veins. They leave the liver and empty blood into the inferior vena cava. Liver cells secrete bile. The bile canaliculi run between the liver cells. The canaliculi join up to form larger bile canals until they form the right and left hepatic ducts which drain bile from the liver.

Liver can be palpated at right costal margins. Normally, liver is not palpable. In abnormal conditions, it extends down to costal arches.

Functions

1. Converts glucose to glycogen by insulin. Gluconeogenesis in the liver is also concerned with maintaining a normal blood glucose concentration.

2. Deamination of amino acids.

   a) formation of urea for removal of ammonia from body fluids.

   b) inter conversions among the different amino-acids and other compounds important to the metabolic processes of the body, uric acid is formed and excreted.

3. Fat metabolism

   a) Desaturation of fats so as to enable the tissues to use and supply energy for other bodily functions.

b) formation of most of the lipo proteins.

c) synthesis of large quantities of cholesterol and phospholipids.

d) conversion of large quantities of carbohydrates and protein to fat.

4. Secretion of bile: The hepatocytes secrete bile. It contains water, bile salts, bile pigments, cholesterol etc.

5. Storage function

   a) Vitamin B_{12}

   b) Water soluble vitamins eg: riboflavin, niacin, pyridoxine, folic acid.

   c) Fat-soluble vitamins: A, D, E and K.

   d) Minerals: iron, copper.

6. Synthesis of vitamin A from carotene derived from carrots and green leafy vegetables.

7. Synthesises of non-essential amino-acids, plasma proteins.

8. Detoxication function of drugs and noxious substances.

9. Inactivates hormones or excretes thyroxines, all steroid hormones such as estrogen, cortisol and aldosterone.

10. Production of heat.

11. Phagocytosis.

12. Vitamin Activation.

Composition of bile

1. Water
2. Bile salts
3. Bilirubin

4. Cholesterol
5. Fatty acids
6. Lecithin
7. Minerals like, Na^+, K^+, Ca^+, Cl^-, HCO_3^-.
8. Mucus

The bile acids, cholic and chenodeoxycholic acid are synthesised by hepatocytes, conjugated (combined) with either glycine or taurine then secreted into bile as sodium or potassium salts. In small intestine, they emulsify fats for digestion. In the terminal ileum, most of the bile salts (Sodium Taurocholate and Sodium glycocholate) are absorbed and return to the liver through hepatic portal vein. Cholesterol is made soluble in bile by bile salts and lecithin.

Bilirubin is one of the end products of haemolysis of erythrocytes by Von Kupffer cells. In its original form, bilirubin is insoluble in water and is bound to albumin. In liver, it is conjugated to glucoronic acid and becomes water soluble before it is excreted in bile. Bacteria in intestine change the forms of bilirubin and excreted as stercobilin in the faeces. The kidneys excrete bilirubin as urobilin in the urine.

Jaundice

In jaundice, yellow colouration of conjunctiva, skin and mucous membranes occurs because of excess of blood bilirubin.

There are three types of jaundice.

1. Haemolytic jaundice
2. Hepatic jaundice and
3. Obstructive jaundice.

Many newborn infants develop a mild form of

jaundice called neonatal (physiological) jaundice. This is because the liver of a newborn functions poorly for the first week. It disappears as the liver matures.

Bile ducts: The right and left hepatic ducts join to form common hepatic duct, just out side the porta hepatis. The hepatic duct passes downwards for about 3 cms. where it is joined by the cystic duct from the gall bladder. The cystic and hepatic ducts together form the common bile duct which passes downward behind pancreas and it is joined by the main pancreatic duct at ampulla of vator. The opening of the combined ducts into the duodenum is controlled by the sphincter of Oddi. The structure of the bile duct have same layers as

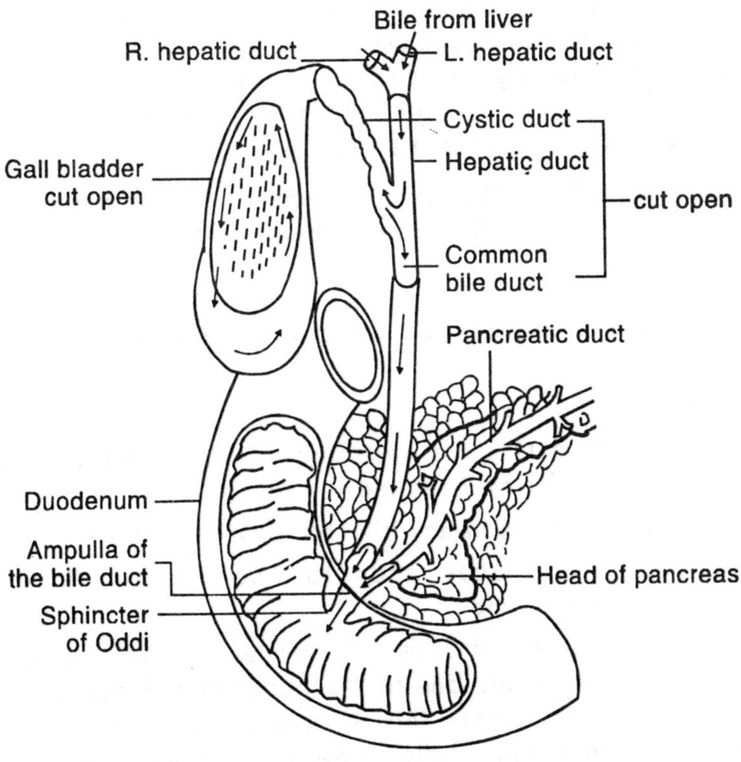

Figure 100. Gall bladder and biliary tract

described by general plan of G-I tract. In the cystic duct, the mucous membrane lining is arranged in irregularly situated circular folds, which have the effect of a spiral valve. Bile passes through the cystic duct twice on its way into the gall bladder and again when it is expelled from the gall bladder to the common bile duct and thence to the duodenum.

Gall Bladder: It is a pear-shaped sac attached to the inferior surface of the liver by loose connective tissue. It has a fundus, a body and a neck, which is continuous with the cystic duct.

Structure: Has same layers as the general plan of G-I tract with some modifications. The peritoneum covers the inferior surface. There is additional layer of oblique layer in the muscle. The mucous membrane displays small rugae when the gall-bladder is empty and disappear when it is distended with bile. There is absence of glands and muscularis mucosa.

Blood supply: By cystic artery which is a branch of hepatic artery. The venous drainage is by cystic vein to hepatic portal vein.

Nerve supply: By autonomic plexuses.

Functions

1. It acts as a reservoir for bile, about 50 to 60 cc is stored.
2. It concentrates bile by absorbing water.
3. The mucus adds to bile by the lining membrane.
4. The contraction of muscles of gall bladder expels the bile to the duodenum. When fatty food enters the duodenum, the duodenal mucosal cells produce cholecystokinin which contracts the muscle of gall bladder.

Questions

1. Draw a neat diagram of digestive system and label the parts.
2. Name and describe the coats that composes of the walls of the oesophagus, stomach and intestines.
3. Differentiate between the mesentery and omentum.
4. Give the names and numbers of temporary teeth and permanent teeth.
5. Draw a neat diagram of the stomach and state the functions of the stomach.
6. Write the composition of gastric juice.
7. What function does the liver perform? Which of these are vital functions?
8. What digestive functions does the pancreas perform?
9. Name the biliary ducts and write the composition of bile.
10. Write short notes on the following:
    a) Salivary glands
    b) Enzymes
    c) Villi
    d) Structure of tooth

Metabolism

Metabolism is the sum total of the chemical changes that is taking place in the body. It consists of anabolism and catabolism.

Anabolism is the process of assimilation of nutritient materials and synthesizing new products (building up process). Catabolism is the process of breaking down substances to provide energy and raw materials for anabolism and substances for excretion as waste.

When nutritional materials are oxidised in the cells of the body, energy is released in the form of heat. Energy may be used immediately to do work or it may be stored in chemical form as adenosine triphosphate (ATP). Abuot 40% of the energy released in catabolism is available for cellular functions. The rest of the energy is converted to heat. Heat is used to maintain the body temperature at the optium level of chemical activity 36.8°C or 98.4°F. Excess heat is lost to the environment. A calorie (capital C) is the amount of heat required to raise the temperature of 1 litre of water through 1 degree celsius.

1 Calorie = 4184 joules (J) = 4.184 Kilojoules (KJ). The nutritional valve of carbohydrates, proteins and fats may be expressed in kilojoules per gram or calories per gram.

1 gram of carbohydrates provides 17 KJ or 4 calories.

1 gram of proteins provides 17 KJ or 4 calories.

1 gram of fats provides 38 KJ or 9 calories.

The metabolic rate is the rate at which energy is released from the nutrients inside the cells. This process requires oxygen and produce carbon di-oxide as waste. The metabolic rate can be estimated by measuring oxygen uptake or carbon di-oxide excretion.

The basal metabolic rate (BMR) is the rate of metabolism when the individual is at rest and is in the post absorptive state i.e., after 12 hours of food intake. The post absorptive state is important because the intake of food, especially, protein, stimulates an increase in metabolic rate, possibly, due to increased energy utilisation by the liver. This is called the specific dynamic action (SDA). In measuring the BMR, the surface area of the body is taken into account because energy in the form of heat is lost through the skin. The surface area in square metres is calculated from the height and weight of a person. Most foods contain a mixture of different amounts of carbohydrates, proteins, fats, minerals, vitamins, roughage and water. Carbohydrates, proteins and fats are the sources of energy and they are obtained from various types of food.

Metabolism of carbohydrates

When food containing carbohydrate is digested, mainly, glucose is absorbed into the blood capillaries of the villi of the small intestine. It is transported to the liver through the hepatic portal circulation.

1. Glucose may be used to provide the energy for the body.
2. The glucose level maintained in circulating blood is 100-200 mg/ 100 ml.
3. Some of the glucose may be converted to the insoluble polysaccharide, glycogen in the liver and stored in the liver and muscles.

   Liver Glycogen constitutes a store of glucose used for liver activity and to maintain the blood glucose level.

   Muscle Glycogen provides the glucose requirements of muscle activity. Adrenalin, thyroxin and glucagon are the main hormones for the conversion of glycogen to glucose.

4. If there is excess of carbohydrate in the body, it is converted into fat and stored in fat depots.

All the body cells require energy to carry out their metabolic processes, including multiplication of cells, for replacement of worn out cells, contraction of muscle fibres and secretions of glands. The oxidation of carbohydrate and fat provides most of the energy required by the body. Complete oxidation of glucose, requires an adequate supply of oxygen. The process of oxidation of carbohydrates in the body, results in the production of energy, carbon di-oxide and water the waste products. Carbon di-oxide is excreted from the body as a gas by lungs, the water is added to the considerable amount of water already present in the body. The excess of water is excreted through kidneys and skin.

Metabolism of proteins

Protein foods taken as part of the diet is made up of a number of amino-acids. About 20 amino-acids have been named and about 8 of these are essential because they cannot be synthesised in the body. The remainder are described as non-essential amino-acids, because they can be synthesised by many tissues. The enzymes involved for this process are called transaminases. The proteins of the diet are broken down into amino-acids.

They are absorbed into the villi of the small intestine, then carried to the liver by portal circulation. From the liver they are carried to general circulation for utilization of all the cells and tissues of the body. Different cells choose particular amino-acids for building or repairing the tissue, or synthesising their secretions, eg. antibodies, enzymes, hormones. The amino-acids are not required for building, are broken down in the liver as the nitrogenous part. It is converted into urea by the process of deamination and excreted in the urine. The remaining part is used to provide energy or stored as fat.

A pool of amino-acids is maintained within the body. This available source is utilized by different cells of the body to synthesise their own materials eg. new cells, secretions, such as, enzymes, hormones and blood proteins.

Sources of amino-acids

1. Exogenous: These are derived from the proteins taken in the diet.
2. Endogenous: These are from break down of body proteins, in the adult 80 to 100 g of proteins are broken down and replaced each day.

Loss of amino-acids

1. Deamination: The amino acids not needed by the body are deaminated, mainly, in the liver. The end product is the urea excreted by the kidneys and the remainder is used to provide energy and heat.
2. Excretion: The faeces contain some amount of protein consisting of desquamated cells from the lining of the alimentary tract.

Endogenous and exogenous amino-acids are mixed up into the pool and the body is said to be in nitrogen-balance, when the rate of removal from the pool is equal to the additions to it. Unlike carbohydrates and fats, the body has no capacity for the storage of amino-acids.

Metabolism of fats

Fats which have been digested and absorbed into the lacteals in the villi of small intestine pass through cisterna chyli and thoracic duct to the blood stream and to the liver. Fatty acids and glycerol circulating in the blood are used by organs and glands to provide energy and in the synthesis of their secretions. In the liver, some fatty acids and glycerol are used to provide energy and heat. Excess fatty acids are taken up by fat cells which change them to neutral fat and stored. When body needs, it is converted back to fatty acids and circulated in the blood and taken up by body cells. The end products of fat metabolism are energy, heat, carbon dioxide and water. Ketone bodies or Ketoacids are produced during the process of oxidation of fats and present in blood in very small amounts. Ketone bodies are acetone, acetoacetic acid and beta-hydroxybutiric acid. They are excreted in the urine and in the expired air as acetone. When the final stages of fat metabolism are blocked due

CITRIC ACID CYCLE OR KREB'S CYCLE

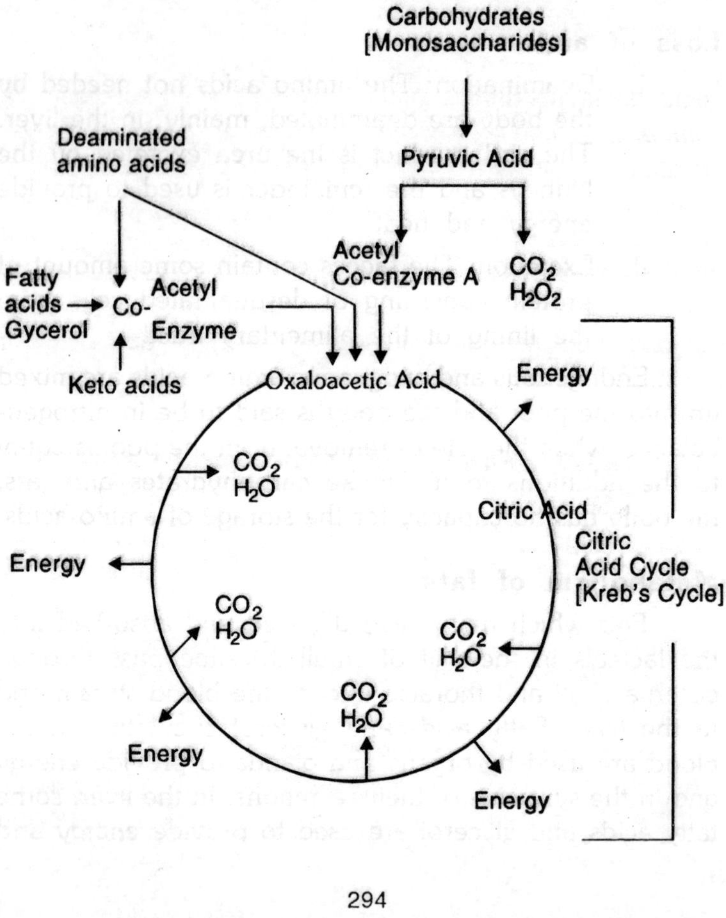

to deficiency in the supply of the products of carbohydrate metabolism, excess keto-acids are formed and a state of ketosis develops. This condition may occur in starvation or in diabetes mellitus when there is deficiency of insulin which helps the movement of carbohydrates into cells. Fat may be synthesised form carbohydrates and proteins, which are taken into the body in excess of its needs and stored in the fat depots i.e., under the skin, in the omentum, around the kidneys.

The degradation of carbohydrates, fatty acids, glyderol and residue after amino-acids are deaminated, occurs inside the cells, releasing energy and forming the waste products, carbo dioxide and water. The catabolism of these materials occurs in a series of steps. Each nutrient passes through a series of separate and distinct stages. Thereafter, they all follow a common pathway which is called the citric acid cycle or Kreb's cycle. The formation of abnormal amounts of ketoacids occurs in starvation and in diabetes mellitus. When excess amounts of fat and amino acids are used to provide energy, excess keto acids are produced. In both these examples, there is an insufficiency of carbo hydrate inside the cells. In diabetes this is due to shortage of the hormone insulin which facilitates the transportation of carbohydrates from the extracellular fluid across the cell membrane and its subsequent metabolism, excess keto acids are excreted in the urine and expired in air as acetone.

The maintenance of body temperature

The normal body temperature is 98.4°F or 36.9°C with a range of from 97° to 99°F or 36.1° to 37.2°C. The diurnal variation is about one degree fahrenheit or half a degree celsius. The lowest level being reached in the early hours of the morning and the highest point between 5 and 7 pm. This normal temperature is maintained by an exact adjustment between heat production and heat lost. This is controlled by the heat regulating centre in the hypothalamus. This centre is very sensitive to the temperature of the blood passing through it, acting like a thermostat.

Summary of Metabolism of Carbohydrates, Proteins and Fats

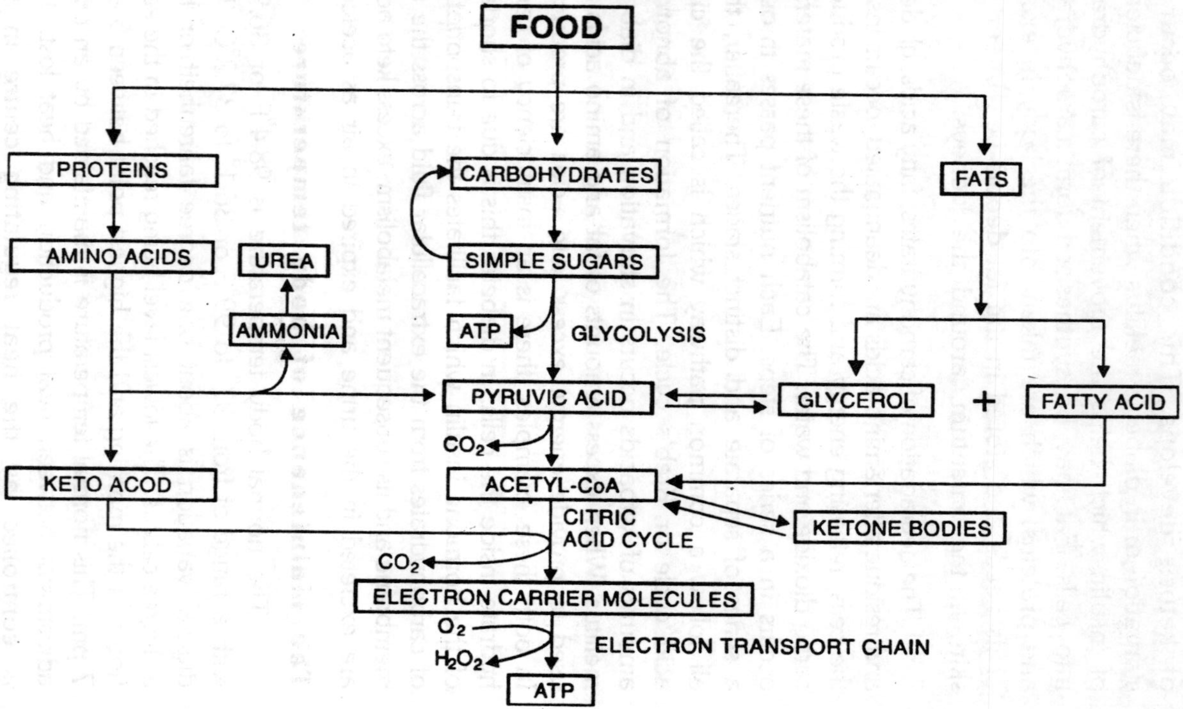

Heat is produced by the metabolic activities in the skeletal muscles and liver. The glycogen stored in the liver is converted into usable glucose and oxidized, with that heat is produced. The metabolic activities must be adjusted to meet the varying demands made, for example by active work, or conditions of rest, the intake of food, at meal times the emotional reactions of the person, the external temperature, the clothing worn and so on. Over heating is, usually, due to a combination of a high external temperature, physical activity and inadequate sweating.

Regulation of body Temperature

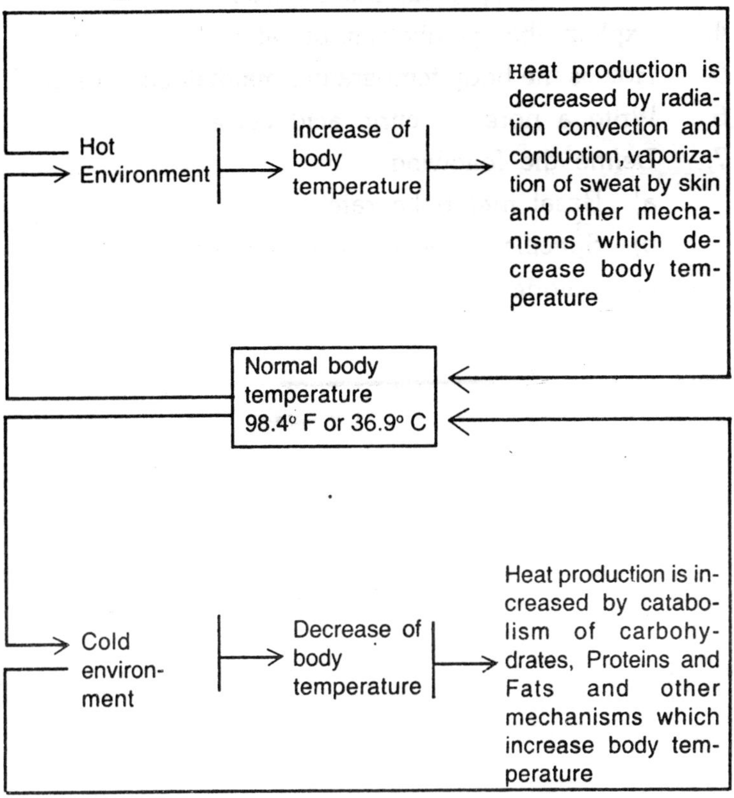

Heat loss is mainly effected by the functional activities of the skin. A certain amount of heat is lost by the evaporation of moisture from the lungs and by sweating. Heat conservation is by vaso constriction and diminished sweating. When the body temperature is lowered in prolonged vaso constriction due to exposure to cold or starvation, shivering and shaking may occur as the muscles contract to warm up the body.

Questions

1. Define metabolism.
2. Explain the metabolism of carbohydrates.
3. How is the protein metabolised?
4. Explain the metabolism of fat.
5. How is the body temperature maintained constant?
6. Write a note on citric acid cycle.
7. Define the following:
   a) Basal metabolic rate
   b) Specific dynamic action of food
   c) Calorie

UNIT 9

The Urinary System

The urinary system consists of the following structures.

2 Kidneys - secrete urine

2 Ureters - convey the urine from the kidneys to the urinary bladder.

1 Urinary bladder-where urine collects temporarily.

1 Urethra through which the urine is discharged from the urinary bladder to the exterior.

Kidneys: The kidneys are situated in the abdominal cavity in relation to posterior abdominal wall, one on each side of the vertebral column, behind the peritoneum and below the diaphragm. They extend from the 12th thoracic vertebra to the 3rd lumbar vertebra. The right kidney is, slightly lower than the left because of the liver on right side.

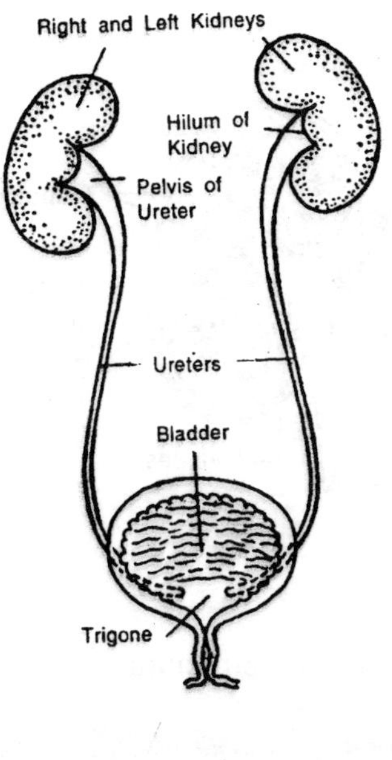

Figure 101. The organs which form the urinary tract.

Relations

Right kidney	: Superiorly: The right adrenal gland.
Anteriorly	: The right lobe of the liver, the duodenum and right colic flexure.
Posteriorly	: The diaphragm, and muscles of the posterior abdominal wall.
Left kidney	: Superiorly: The left adrenal gland.
Anteriorly	: The spleen, stomach, pancreas, jejunum and left colic flexure.
Posteriorly	: The diaphragm and muscles of the posterior abdominal wall.

An adult kidney is about 10-12 cm (4-5 in.) long, 5-7 cm (2-3 in.) wide and 2.5 cm (1 in.) thick.

Gross structure: When the longitudinal section of a kidney is viewed with naked eye, the following structures are seen. Each Kidney is surrounded by three layers of tissue.

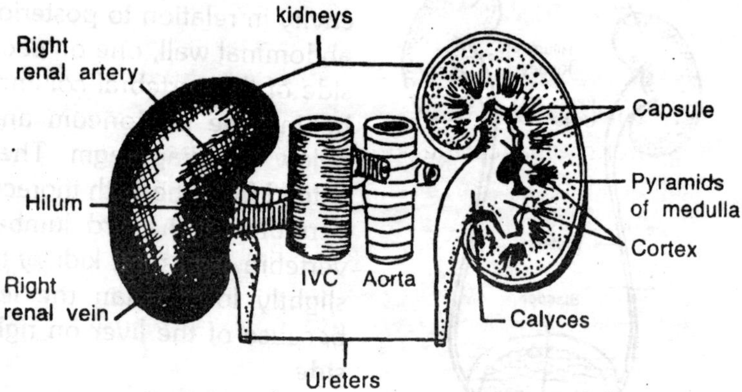

Figure 102. Kidneys- Gross structure.

1. The deep layer is a fibrous capsule. The intermediate layer is adipose tissue which surrounds the renal capsule. It offers protection to the kidney and holds it firmly in place within the abdominal cavity. The outer layer is the renal fascia which anchors the kidney to its surrounding structures and to the abdominal wall.
2. The cortex is the reddish layer below the capsule and between the pyramids.
3. The medulla is the inner most layer consisting of a deep reddish brown region called the renal medulla. It contains 8-18 cone shaped structures called renal pyramids.

Hilum is the concave medial border of the kidney where the renal blood vessels, lymphatic vessels and nerves enter and leave. The renal pelvis is the funnel-shaped structure which receives urine from the major calyces (2 to 3). Urine is formed in the kidney and passes through a papilla at the apex of a pyramid into a lesser calyx, then into greater calyx, from there to pelvis of ureter. It is lined by transitional epithelium and contains smooth muscle. A wave of contraction, propels urine through the pelvis of ureters to the bladder through the ureters.

Microscopic structure of the kidneys

The cortex and pyramids of the kidney constitute the parenchyma of the kidney. Within the parenchyma of each kidney there are two types of nephrons. They are cortical nephrons (80-85%) and juxtameduallary nephrons (15-20%). Each kidney contains about 1 million nephrons which are the functional units of the kidney and a small number of collecting tubules. The uriniferous tubules are supported by a small amount of connective tissue, containing blood vessels, nerves and lymph vessels. A nephron consists of a tubule at one end opening into a collecting tubule. The closed or blind end is indented to form the cup-shaped glomerular capsule (Bowman's capsule). The Bowman's capsule almost encloses a net work of arterial capillaries, the glomerulus. The ramainder of the naphron has the proximal convoluted tubule, the loop of Henle and the distal convoluted tubule, leading into a collecting tubule. The renal artery enters the kidney through the hilum and divides into smaller arteries and arterioles. In the cortex, an afferent arteriole enters each glomerular capsule to form capillary net work. Between

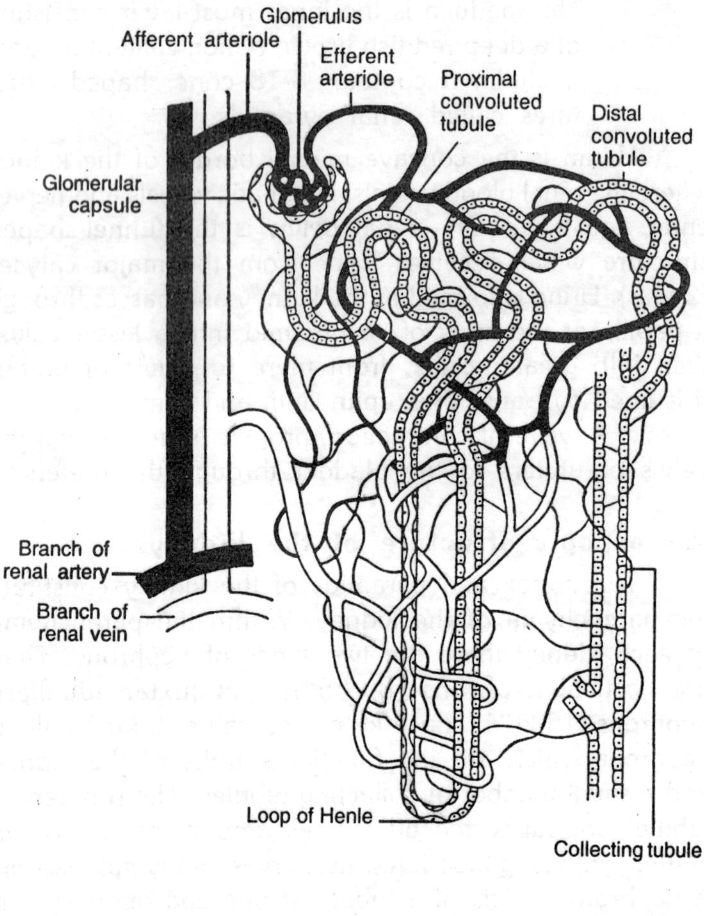

Figure 103. Diagram of a nephron microscopic structure

the capillary loops, there are phagocytic mesangial cells and for the most part they are separated from capillary lamina by endothelial cells. The efferent arteriole comes out from the glomerulus. It breaks up into a second capillary net work (Peritubular capillary net work) to supply oxygen and nutritional materials. The peritubular capillaries supply blood to the cortical nephrons. The peritubular capillaries and vasa recta that arise from some efferent arteriols supply blood to the juxtamedullary nephrons. The venous blood leaves the kidney through the renal vein which joins the inferior vena cava. The blood pressure in the glomerulus is higher than in other capillaries because the caliber of the afferent arteriole is greater than that of the efferent arteriole.

The afferent artiole before entering the Bowman's capsule (which is near the final portion of ascending limb of loop of Henle) contains special cells called juxtaglomerular cells. They secrete an enzyme called renin. It converts angiotensinogen into angiotensin I which is converted into angiostensin II. Angiotension II stimulates the secretion of altosterone from the adrenal cortex.

The parietal layer of Bowman's capsule is lined by a simple flattened epithelial cells. The visceral layer of Bowman's capsule surrounds the glomerulus and consists of specialized cells called podocytes. The glomerular capillaries have pores in their walls. Each podocyte has thousands of cytoplasmic extensions called pedicles which have gaps between them.

The pores in the walls of the glomerular capillaries, basement membrane between the pedicles and the slit membranes between pedicles form a filtration membrane.

Renal tubules: From the capsular space, filtered fluid passes into the renal tubule, which has three main sections. The proximal convoluted tubule is lined by cuboidal epithelium with brush border. The distal convoluted tubule is lined by simple cuboidal epithelium and loop of Henle is lined by simple squamous epithelium. It continues as distal convoluted tubule.

The distal convoluted tubules of several nephrons empty into a single collecting tubule. Collecting tubules open into apices of renal pyramids which drain into minor calyces.

The kidneys receive 20 to 25% of the cardiac output. This amounts to about 1200 ml of blood per minute.

Blood supply

Kidneys receive blood from the right and left renal arteries which are the branches of abdominal aorta. Each renal artery divides as follows.

Renal Artery
↓
Segmental artery
↓
Interlobar artery
↓
arcuate artery
↓
Interlobular artery
↓
Afferent arterioles
↓
Glomerulus
↓
Efferent artiole

↓ Peritubular cappillaries

↓ Vasa recta (Long loop shaped capillaries)

Renal Veins

Peritubular capillaries and/or vasa recta

↓

Peritubular venules

↓

Interlobular veins

↓

Arcuate veins

↓

Interlobar veins

↓

Segmental veins

↓

Renal vein

The right and left renal veins join the inferior vena cava.

Nerve supply: By renal plexus of the sympathetic division of the autonomic nervous system.

Functions of the kidney

There are three phases in the formation of urine.

1. Simple filtration
2. Selective reabsorption
3. Secretion

1. Simple filtration

Simple filtration takes place through the semipermeable walls of the glomerulus, the basement membrane of the glomerulus and slit membrane between pedicles. Water and a large number of small molecules pass through some of which are reabsorbed later. Blood cells, plasma proteins and other large molecules are not filtered and remain in the capillaries. Another factor for filtration is difference between the blood pressure in the glomerulus and the pressure of the filtrate in the glomerular capsule. The other factor is the calibre of the efferent arterioles is less than that of the afferent arteriole. A capillary hydrostatic pressure about 70 mm Hg builds up in the glomerulus. This pressure is opposed by the osmotic pressure of the blood, about 30 mm Hg and by filtrate hydrostatic pressure of about 5 mm Hg in the glomerulus capsule. The net filtration pressure is 70- (30+5) = 35 mm, Hg. About 180 litres of dilute filtrate are formed each day by the two kidneys. Of these 1 to 1.5 liters are excreted as urine. The difference in volume and concentration is due to selective reabsorption, of some constituents of glomerular filtrate.

Two hormones regulate the glomerular filtration rate are angiotensin II and atrial natriuretic peptide. Angiotensin II stimulates the adrenalin cortex to secrete aldosterone and stimulate the posterior pituitary gland to secrete antidiuretic hormone. The atrial natriuretic peptide is secreted by cells in the atria of the heart. It promotes excretion of water and sodium.

Glomerular filtration rate is influenced by neural regulation.

2. Selective reabsorption

Selective reabsorption is the process by which the composition and volume of the filtrate are altered while passing through the renal tubules. The purpose of this reabsoption is to maintain fluid and electrolyte balance and blood alkalinity. Substances useful to the body such as water, glucose, amino-acids, sodium and chloride ions are reasbsorbed by the tubular cells and passed back into the blood in the capillary network round them. some substances are reabsorbed completely and others are absorbed partially. Proximal convoluted tubule reabsorbs most of the substances. Waste materials like urea, uric acid or creatinine and unwanted electrolytes pass out of the collecting tubule. By the time the glomerular filtrate reaches the end of the distal convoluted tubule about 90% of water is reabsorbed. (Obligatory water reabsorption) and solutes are returned to the blood stream. The principal cells which are located in the final portion of the distal convoluted tubule and through out the collecting tubule reabsorb the remaining 10% of water (facultatine water reabsorption). This water reabsorption is regulated by A.D.H. The remaining 10% of solutes are also reabsorbed. If the level of glucose rise above renal threshold (160 mg/100 ml), it appears in the urine becuase the mechanism for active transfer out of the tubules is over loaded.

The renal threshold of some substances varies according to the body's need for them at that time. In some instances, reapsorption is regulated by hormones. Antidiuretic hormone (ADH) from the posterior lobe of the pituitary gland affects the permeability of the distal convoluted tubules and collecting tubules, regulating water reabsorption. Parathormone from parathyroid glands and calcitonin from thyroid gland, together regulate reabsorption of calcium and phosphate.

Aldosterone secreted by the cortex of the supra renal glands regulate the reabsorption of sodium and excretion of potassium. The substances that are not normal blood constituents are not reabsorbed.

Filtrate produced	100%
Filtrate reabsorbed	
Proximal convoluted tubule	65%
Descending loop of Henle	15%
[Ascending loop of Henle is not permeable to water. It functions to dilute the filtrate by removing solutes]	
Distal convoluted tubule	19%
	99%

Filtrate passed as urine 1%

3. Secretion

The movement of materials from the blood into tubular fluid is called secretion. It can be either active or passive. The substances not required by the body including by products of metabolism that become toxic in high concentration, foreign materials eg: drugs may not be filtered through the glomerulus because of their short stay in the glomerulus.

Hydrogen ions are actively secreted in proximal convoluted tubule. It plays an important role in the regulation of the body fluid pH.

In the proximal convoluted tubule, potassium ions are actively reabsorbed. In the distal convoluted tubule and collecting tubule, potassium ions are secreted and passed out with urine.

Urine is amber in colour due to the presence of urobilin, a bile pigment altered in the intestine. The specific gravity is 1020 and 1030, and the reaction is acid. A healthy adult passes 1000-1500 ml. per day. the amount of urine secreted and the specific gravity vary according to the fluid intake and the amount of solute excreted.

Composition of normal urine

Water-96%, urea-2% and remaining excretion forms 2% ie, uric acid, creatinine, ammonia, sodium, potassium, calcium, chlorides, phosphates, sulphates, oxalates and urinary pigments.

Normal physical characteristic of Urine

Volume	–	1.0 to 1.5 litres in 24 hours
Colour	–	Yellow or amber colour
Turbidity	–	Transparent when freshly passed, becomes turbid after standing
Odour	–	Midly aromatic
pH	–	4.5 to 7.8 Average 6.0
Specific gravity	–	1.015 to 1.025

A small amount of protein (albumin) may normally be excreted in the urine in 24 hours. If the hormones are in excess, they are also passed out in urine.

Traces of ketone bodies are normally passed in the urine.

Abnormal constituents of urine

1. Protein especially albumin (albuminuria)
2. Glucose (glucosuria)
3. Ketone bodies - large amounts (Ketonuria)
4. Blood in the urine (Haematuria)

   R.B.C's and W.B.C's are seen under microscope.
5. Pus in the urine (Pyuria)
6. Bile Pigments
7. Casts. (hyaline casts and granular casts). They are the shed cells from the lining of the renal tubules and R.B.C and W.B.C. casts.
8. Microbes : They are identified by microscopic examination.

Water balance and urine output

Water is taken into the body through the alimentary canal. Water is excreted in saturated expired air, with faeces, through the skin as sweat and as the main consitutent of urine. The amount of sweat production is associated with the maintenance of normal body temperature. The balance between fluid intake and output is controlled by the kidneys. This water balance is controlled, mainly, by the antidiuretic hormone (ADH) released into the blood by the posterior lobe of the pituitary gland. There is a close link between the posterior pituitary and the hypothalamus. In hypothalamus, some specialised cells (osmoreceptors) are sensitive to the changes in the osmotic pressure of the blood. The osmoreceptors stimulate the posterior lobe of the pituitary gland to release

ADH. When the osmotic pressure is raised, ADH output is increased, as a result, water reabsorption is increased. When the osmotic pressure is reduced, this feed back mechanism maintains the blood concentration within normal limits. Excess of urine formation is called polyurea. This condition may lead to dehydration in spite of increased production of ADH but it is usually accompanised by acute thirst and increased water intake.

Electrolyte balance: Changes in the concentration of electrolytes in the body fluids may be due to changes in the amounts of water or of electrolytes.

Sodium is the most common cation (postively charged ion) in extracellular fluid and potassium is the most common intracellular cation. Sodium is present in all the foods and even added during cooking. If the intake of sodium exceeds the body's needs, it is excreted in urine and sweat. Sodium excretion is regulated by the hormone aldosterone, secreted by the cortex of adrenal gland. Cells in the afferent arteriole of the nephron are stimulated to produce an enzyme Renin by sympathetic nerves or low arterial blood pressure. This enzyme converts angiotensinogen (produced by the liver) to angiotensin I which is converted into angiotenson II which stimulates the adrenal cortex to secrete aldosterone. Water is reabsorbed with sodium, so, increase the blood volume. When sodium reabsorption is increased, potassium excretion is increased indirectly reducing intracellular potassium. The amount of sodium excreted in sweat is insignificant except when sweating is excessive. In order to maintain the normal blood pH. Hydrogen ions are secreted by the cells of the convoluted tubules and are excreted in urine. They are secreted in combination with bicarbonate as carbonic acid, with ammonia as ammonium chloride. The normal pH of urine varies from 4.5 to 7.8, average pH is 6, depending on the diet and a number of other factors.

In addition to the kidneys, the circulatory system with three principal classes of buffers and the respiratory system take part in the regulation of acid base balance in the body.

Abnormalities of acid base balance

1. Acidosis is a condition characterised by a lower than normal blood pH (below pH of 7.35 or lower). There are two types, respiratory acidosis and metabolic acidosis.
2. Alkalosis is a condition characterized by a higher than normal blood pH (pH of 7.45 or above). There are two types, respiratory alkalosis and metabolic alkalosis.

Dialysis

Dialysis means the separation of large particles from smaller ones through the use of a selectively permeable membrane.

In certain diseases or injury to the kidneys nitrogenous waste, are not excreted, pH is altered and concentration of various ions in blood plasma is not adjusted. Then blood must be cleansed artificially by dialysis (haemrodialysis or peritoneal dialysis).

URETERS

The ureters are the tubes that convey urine from the kidneys to the urinary bladder. They are about 25 cms in length with a diameter of about 3mm. They are closely related to the posterior abdominal wall. The ureter starts from funnel - shaped renal pelvis, passes downwards the posterior abdominal wall in the abdominal cavity behind the peritoneum to the pelvic cavity and enters the bladder obliquely through the posterior wall of urinary bladder. Because of this arrangement, ureters are compressed and the opening occluded when urine accumulates and the pressure rises in the bladder and also prevents reflux of urine as the bladder fills and during micturition the pressure increases as the bladder wall contracts.

Structure

1. An outer fibrous layer, continuous with the fibrous capsule.
2. Muscular layer: It is thick having circular and longitudinal smooth muscle fibres to propel the urine to bladder.
3. An inner layer of transitional epithelium, (non-absorbable epithelium).

Function: The ureters propel the urine from kidneys into the bladder by peristaltic contraction of the muscular wall. This is not under nerve control, the wave of contraction originate in a pace maker in a minor calyces. Peristaltic waves occur at about 10 second intervals, sending drops of urine into the bladder.

Urinary bladder

It is situated in pelvic cavity almost in the median plane. Its size and shape vary, depending on the amount of urine it contains. When distended, the bladder rises into the abdominal cavity.

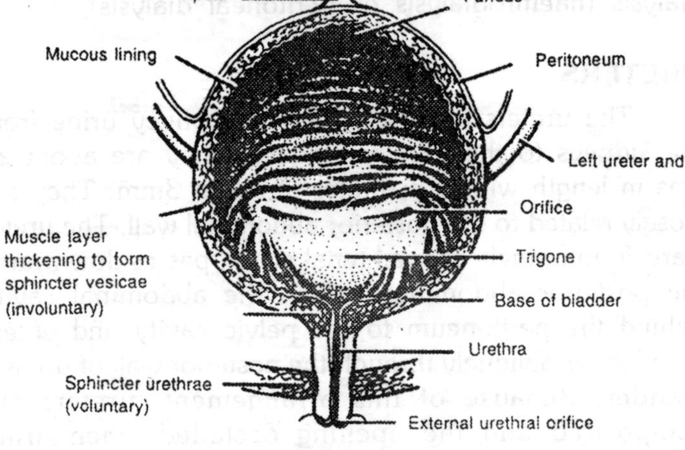

Figure 104. Urinary blader.

Relations in the female

Anteriorly	:	the pubic symphysis.
Posteriorly	:	the uterus and upper part of the vagina.
Superiorly	:	the small intestine.
Inferiorly	:	the urethra and the muscles forming the pelvic floor.

In the male

Anteriorly	:	the pubic symphysis
Posteriorly	:	the rectum and seminal vesicles
Superiorly	:	the small intestine.
Inferiorly	:	the urethra and prostate gland.

The bladder is roughly pear-shaped, but becomes more oval as it fills with urine. It has anterior, superior and posterior surfaces. The posterior surface is the base. The bladder opens into the urethra at its lowest point, the neck. It is a freely movable organ held in position by folds of the peritoneum. Peritoneum covers the superior surface and it is reflected to abdominal wall as parietal peritoneum. Posteriorly, it is reflected on to the uterus in the female, and on to rectum in the male.

Structure

1. Outer layer of loose connective tissue.
2. Middle layer, thick muscles arranged in 3 layers.
3. Inner layer is transitional epithelium.

When the bladder is empty, the inner lining layer is thrown into folds and these gradually disappear as the bladder fills. Three openings or orifices in the bladder will form a triangle or trigone. The trigone has a smooth appearance because its mucosa is firmly bound to the muscularis. It has a rich blood supply and nerve supply. The upper two orifices on the posterior wall are the openings of the ureters. The lower orifice is the point of origin of the urethra, where the urethral orifice is surrounded by thick smooth muscle layers to act as a sphincter and controls passage of urine from the bladder into the urethra. This sphincter is under the autonomic nerve control.

Urethra: The urethra is a canal extending from the neck of the bladder to the exterior. Its length differs in the male and in the female. The male urethra is associated with reproductive system.

The female urethra is about 4 cms long, runs downwards and forwards behind the pubic symphysis and opens at the external urethral orifice above the vaginal opening in the vestibule. The external urethral orifice is guarded by the external sphincter which is under voluntary control.

Structure

1. A muscular layer is continuous with the bladder. At origin, there is an internal sphincter. It is under autonomic nerve control. Near the external urethral orifice, the smooth muscle is replaced by striated muscle which forms the external sphincter which is under voluntary control.
2. A thin spongy coat, or lamina propria contains blood vessels.
3. A lining of mucous membrane, transitional epithelium is in the upper part of the urethra. In the lower part these is stratified squamous epithelium which is externally continuous with skin of the vulva.

Mechanism of micturition

The urinary bladder acts as a reservoir for urine. When 200 to 300 ml, of urine have accumulated, autonomic nerve fibres in the bladder wall, sensitive to stretch are stimulated. In an infant, this initiates a spinal reflex action and micturition occurs. When the nervous system is fully developed the micturition reflex is stimulated but sensory impulses pass upward to the brain and there is an awareness of the desire to micturate. By conscious effort, reflex contraction of the bladder wall and relaxation of the internal sphincter can be inhibited for a short time. Micturition occurs when the muscular wall of the bladder contracts, reflex relaxation of the internal spincter occurs. It can be assisted by increasing the pressure within the pelvic cavity. It is achieved by lowering the diaphragm and contracting the abdominal muscles. Over distension of the bladder is extermely painful. When this stage is reached, there is a tendency for involuntary relaxation of the external sphincter to occur and a small amount of urine escapes.

Questions

1. Draw a neat diagram of the urinary system.
2. Explain the kidneys, the relations to other structures including gross structure.
3. Draw a neat diagram of the nephron and label the parts.
4. Write the process of urine formation in the urinary system.
5. Give a brief description of urinary bladder and its function.
6. State the mechanism of micturition.
7. Write short notes on the following:
   a) The ureters
   b) Trigone of the urinary bladder
   c) Composition of urine.

UNIT 10

The Endocrine System

The endocrine glands or ductless glands, secrete the hormones. They pass directly to the blood stream. A hormone is a chemical messenger secreted by an endocrine gland and carried through the blood to act on another organ or target organ or tissue. The internal environment of the body is controlled and regulated partly by hormones and partly by autonomic nervous system. Endocrine glands are

1 Pituitary gland
1 Thyroid gland
4 Parathyroid glands
2 Adrenal (supra renal) glands.
   Islets of langerhan's of pancreas
1 Pineal gland or body
2 Overies in the female
2 Testes in the male

PITUITARY GLAND (HYPOPHYSIS)

The pituitary gland was called the master of the endocrine glands for many years becaue it secretes several hormones that control other endocrine glands. It is now known that the pituitary gland itself has a master, the hypothalamus. The hypothalamic cells synthesize nine different hormones. The pituitary gland, anterior lobe secretes seven hormones and the posterior lobe secretes two hormones. The hypothalamus controls the pituitary gland in two ways.

1. The releasing hormones from the hypothalamus stimulates the anterior lobe to release hormones. The inhibiting hormones from the hypothalamus suppresses the secretion of hormones of the anterior lobe.

The hypothalamic pituitary portal system consists of the primary plexus and secondary plexus of capillaries and the hypophyseal viens that transport the hormones from the hypothalamus and anterior pituitary lobe.

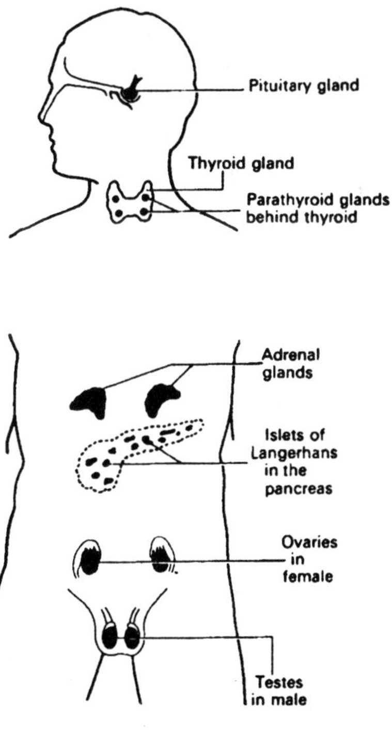

Figure 105. Endocrine glands in the body

2. The hormonal secretion from the posterior lobe is controlled by nervous system stimulation of nerve cells with the hypothalamus.

Within the hypothalamus and the pituitary gland, the nervous and endocrine systems are closely interrelated.

The pituitary gland lies in the sella turcica (hypophyseal fossa) of the sphenoid bone. It is connected to the hypothalamus by a stalk called infundibulum. It is a pea shaped gland measures about 1 to 1.5 cm (½ in.) in diameter. It has two lobes, the anterior and the posterior. The adenohypophysis (anterior lobe) is made up of epithelial cells and is an out growth from the embryonic oral cavity. It weighs about 75% of the total weight of the gland. The neurohypophysis (posterior lobe) is a down growth from the forebrain. The nerve fibres run between the hypothalamus and the neurohypophysis and the adeno hypophysis. Between these lobes, there is a thin slip of tissue called the intermediate lobe (Pars intermedia). It atrophies during foetal development and ceases to exist as a separate lobe in adults.

Blood supply : By branches from the internal carotid artery. The anterior lobe of the pituitary gland is supplied indirectly by blood capillaries from the hypothalamus. This network of blood vessels and the pituitary portal system, convey blood to vascular sinusoids in the anterior lobe. The blood pressure in the sinusoids is lower than in the portal system. This blood conveys the releasing and inhibiting hormones, secreted by the hypothalamus that influence the secretion and release of hormones formed in the anterior lobe. The posterior lobe is supplied directly by a branch from the carotid artery.

Venous blood from the lobes, containing hormones, leaves the gland in short veins and enter into the venous sinuses.

Adenohypophysis (Anterior lobe)

Some of the hormones secreted by the anterior lobe. stimulate or inhibit secretions by other endocrine glands (target glands). While others have a direct effect on target tissues. Hypothalamus stimulates the anterior lobe to release hormones. The releasing hormones from hypothalamus pass through the portal system. The whole system is controlled by a negative feed back mechanism. The blood level of that hormones rises and inhibits the secretion of releasing factor by the hypothalamus.

1. Growth Hormone (GH) is synthesised by somatotrops of the adenohypophysis. Its release is stimulated by GHRF (Somatotrophin) and inhibited by GHRIH (Somatostatin). Both are secreted by the hypothalamus. Growth Hormone (GH) is the most abundant anterior pituitary hormone. It promotes growth of skeleton, muscles, connective tissues and organs such as liver, kidneys, intestines, pancreas and adrenal glands. It has many effects on metabolism. It stimulates protein synthesis and inhibit protein break-down. Somatostatin inhibits secretion of GH, TSH, ACTH, gastrin, CCK (cholecystokinin), glucogon, insulin and renin. It also inhibits secretion of gastric juice, emptying of the stomach, platelet aggregation and it diminishes the transmission of nerve impulse. Increased secretion is stimulated by exercise, anxiety, sleep and hypoglycaemia.

2. The thyrotrophs secrete the thyroid stimulating hormone (TSH)

   Its release is stimulated by TRH secreted from the hypothalamus. TRH passes on to the anterior lobe to synthesise and release TSH. It acts on growth and activity. The thyroid gland secretes hormone thyroxine (T4) and tri-iodothyronine (T3). It is highest between 4 p.m. and 7 p.m. Secretion is also regulated by a negative feed back mechanism. When the blood level of thyroid hormones is high, secretion of TSH is reduced and vice versa.

3. Adrenocorticotrophic hormone (ACTH)

Cortico trophin releasing factor (CRF) from the hypothalamus promotes the synthesis and release of ACTH by corticotrophs of the adenohypophysis. This stimulates the flow of blood to the adrenal cortex, increases the concentration of cholesterol and steroids within the gland and increases the output of steroid hormones especially, cortisol. The production of CRF is believed to be influenced by 1) Nerve impulse from the higher centres. 2) A low blood level of cortisol, 3) Physical stress i.e., exercise 4) Emotional stress, 5) Hypoglycaemia, 6) Negative feed back mechanisms stimuulated by increased blood ACTH and cortisol. ACTH levels are highest at about 8 a.m. and fall to their lowest about mid night. Although high levels sometimes occur at mid day and 6 p.m. this circadian rhythm is maintained throughout life.

4. Prolactin

This hormone has a direct effect on the breasts immediately after parturition. The blood level of prolactin is not dependent on a hypothalamic releasing factor, but it is lowered by the inhibiting factor, dopamine and by an increase in blood level, of prolactin Suckling stimulates prolactin secretion and resultant high blood level is a factor in reducing the incidence of conception during lactation. Emotional stress increases production of prolactin. Prolactin together with estrogens, cortico steroids, insulin and thyroxine are involved in initiating and maintaining lactation.

5. Gonadotrophic hormones

The anterior lobe (gondotrops) secretes two Gonadotrophic hormones in females and males.

Follicle-stimulating hormone (FSH) and luteinizing hormone (LH).

Female gonadotrophic hormones:-

The follicle-stimulating hormone stimulates the development and ripening of the ovarian follicle. During its development, the ovarian follicle secretes its own hormone, estrogen. As the level of estrogen increases in the blood, FSH secretion is reduced. The luteinizing hormone promotes the final maturation of the ovarian follicle and promotes ovulation. Its other function is to promote the formation of the corpus-luteum which secretes the second ovarian hormone, progesterone. As the level of progesterone in the blood increases, there is a gradual reduction in the production of the luteinizing hormone.

Male gonadotrophic hormones:-

The gonadotrophs synthesize gonadotrophic hormones. The follicle stimulating hormone (FSH) stimulates the primordial germ cells of the seminiferous tubules in the testes to produce spermatozoa. The luteinizing hormone stimulates the interstitial cells in the testes to secrete the hormone testosterone.

Neurohypophysis (posterior lobe)

The posterior lobe of the pituitary gland is composed of neuroglial cells called pituicytes and nerve fibres (axons and axon terminals) which arise from more than 10,000 cell bodies which are located in supra-optic and paraventricular nuclei of the hypothalamus. The hormones released by the neurohypophysis are oxytocin and antidiuretic hormone (ADH or vasopressin). They are synthesised by the cells of the hypothalamus and pass along nerve fibres to the posterior pituitary gland where they are stored in the nerve endings.

Oxytocin

Oxytocin promotes contraction of uterine muscle and contraction of myoepithelial cells of the lactating breast, squeezing milk into the large ducts behind the nipple. The uterus becomes sensitive to oxytocin in later months of pregnancy. The amount secreted is increased just before and during labour and by the suckling baby.

Antidiuretic hormone (ADH) or vasopressin

1. Antidiuretic effect

It increases the permeability to water of the distal convoluted and collecting tubules of the nephrons of the kidneys. Then the reabsorption of water from the glomerular filtrate is increased. ADH secretion is influenced by the osmotic pressure of the blood circulating to the osmoreceptors in the hypothalamus. As the osmotic pressure rises, the secretion of ADH increases and more water is reabsorbed. When the osmotic pressure of the blood is low, the secretion of ADH is reduced, less water is reabsorbed and more urine is produced.

2. Pressor effect

In pharmacological doses, ADH stimulates contraction of smooth muscle, especially in blood vessel walls of the skin and abdominal organs, raising the blood pressure.

Effects of secretion of pituitary hormones especially human growth hormone or somatotropin

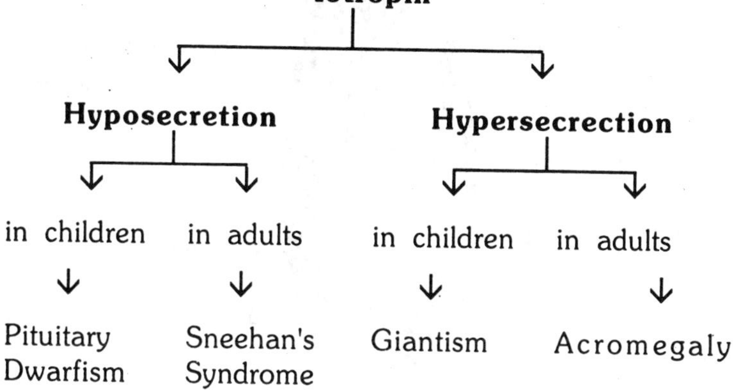

Excess secretion of human growth hormone may have a diabetogenic effect and it causes diabetes mellitus.

Diabetes Insipidus

It is a pathological condition in which the posterior pituitary fails to secrete Antidiuretic hormone (ADH). Two types of problems can cause diabetes Insidipidus,

1. Neurogenic: For Eg: – a brain tumour or head injury that damages the posterior pituitary gland.
2. Nephrogenic – The kidneys do not re spond to ADH.

THYROID GLAND

It is situated in the neck in front of the larynx and trachea at the level of the 5th, 6th and 7th cervical and 1st thoracic vertebrae. It consists of two lobes connected by narrow part isthmus. It is a highly vascular gland surrounded by a fibrous capsule. This capsule is firmly connected to the trachea, so, it moves with the trachea. The lobes are roughly cone-shaped, about 5 cms long and 3 cms wide. It weighs about 30 gms (1 oz.).

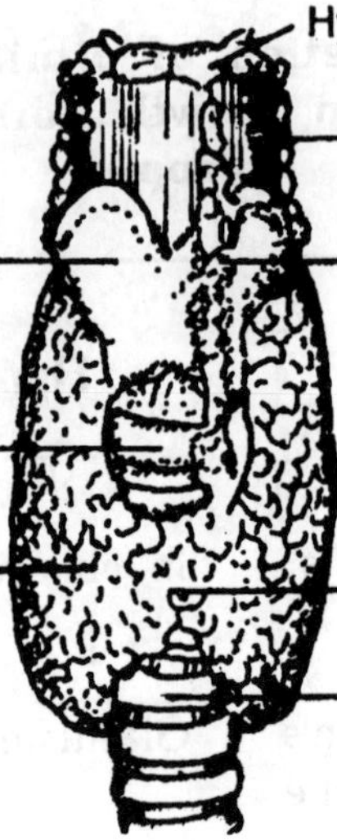

Figure 106. The Thyroid Gland.

It has a rich blood supply. it receives 80-120 ml. of blood per minute. The arterial blood supply to the gland is through the superior and inferior thyroid arteries. The superior thyroid artery is a branch of external carotid artery and the inferior thyroid artery is a branch of the subclavian artery. The venous drainage is by the thyroid veins into the internal jugular veins. Two parathyroid glands lie against the posterior surface of each lobe and are sometimes embedded in thyroid gland tissue. The recurrent laryngeal nerve passes upwards between the lobes and esophagus. At the inferior pole of the gland enters the inferior thyroid arteries. At the superior pole, the superior thyroid arteries enter. The gland is composed of epithelial cells. They form closed spherical follicles, containing sticky semifluid called colloid, in conjunction with which thyroid hormones are stored. The follicular cells secrete triiodothyronine (T3) and thyroxine (T4). Between the follicles, there are parafollicular cells (C-cells) which secrete the hormone calcitonin.

Functions

The iodine is ingested in food and most of it is taken up by the thyroid gland and used in hormones formation i.e., thyroxine (T4) and tri-iodothyromine (T3). Thyroid hormones are stored with colloid as thyroglobulin. The thyroid gland stores its secretion in a large quantity (about a 100 day supply). Their release into the blood is regulated by thyroid stimulating hormone (TSH) from the adenohypophysis. Secretion of TSH is stimulated by the thyroid releasing hormone TRH from the hypothalamus and secretion of TRH is stimulated by exercise, stress, low plasma glucose, malnutrition and sleep. The level of secretion of TSH depends on the plasma levels of T3 and T4. Increased levels of T3 and T4 decrease TSH secretion and vice versa. When the supply of iodine is deficient, excess TSH is secreted and there is proliferation of thyroid gland cells and enlargement of the gland, that condition is called goitre. Secretion of T3 and T4 begins about the 3rd month of foetal life and is increased at puberty, and in women, during the reproductive years, especially during pregnancy.

The effect of T4 and T3 is with growth and development of tissues, especially, the nervous system and the regulation of metabolism. (Oxygen use and basal metabolic rate and cellular metabolism). Oxygen is used to prepare the ATP. As cells use more oxygen to produce ATP, more heat is given off and body temperature rises, This phenomenon is called the calorigenic effect of the thyroid hormones.

Calcitonin acts on bone and the kidneys to reduce the blood calcium level. It reduces the reasorption of calcium from bones and inhibits reabsorption of calcium by the renal tubules. Its effect is opposite to that of parathormone secreted by parathyroid glands. Release of calcitonin is stimulated by an increase in ionised calcium in the blood.

Conditions of the thyroid gland

Goitre is any enlargement of thyroid gland. Deficiency of iodine in the gland causes goitre. When iodine is deficient thyroid hormone production is also deficient. This stimulates secretion of TSH in the anterior pituitary, which causes an enlargement of thyroid gland.

Effects of secretion of thyroid hormones

- Hyposecretion
  - in children at birth or infancy → creatinism
  - in adults → Mxyoedema
- Hypersecretion → Thyrotoxicosis or exophthalmic goitre (grave's disease

Parathyroid glands

There are four small parathyroid glands. Two glands are embedded in posterior surface of each lobe of the thyroid gland. The epithelial cells forming the glands are spherical in shape and are arranged in columns with channels containing blood between them. There are two kinds of cells. The principal (chief) cells. They are numerous. They secrete parathyroid hormone - parathormone. The other kind of cells are oxyphil cells. Their function is not known.

Functions

The parathyroid glands secrete the hormone parathormone (PTH). The secretion is regulated by the blood levels of ionised calcium. When this falls, the secretion of PTH is increased and vice versa.

Function of PTH is to maintain the blood concentration of calcium within normal limits. This is achieved by influencing the amount of calcium absorbed from the small intestine and reabsorbed from the renal tubules. If these sources provide inadequate supplies, PTH stimulates increase in number and activity of osteoclasts to reabsorb calcium from bones. PTH from the para thyroid and calcitonin from the thyroid gland act together to maintain the blood calcium level within normal limits. PTH also stimulates the kidneys to release another hormone called calcitriol (Vit. D).

Effects of secretion of PTH

- Hyposecretion → Tetany
- Hypersecretion → Osteitis fibrosa cystica

Adrenal or Supra renal glands

There are two supra renal glands. Each is situated on the upper pole of each kidney, enclosed within renal fascia. Each is about 4 cms long and 2 to 3 cms in width and weighs about 3.5 to 5 gms.

Blood supply is by the branches from abdominal aorta and renal arteries. The venous drainage is by supra renal veins. The right gland drains into the inferior vena cava and the left gland drains into the left renal vein.

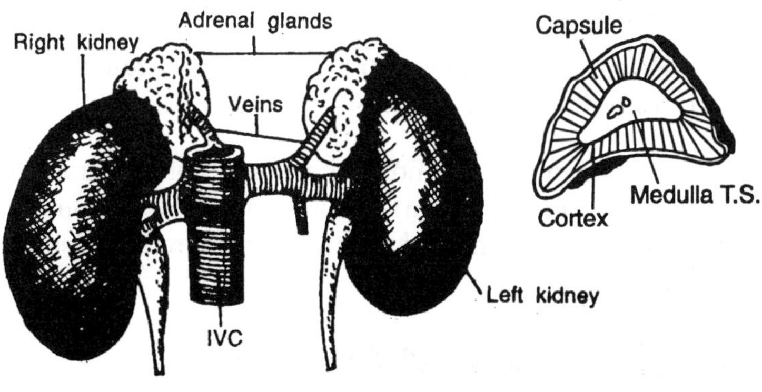

Figure 107. The Adrenal Glands.

On cut section, it has two parts which differ both anatomically and psysiologically. The outer part is the cortex and the inner part is the medulla. Adrenal cortex produces 3 groups of hormones;

1. Gluco corticoids secreted by zona glomerulose (outer zone)
2. Mineralo corticoids secreted by zona fascicolata (middle zone)
3. Small amounts of Androgens (Male Sex hormones) secreted by zona reticularis

Glucocorticoids

Cortisol (hydrocortisone), corticosterone and cortisone are the main gluco corticoids. The secretion is stimulated by ACTH from the anterior pituitary and by stress. The highest level of hormones occurs between 4 am and 8 am and the lowest between mid night and 3 a.m. The hormones have wide spread effects on body system.

1. Regulation of carbohydrate metabolism
2. Promotion of the formation and storage of glycogen
3. Gluconegenesis from protein, raising the blood glucose level.
4. Promotion of the sodium and water reabsorption from the renal tubules.

In pathological and pharmacological quantities gluco corticoids have an anti-inflammatory action, and suppress the response of the tissues to injury, delaying healing.

Mineralocorticoids (Aldosterone)

Aldosterone is the main mineralocorticoid. Its action is the maintenance of the electrolyte balance in the body.

It stimulates the reabsorption of sodium by the renal tubules and when the amount of sodium reabsorbed is increased, the amount of potassium excreted is increased. The aldosterone production is influenced by the sodium level in the blood. If there is a fall in the sodium level in blood, more aldosterone is secreted and more sodium is reabsorbed.

Renin-angiotensin system: When renal blood flow is reduced, the enzyme renin is secreted by kidney cells. This promotes the conversion of angiotensinogen, produced by the liver, to angiotensin I which is converted into angiotensin II, which stimulates the production of aldosterone by the adrenal cortex. Aldosterone increases the reabsorption of sodium and water and the excretion of potassium by the kidneys. This raises the blood volume and the flow of blood through the kidneys, suppressing renin production and reducing aldosterone secretion.

Androgens

Male sex hormones produced by zona reticularis of the adrenal cortex are believed to have little significance compared to those produced by the gonads. Its effect may be deposition of proteins in muscles and retention of nitrogen, especially, in males.

Adrenal Medulla

The medulla is completely surrounded by the cortex. It is derived from the nervous system. Its function resembles to sympathetic part of autonomic nervous system. The medulla consists of chromaffin cells which produce adrenaline and noradrenaline. Adrenaline constitutes about 80% of the total secretion of the gland. The noradrenaline is the chemical transmitter of the sympathetic nervous system. The main function of noradrenaline is maintenance of blood pressure by causing general vaso-constricton, except for the coronary arteries. Other functions of adrenaline and noradrenaline are,

1. Constricting skin blood vessels
2. Dilating blood vessels of muscles of limbs.
3. Increasing heart rate and force of contraction.
4. Converting glycogen to glucose.
5. Increasing the metabolic rate.
6. Dilating the branchioles.
7. Dilating the pupils.
8. Decrease the rate of digestion.

Islets of Langerhans of pancreas

The islets of langerhans are islets in the pancreatic tissue. These groups of cells are endocrine glands. There are four types of endocrine cells. Alpha cells constitute about 20%, beta cells constitute about 70%, delta cells constitute about 5% and F cells constitute about 5% of islet cells of pancreas. Their secretions pass to the blood

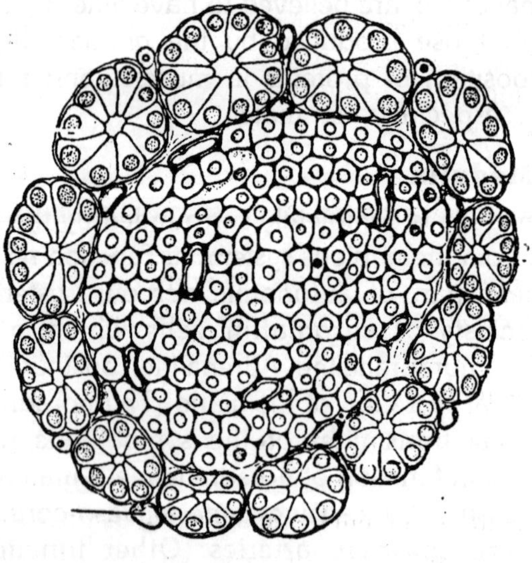

Figure 108. Diagram of a pancreatic islet

vessels and circulate through out the body. Alpha-cells secrete glucogon, Beta-cells secrete insulin, Delta-cells secrete somatostatin and F cells secrete pancreatic polypeptide. Glucogon tends to raise the blood glucose level and insulin reduces it. Clinically, deficiency of insulin results in hyperglycaemia, a high blood sugar, loss of weight, fatigue and polyuria, later stages, accompanying thirst, hunger, dry skin, dry mouth and tongue. Further, if not treated, it may go into a stage of ketosis and acidosis and an increased rate of respiration.

The opposite condition is hypoglycaemia, a low blood sugar level may produce due to over dose of insulin or the patient has not taken food after his insulin injection. Excess insulin in blood may lead to hypoglycaemic coma. Diabetes mellitus may be due to lack of insulin, if untreated it may lead to diabetic coma. These patients are treated with insulin. Too much insulin intake causes hypoglycaemic coma which is treated with glucose.

Normal blood glucose level is about 80-100 mg/ 100 ml. of blood. The normal blood glucose may fall below the normal range, when there is excessive exercise or insufficient intake of carbohydrates. When this happens, glucogon raises the blood glucose level by mobilising the glycogen stores in the liver. Insulin is generally, anticatabolic and it maintains homeostasis but when intake of nutrients is in excess, it promotes storage. It acts on cell membranes stimulating the uptake of glucose, amino-acids and fats. In addition, it is associated with conversion of glucose into glycogen in liver and muscles, synthesis of DNA and RNA, storage of fat in adipose tissue and prevention of gluconeogenesis.

Secretion of insulin is stimulated by increased blood glucose and aminoacids levels, gastro-intestinal hormones such as gastrin, secretin and pancreozymin. Secretion is inhibited by sympathetic stimulation, adrenalin and somatostatin (GHIF) secreted by delta cells of the islets of langerhans. Amounts of insulin are expressed in units and 1 unit is about 40ug.

Ovaries and tests (Gonads)

The female gonads are the ovaries. They are paired glands. They produce female sex hormones, called oestrogen and progesterone. They affect sexual characteristics. These hormones together contribute to the development and function of female reproductive structures and development and maintenance of female secondary sex characteristics. Along with the gonadotropic hormones of the pituitary gland, these hormones regulate the female reproductive cycle, maintain pregnancy and prepare the mammary glands for lactation.

The male gonads are the testes that produce testosterone. It is responsible for the growth and development of the male reproductive structures, muscle enlargement, growth of body hair, voice changes and increased male sex drive.

PINEAL GLAND OR BODY

The pineal gland is situated under the brain and behind the 3rd ventricle. It is connected to the brain by a short stalk containing nerve fibres which end in hypothalamus. It is reddish brown in colour and it may be about 10 mm long. It consists of masses of neuroglia and secretory cells called pinealocytes. It secretes an hormone called Melatonin. Its action may be co-ordination of the circadian and diurnal rhythms of many tissues through the hypothalamus and inhibition of growth and development of the sex organs before puberty. The gland tends to atrophy after puberty and may become calcified in later life.

Thymus Gland

The thymus gland secretes four hormones namely thymosin, thymic humoral factor (THF), thymic factor

(TF) and thymopoietin. They promote the proliferation and maturation of T lymphocytes which destroy microbes and foreign substances. The thymus gland may retard the aging process.

LOCAL HORMONES

1. Histamine is synthesised by mast cells in the tissues and basophils in blood. When there is inflammation in the tissues, it is released and there will be increased capillary permeability and dilatation and it also causes contraction of smooth muscle of the bronchi and alimentary tract and stimulate the secretion of gastric juice.

2. SEROTONIN (5-hydroxy tryptamine)

   It is present in platelets, in the brain and in the intestinal wall. It causes intestinal secretion and contraction of smooth muscle.

   PROSTAGLANDINS: They are produced by the cells in most tissues. The members of the group are,

   a) THROMBOXANES are synthesised by platelets and when released, they cause vaso constriction and platelet aggregation, thus increasing the process of coagulation.

   b) LEUKOTRIENS are produced from mast cells, may assist in promoting allergic responses and inflammatory reactions. They may cause broncho spasm; vaso constriction, increases capillary permeability and attract neutrophils and eosinophils to sites of inflammation. In rheumatoid arthritis, the concentration is high in joints.

   c) PROSTACYCLIN: Is synthesised by endothelial and smooth muscle cells in the walls of blood vessels, causing vasodilatation and inhibition of platelet aggregation.

In addition, the prostglandins have other wide ranging effects, e.g., they are believed to influence: the response of the pituitary gland to hypothalamic hormones, the regulation of the female reproductive cycle, maintain body temperature in some inflammatory conditions, production of renin by the kidneys, and the effects of neurotransmitters.

There are several recently discovered hormones. They are called growth factors. They act locally as autocrines or paracrines.

Questions

1. What do you understand by "Endocrine glands"?
2. Name the endocrine glands of the human body.
3. List the hormones secreted by the anterior and posterior lobes of pituitary gland.
4. List the functions of thyroid gland.
5. Name three hormones secreted by the adrenal cortex.
6. Write short notes on the following:
   a) Islets of Langerhans of pancreas
   b) Antidiuretic hormone
   c) Pineal gland or body
   d) Male and female sex hormones

UNIT 11

The Integumentary System

THE SKIN

The skin is the general sensory organ. It completely covers over the body and it is continuous with the mucous membrane lining the orifices. This junction of skin with mucous membrane is called muco-cutaneous junction. It has many functions. It protects the body from external environment. It contains the tactile nerve endings, helps to regulate the body temperature, to control the loss of water from the body and possesses some excretory, secretory and absorptive properties.

Structure: The skin is divided into two layers,

1. Outer or epidermis (superficial)
2. Inner or dermis or corium (deep)

Epidermis: It is the superficial layer composed of keratinized stratified squamous epithelium, which varies in thickness in different parts of the body. It is thickest on the palms of the hands and soles of the feet. There are 5 layers in epidermis from superficial to deep. They are stratum corneum, stratum lucidum, stratum granulosum, stratum spinosum and stratum basale. The first 3 layers form the horny zone and the other two layers form the germical zone.

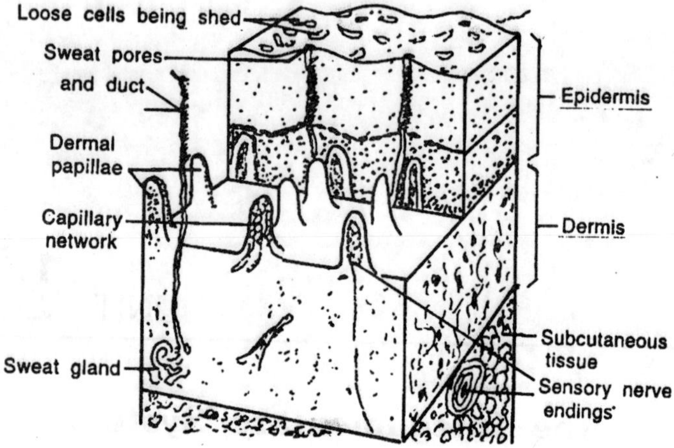

Figure 109. Skin Structures

Horny layer

1. The stratum corneum consists of 25-30 layers of flat scale-like cells which are constantly being cast off and replaced by cells from deeper layers. They are non-nucleated dead cells. This layer forms an effective barrier against light, heat, bacteria and many chemicals.

2. Stratum lucidum consists of 3 to5 layers of clear flat, dead cells that contain droplets of an intermediate substance (eleidin) that is eventually transformed to keratin.

3. Stratum granulosum contains (granular layer) three to five layers of well defined cells containing nuclei and also granules of keratin. Keratin molecules form intermediate filaments that protect deeper layers from injury and microbial invasion and make the skin waterproof. The nucleui of cells are under degeneration.

4. Stratum spinosum or prickle cells. It consists of 8 to 10 layers of polyhedral cells. These cells have minute fibrils which connect one cell with another

cell in the same layers. Because of these processes the cells are called prickle cells.

5. **Stratum basale:** Stratum germinativum This layer consists of cuboidal columnar cells that form the base and are constantly reproduced to replace the superficial cells. This layer also contains tactile (Merkel) discs that are sensitive to touch. The epidermis does not contain blood vessels. The ducts of sweat glands pass through it and also the hair follicles. Epidermal cells line the hair follicles. The surface of the epidermis is marked by lines and ridges. These correspond to the dermal papillae. Beneath the lines on the tips of the fingers and thumbs are distinct patterns, which differ in each individual. To identify the person or criminals, they study the finger prints in criminology. The colour of the skin depend on 3 factors.

1. Melanin, a dark pigment secreted by Melanocytes in the germinative layer. The colour depends on the amount of melanin secreted by melanocytes. The amount varies between different parts of the body. Sunlight darkens existing melanin and promotes its secretion.

   Deficiency or absence of melanin production in the germinative layer gives rise to a condition called albinism. It may be an hereditary condition or due to endocrine dysfunction.

   The epidermis below stratum lucidum contains four principal types of cells. They are keratinocytes (90%) which produce keratin, melanocytes which produce the pigment melanin, Langerhans cells interact with helper Tcells in immune responses, and Mercel cell (Tactile disc) which functions in the sensation of touch.

2. Pink colour of the skin is due to level of oxygenated blood and amount of blood circulating in the dermis.

3. Yellow colour is due to presence of biie pigments in the blood.

Dermis

It is made up of areolar, fibrous and elastic tissues. The papillary (superficial) layer contains areolar tissue. They are:

Blood vessels

Lymphatic vessels

Sensory nerve endings

Hair roots, hair follicles and hairs

Sweat glands and their ducts

Sebaceous glands

The arrectores pilorum muscles and a small quantity of adipose tissue

1. **Blood vessels:** Arterioles form the capillary net work supplying the contents of dermis. The epidermis has no blood vessels. It gets its nutrition and oxygen from interstitial fluid, derived from the papillae of the dermis.

2. **Lymphatic vessels** form a net work in dermis and deep to epidermis.

3. **Sensory nerve endings:** The skin is a sensory organ carrying sense of touch, change in temperature, (heat or cold) pain and pressure. The sensory nerve endings are widely distributed in the dermis. The following nerve endings are found in the dermis and subcutaneous layer. They are (1) Corpuscles of touch (Meissner's corpuscles) (2) Lamellated or pacinian corpuscles are sensitive to pressure (3) Nerve endings sensitive to cold are found in and just containing fine elastic fibres. Its surface area is greately increased by dermal papillae. The deeper portion of the dermis is called the reticular region

(layer). It is contains bundles of collagen and some course elastic fibres. This layer also contains other structures, deep to the dermis and (4) Nerve endings sensitive to heat are found in the intermediate and superficial dermis. Nerve impulses are conveyed to spinal cord and then to sensory area of the cerebrum.

4. **Sweat (Sudoriferous) glands:** They are widely distributed through out the skin and more numerous in the palms of the hands, soles of the feet, axilla. They are simple coiled tubular glands. The tubes open on the surface of the skin as pores and some open into hair follicles. In the axilla, they secrete odourless fluid. Sweat glands are stimulated by sympathetic nerves in response to raised body temperature and fear. The secretion of the sweat glands assists in the regulation of the body temperature. The temperature regulation centre is situated in the hypothalamus. Excessive sweating may lead to dehydration.

   There are two types of sweat glands, ecrine and apocrine sweat glands.

   Ceruminous Glands: They are, modified sweat glands found in the external auditory canal. Mammary glands are specialised sudoriferous glands. They secrete milk.

5. **Hair follicles:** They are the down-growth of epidermal cells into the dermis. At the base of each follicle, is a hair bulb where the multiplication of cells for the growth of the hair occurs. Next is the hair root and above the skin is the shaft. The colour of the hair depends on the amount of melanin present and the white hair is due to replacement of melanin by tiny air bubbles.

6. **The sebaceous glands:** They are developed from epidermis and pour their secretion, the sebum, into

the hair follicles. They are present all over the skin except where the hairs are absent. They are more numerous in the skin of the scalp, face, axillae and groins. In certain areas, their secretion is poured on to surface of that area. They are eyelids, nipple, labia minora and glans penis. Sebum is an oily substance that keeps the hair soft and pliable and gives a shiny appearance. On the skin, it provides water proof and acts as bactericidal and also prevents drying and cracking of skin, especially, on exposure to heat and sunshine.

Clinically, the dermis is sometimes the site of injections such as the tuberculin skin test.

The arrector pilorum muscles are tiny bundles of involuntary smooth muscle fibres attached to the hair follicles. In sympathetic stimulation due to fear and cold, the hair stand erect and raises the skin around the hair causing 'goose flesh'.

Appendages of the skin are,

1. The hairs and nails.

Nails: They are derived from stratum lucidum of epidermis and consist of a hard horny type of keratinised dead cells. They protect the tips of the fingers and toes. The root of the nail is embedded in the skin. It is covered by the cuticle and forms the hemispherical pale area called the lunula. The body of the nail grows out from the germinative zone of the epidermis, called the nail bed. The finger nails grow more quickly than toe nails.

Functions of the skin

1. **Protection:** It protects the deeper structures against the invasion of microbes and other harmful agents.

2. **Sensory organ:** The skin carries sensory impulse of pain, temperature and touch to the brain.

3. **Formation of Vitamin D_3:** The ultra violet rays from the sun begins to convert the fatty substance, 7-dehydrocholesterol (Ergosterol) into vitamin-D. This is finally synthesised into the most active form of vitamin D by the enzymes in the liver and kidneys. Vitamin D can be called an hormone as it is produced in one location in the body, carried by the blood and exerts its effect in another location. For this reason, skin can be considered an endocrine gland.

4. **Regulation of body temperature**: The body temperature is fairly constant at about 36.9°C or 98.4°F. The diurnal variation may be 1-4°F. The temperature may be raised in exercise. If the temperature is raised, the metabolic rate is increased. If the temperature is lowered the metabolic rate is reduced. To have constant temperature, a fine balance is maintained between heat production and heat lost in the body.

5. **Storage:** Skin acts as storage for water and the adipose tissue beneath the epidermis. It is one of the principal fat depots of the body.

6. **Immunity:** Certain epidermial cells protect the body against foreign invaders thus act as a part of immune system.

7. **Reservoir of blood** : The dermis carries 8 to 10 percent of the total blood flow in a resting adult. Skin blood flow increases in moderate exercise. Skin blood vessels constrict somewhat during strenuous exercise and this allows more blood to circulat through contraction of muscles.

Questions

1. Define the structure of the skin with a neat diagram.
2. List the functions of skin.
3. Write short notes on:
   a) Formation of Vitamin D
   b) Function of different nerve endings of the skin and maintenance of body temperature.

UNIT 12

The Special Senses

SENSE OF SMELL

The sense of smell is carried through the olfactory nerves to the brain. Their origin is in special cells in the nasal epithelium of the superior protion of the nose which contains between 10 and 100 million receptors for the sense of smell. The total area of the olfactory epithelium is a little less than one square inch ($5cm^2$). It extends along the superior nasal concha and upper part of the middle nasal concha. The olfactory epithelium consists of three kinds of cells : olfactory receptors, supporting cells and basal cells.

Olfactory receptor's are the first order neurons of the olfactory pathway. They are bipolar neurons. From the dendrites (knowb-shaped) of these neurons several cilia (olfactory hairs) project into a thin mucous film on the epithelial surface. The cilia are sites of olfactory interaction. Odorant molecules become dissolved in the fluid on the surface of the epithelium. They bind to the receptor molecules of the ciliary membrane. The molecules are dissolved first in fluid inorder to reach the olfactory receoptors. When they reach the olfactory receptors they cause the olfactory neurons to depolarize, very few molecules are required to initiate an action potential. The olfactory receptors can detect only seven types of odours (or combination of odours). Axons from olfactory neurons form the olfactory nerves.

There are 15-20 olfactory nerves. They pass upwards through the cribriform plate of the ethmoid bone to join the olfactory bulb. Bundles of nerve fibres form the olfactory tract. They pass backwards to the lateral olfactory area in the temporal lobe of the cerebral cortex in each hemisphere. The lateral surface area is considered the primary olfactory area because many olfactory tract axons terminate there. In this area conscious awareness of odours begins.

SENSE OF TASTE

The receptors for the sensation of taste are located in the taste buds. Taste buds are found in the papillae of the tongue and are widely distributed in the epithelium of the tongue, soft palate, pharynx and epiglottis.

The tongue of a young adult contains nearly 10,000 taste buds. Each taste bud is a oval structure which consists of three kinds of epithelial cells. They are the taste (gustatory) receptor cells, the supporting cells and the basal cells. Each taste bud contains about forty taste receptor cells. Each taste cell contains hairlike processes called taste hairs, that extend into a tiny opening in the epithelium of the taste bud, called a taste pore.

Taste buds are found in elevations of the tongue called papillae.

The different papillae are

1. **Circum Vallate papillae** are usually 10-12 in number and are arranged in rows of inverted V-shaped towards the base of the tongue. There are the largest papillae and are easily seen on the tongue. It contains many taste buds.

2. **Fungiform papillae**: They are more numerous, situated mainly at the tip of the tongue, and most of them contain tase buds.

3. **Filiform papillae**: They are the smallest of the three. They are situated on the surface of the anterior two-thirds of the tongue. They are whitish and contain no taste buds.

Nerve supply

The hypoglossal nerve (12th cranial nerve) is motor supply to the tongue.

The lingual branch of the mandibular nerve is the sensory nerve.

The facial and glossopharyngeal nerves (7th & 9th cranial nerves) are the nerves of the special sensation of taste.

Physiology of taste

Chemical (food) substance is first dissolved in saliva. Then it makes contact with the plasma membrane of the

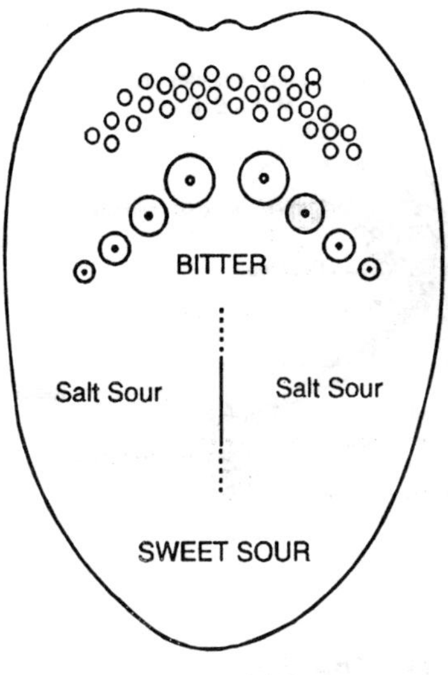

Figure 110. Diagram showing the parts of the tongue in which the various sensations of taste are appreciated

taste hairs that extend into the taste pores and initiate action potentials. These action potentials are propogated as taste impulse which passes through the facial, glossophyrangeal and vagus. nerves. The nerve impulses are transmitted to the thalamus, then to the primary taste area in the parietal lobe of the cerebral cortex, one in each hemisphere, where the taste is perceived. There are four types of sensation of taste. They are sweet, sour, bitter and salt.

SENSE OF HEARING AND BALANCE

The ear is the organ of hearing, the nerve supplying this, is the 8th cranial nerve or vestibulo cochlear nerve. The ear is divided into three parts, external, middle and internal ear.

External Ear

External ear consists of the auricle or pinna. It is an expanded portion projecting from the side of the head. It is composed of elastic cartilage covered on both sides

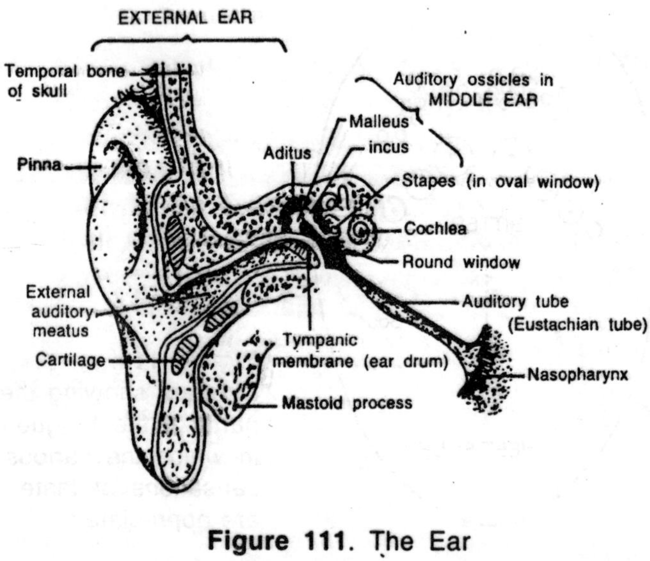

Figure 111. The Ear

by skin. The helix forms the rim of the auricle. The lobule is the soft pliable part composed of fibrous and adipose tissue. It has a very rich capillary network and bleeds freely if it is cut or pricked. This area is used to take small samples of blood.The pinna collects the vibrations of the sound, and passes them inward to the tympanic membrane through the external auditory meatus.

The external auditory canal has to be straightened while examining the tympanic membrane. This is done by pulling the pinna backwards and upwards in adults. The pinna is pulled backwards and downwards in children.

External acoustic meatus: It is the S-shaped canal. It starts from the pinna and conveys the vibrations of sound to the tympanic membrane. The canal is about 2.5 cms long extending from the auricle to tympanic membrane. The lateral third is cartilagenous and remainder is the bony portion in temporal bone. The meatus is lined by hairy skin and numerous sebaceous and ceruminous glands in the lateral third. They secrete cerumen (wax), a sticky material which prevents dust and insects reaching the tympanic membrane. (Cerumen is a combined secretion of sebaceous and ceruminous glands)

The timpanic membrane (Ear drum)

It is a thin, circular, semitransparent membrane which separates the external acoustic meatus from the middle ear. It is composed of fibrous connective tissue. The handle of the malleus is attached to it. On examination with an otoscope it appears grey in color, the handle of the malleus and a cone of light can be seen. It receives the sound waves through the external acoustic meatus and conveys them to the malleus.

Middle ear or tympanic cavity

It is an irregular-shaped cavity within the petrous portion of the temporal bone. It communicates with the nasopharynx through the Eustachian tube. This tube consists of both bone and hyaline cartilage. It is normally closed at its pharyngeal end. It opens during swallowing and yawning. Pathogenic microbes may travel from the nose and throat to the middle ear through this tube. The tube and cavity is lined by simple squamous epithelium. The presence of air at atmospheric pressure on both sides of the tympanic membrane, enables it to vibrate when sound waves strike it. The lateral wall is formed by the tympanic membrane. The posterior and inferior walls are formed by the temporal bone.

There is an opening in the superior part of the posterior wall which is called as the tympanic antrum. It communicates with the mastoid air 'cells' of the temporal bone. Through this infection from the middle ear may spread to the mastoid air cells causing mastoiditis.

The medial wall is formed by a thin layer of temporal bone in which two openings are present. The oval window (fenestra vestibuli)to which the footplate of the ossicle stapes is attached. Another opening, round window (fenestra cochlea) is closed by a membrane called secondary tympanic membrane. The middle ear contains three auditory ossicles.

Auditory ossicles: These three small bones are malleus, incus and stapes. They extend from the tympanic membrane to the oval window. Between these ossicles, are the synovial joints. The malleus is the lateral hammer-shaped bone. The handle is in contact with the tympanic membrane and the head forms the movable joint with incus.

The incus: It is the middle bone, the body articulates with the malleus, the long process with the stapes. It is stabilised by short process, fixed by fibrous tissue to the posterior wall of the cavity.

The stapes is the medial stirrup-shaped bone. Its head articulates with the incus and its base fits into the oval window of the vestibule of the internal year.

Internal ear

It is also called the labyrinth. It contains the organs of hearing and balance. It is described in two parts, the bony labyrinth and the membranous labyrinth.

Bony labyrinth

This is a cavity within the temporal bohe and is larger than the membranous labyrinth of the same shape which fits into it. Between the bony and membranous labyrinth, is a fluid called perilymph,which is chemically similar to C.S.F. Within the membranous labyrinth is a similar fluid called Endolymph which is chemically similar to intracellular fluid. The bony labyrinth consists of one vestibule, one cochlea and three semicircular canals. The vestibule is the central expanded part nearest to the middle ear. It contains the oval and round windows. The cochlea resembles a snail's shell. Its broad base is continuous with the vestibule and a narrow apex and it spirals round a central bony column. The semi-circular canals are three tubes arranged so that one is situated in each of the three planes of space. They are continuous with the vestibule.

Membranous labyrinth

Membranous labyrinth is lined with epithelium. It is as the same shape of its bony labyrinth and is separated

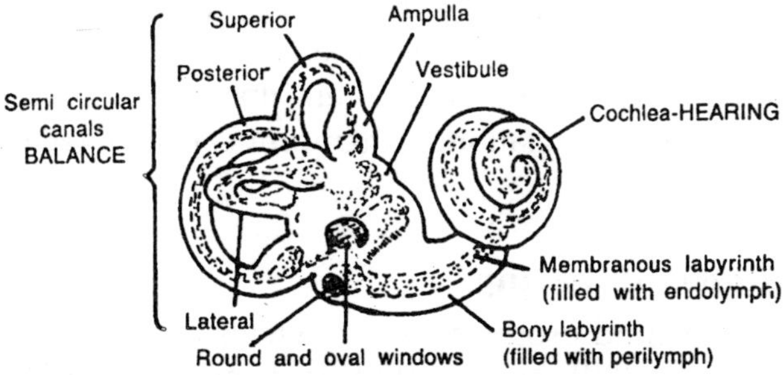

Figure 112. Cochlea and semicircular canals

by perilymph. It contains endolymph. It is divided into the same parts: (1) the vestibule which contains the utricle and saccule, (2) the cochlea and (3) three semicircular canals.

The cochlea

It is anterior to the vestibule. It resembles a snail's shell and makes two and a half turns around a central bony core called the modiolus. The threads of the turns are called the spiral lamina. A cross section of the cochlea shows a Y shaped membranous complex which divides the cochlea into three portions. The stem of the Y is the spiral lamina (a bony shelf) that protrudes into the vestibular membrane and the other branch is basilar membrane. The cochlear duct (scala media) is in between these membranes. This complex is the membranous labyrinth which is filled with endolymph. The space above the Y is called the scala vestibuli and that below the Y is the scala tympani. These two spaces are filled with perilymph. The scala vestibuli extends from the oval window to the tip of the cochlea. The scala tympani extends from the apex to the round window. The two scalae are completely closed except for an opening at the apex of the cochlea called the helicotrema.

The organ of hearing is the spiral organ (organ of corti) which is contained within the cochlear duct. It contains the specialised sensory cells called hair cells (about 16,000) which are the receptors for auditory sensations. On the surface of these hair cells are hairlike projections called microvilli. Their tips are embedded within a delicarte gelatinous membrane called tectorial membrane.

Physiology of haring

Every sound produces sound waves in the air. They travel at about 332 meters (1088 feet) per second. They are collected by the auricle and directed into the external auditory canal toward the tympanic membrane. The sound waves strike the tympanic membrane and it vibrates. The vibration is transmitted to the ossicles of the middle ear. In the ossicles the force of vibration is amplified and directed to the oval window. The vibration of the oval window set up fluid pressure waves in the perilymph of the cochlea. The oval window bulges inward and pushes on the prilymph of the scala vestibuli. From here pressure waves are transmitted to the scala tympani and then to the round window causing it bulge outward into the middle ear.

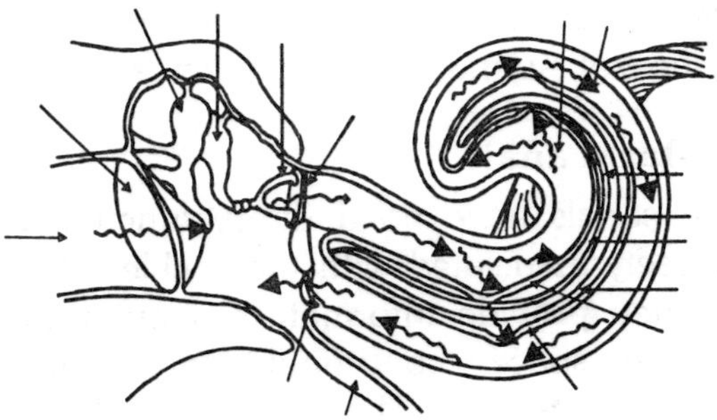

Figure 114. Effect of sound waves on cochlear structures.

Sound waves produced in the perilymph cause the vestibular membrane to vibrate. As a result, fluid pressure waves are created in the endolymph within the cochlear duct. This causes vibration of the basilar membrane slightly, when the basilar membrane vibrates, the hair cells of the spiral organ (organ of corti) move against the tectorial membrane. The bending of the mocrovilli stimulates the hair cells which produce action potentials that ultimately lead to the generation of nerve impulses in cochlear nerve fibres. [Hair cells convert a mechanical force (stimulus) into an electrical signal (recepor potential)].

(The basilar membrane is not uniform throughout its length. This arrangement can be compared to the strings in a piano. Different hair cells are stimulated in each case. So the person is able to detect variations in pitch.)

The nerve fibres combine to form the auditory part of the vestibulo-cochlear nerve (the 8th cranial nerve). It passes through the internal acoustic meatus and conduct the impulses over their normal pathways to the primary auditory area in the temporal lobe of the cerebral cortex. (located in the superior part of the temporal lobe near the lateral cerebral sulcus) It interprets the basic characteristics of sound such as pitch and rhythm.

Semicircular canals

These canals have no auditory function although they are closely associated with the cochlea through the vestibule. They provide information about the position of the head in space contributing to maintenance of equilibrium and balance. They are situated above and behind the vestibule and open into it. These canals one lying in each of the three planes of space.

Structure

The semicircular canals, like the cochlea, are made up of outer bony wall and inner membranous tubes. The membranous tube is separated by the bony wall by perilymph and the inner tube contains endolymph.

A sac like dilation at the base of each semicircular canal is called ampulla. In each ampulla there is a small elevation called crista. Each crista contains a group of hair (receptor) cells and supporting cells. They are covered by a mass of gelatinous material called the cupula. (There are no otoliths in the cupula)

VESTIBULE

The utricle is a membranous sac and is part of the vestibule and the three membranous ducts open into it at their dilated ends, the ampullae. The saccule is a part of the vestibule and communicates with the utricle and the cochlea. In the walls of the utricle and saccule. There are structures called maculae. Each macula contains hair cells (receptor cells). These hair cells contain microvilli on their surface which are embedded in a otolithic membrane (contains otoliths). Minute nerve endings start from these hair cells (8th cranial nerve) and form the vestibular part of the vestibulo-cochlear nerve.

Physiology of equilibrium

There are two kinds of equilibrium or balance. One is the static equilibrium and the other is the dynamic equilibrium. The receptor organs for the two kinds of equilibrium are collectively known as the vestibular apparatus which includes the saccule and utricle and the semicircular canals.

1. The static equilibrium is associated with the vestibule (saccule and utricle) and is involved in evaluating the position of the head relative to gravity.
2. The dynamic equilibrium is associated with the semicircular canals and is involved in evaluating the change in rate of head movements.

Any change of position of the head causes movement in the perilymph and endolymph which stimulate the nerve endings and the hair cells in the utricle, saccule and ampullae. The impulses are transmitted by the vestibular nerve which joins the cochlear nerve to form the vestibulo-cochlear nerve. Then the impulse is carried to cerebellum. The cerebellum also receives nerve impulse from the eyes, the muscles and joints. The co-ordinated and efferent nerve impulses are carried to the cerebrum where position in space is perceived and to muscles to maintain posture and balance.

THE SENSE OF SIGHT – VISION

The eye is the organ of the sense of sight (vision). The structures related to the sense of sight may be divided into

1. Organs of the visual apparatus, namely, the eyeball, the optic nerve and the visual centres in the brain.
2. Accessory organs of the eye.

THE EYE BALL

The eyeball is situated in the orbital cavity and is supplied by optic nerve. It is spherical in shape and is about 2.5 cms in diameter. The space between eye ball and orbital wall is filled with fat and extra ocular muscles. The two eye balls are separate but their activities are co-ordinated, so that, they function as a pair.

Structure of the eye ball: It has three layers.

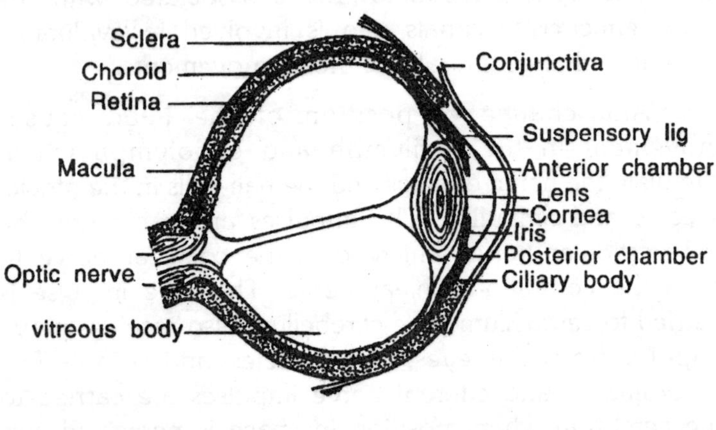

Figure 114. The Eye Ball.

1. The outer fibrous layer, sclera and cornea.
2. The middle vascular layer, choroid, ciliary body, and iris.
3. The inner nervous layer - Retina.

Structures inside the eye ball are, aqueous humour, the lens, and vitreous body.

Sclera: It is the outer fibrous, white, non transparent posterior layer. Anterior 1/6th of the layer is a transparent layer called cornea. The fibrous layer maintains the shape of the eye ball and gives attachment to the extra ocular muscles of the eye ball. The light rays pass through the cornea to reach the retina. The anterior surface of the cornea is convex and involved in refracting or bending light rays to focus them on the retina.

There is an opening called the canal of Schlemn at the junction of the sclera and cornea.

Choroid: It is the middlelayer of the eye ball. The choroid lines the posterior five - sixth of the inner surface of the sclera. It contains rich capillary bed and is deep chocolate brown in colour. Melanin produced by melanocytes gives this colour. It provides nourishment to the posterior surface of the retina. It forms the ciliary body and iris in front. The opening in the iris is called pupil. The light rays enters through the pupil to the retina.

Ciliary Body: It is the anterior continuation of the choroid, contains smooth muscle fibres (Ciliary Muscle) and secretary epithelial cells. The ciliary muscle gives attachment to suspensory ligaments. Other ends are attached to the capsule of the lens. Contraction and relaxation of the ciliary muscle, changes the thickness of the lens which refracts light rays entering the eye to focus. The epithelial cells secrete aqueous fluid into the anterior segment of the eye i.e., to posterior chamber.

Iris: The anterior extension of ciliary body is called the iris which is in front of the lens and behind the cornea. It divides the anterior segment into anterior chamber and posterior chamber, that contain aqueous humour. It is a circular body or diaphragm containing pigment cells which gives the colour of iris. It contains circular and radiating muscle fibres. In the centre, there is an aperture, the pupil. The function of the iris is to regulate the amount of light entering the eyeball through the pupil. In bright light, the circular muscle fibres contract and constrict the pupil. In dim light the radiating muscle fibres contract to dilate the pupil. The iris is supplied by autonomic nerves, parasympathetic through the oculo motor, and sympathetic from the superior cervical ganglion. Sympathetic stimulation dilates and parasympathetic stimulation constricts the pupil. The colour of the iris depends on the number of pigment cells present. Albinism is the absence of pigment cells in the iris and skin of the body.

Lens: The lens is biconvex, elastic, transparent body situated behind the pupil. The lens is made up of proteins called crystallins, arranged like the layers of an onion. It is suspended by suspensory ligaments from the ciliary body. It is enclosed within a transparent capsule. The lens can vary its refractory power by changing thickness. When the ciliary muscle contracts the thickness of the lens increases. When the objects are nearer the lens becomes thicker to bend the rays toward the central fovea. This adjustment in the convexity of the lens for near or far vision is called accommadation.

Retina: It is the inner most layer of the eye ball. It is composed of 10 layers made up of bipolar cells, nerve fibres and pigment layer. The outer pigment layer is attached to choroid layer. The layer of rods and cones (photoreceptors) are highly sensitive to light. Horizontal cells and amacrine cells are also present in retina. The retina lines about three quarters of the eyeball. It is thickest at the posterior part and thins out anteriorly to end just behind the ciliary body. Near the centre of the posterior part, there is an area of yellow colour called Macula lutea. In the centre of this area, there is a depression called the fovea centralis, consisting of only cone cells. Towards the anterior part of the retina, there are fewer cones than rod cells. The rods and cones contain photo sensitive pigments involved in the conversion of light rays into nerve impulses. Rhodopsin is a pigment present in rods. It is bleached when exposed to light. Other pigments present in cones, respond to different wave lengths of visible light and are responsible for colour vision. About 0.5 cms to the nasal side of the macula lutea, all the nerve fibres of the retina converge to form the optic nerve. It passes out through the choroid and sclera and to reach the cerebral cortex in the occipital lobe. The small area of retina where the optic nerve leaves the eye ball is the optic disc or the blind spot, it has no light sensitive cells (rods and cones).

Blood supply: The eye ball is supplied by the branches of ophthalmic artery. The branches are ciliary artery and the central artery of retina. It is the end artery supply to retina. The occlusion of central artery of retina in a person causes blindness. This artery enters the eye ball through the optic nerve. The venous drainage is into cavernous sinus.

Interior of the Eyeball

The anterior segment of the eye is divided by iris into anterior and posterior chambers containing aqueous humour. The anterior segment is the space between cornea and lens, the aqueous fluid is secreted in the posterior chamber, passes into the anterior chamber through the pupil. The fluid is absorbed into the venous circulation through the canal of schlemm An increase in intra ocular pressure is called glaucoma. The aqueous fluid supplies oxygen and nutrients to the lens and cornea and remove the waste products. Behind the lens, the space is filled with vitreous body. It is a soft, colourless, transparent, jelly like substance. It contains water, some salts and mucoprotein. It maintains intra ocular pressure and holds the lens in place, support the retina against the choroid preventing the walls of the eye ball from collapsing. The shape of the eye ball is maintained by the intra ocular pressure exerted by the vitreous humour mainly and partly by aqueous humour, constantly throughout life. Both aqueous humour and vitreous humour function to refract the light rays on the retina.

Function of Retina

The retina is the photo sensitive part of the eye. The light sensitive cells are the rods and cones. The rods are more sensitive than the cones. They are stimulated by dim light. So Rods provide the vision of shades of gray in dim light. They all provide the vision of shapes and movement. The cones are sensitive to bright light and colour. The photo sensitive pigment is in the cones resulting in the perception of different colours. There are three types of cones. Each is sensitive to a different colour blue, green or red. More rods are present at the periphery of the retina. Rod cells contain a photosensitive pigment called rhodopsin. Rhodopsin is made up of the protein opsin in loose chemical combination with a pigment called retinol. The rhodopsin (visual purple) is quickly reconstituted when an adequate supply of vitamin A is available. Vitamin A is stored in a large quantity in the pigment epithelium, adjacent to the photoreceptors. When a person moves from an area of bright light to one of dim light, certain period of time he feels difficulty to see. The rate at which dark adaptation takes place is dependent upon the rate of reconstitution of Rhodopsin. Deficiency of Vitamin A in a person develops a condition called night blindness (nyctalopia).

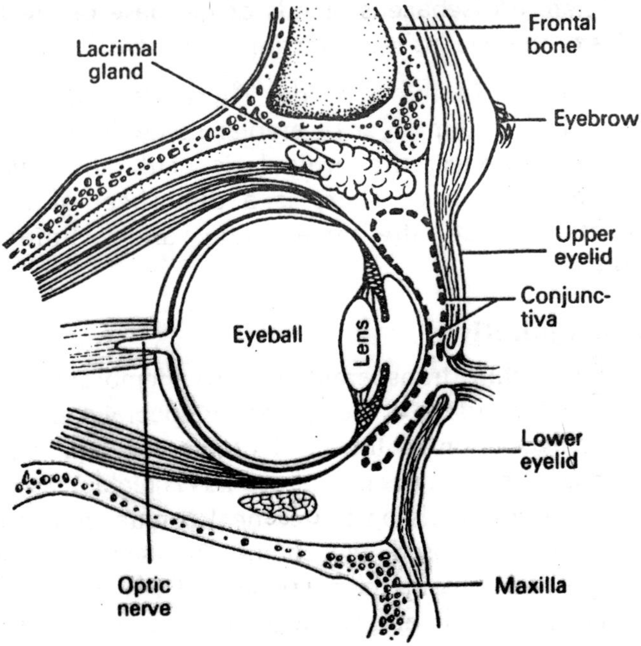

Figure 115. Section of the Eye and its accessory structure

Accessory organs of the eye

Eye brows

Eyelids and eyelashes

Lacrimal apparatus.

Eye brows

These are two arched ridges of the supraorbital margins of the frontal bone. Numerous hairs project from the skin and they prevent dust and other foreign bodies falling on the eye ball.

Eye lids: These are the two movable folds situated above and below the front of each eye, and on their margins, they are short curved hairs called eyelashes.

There are sebaceus glands at the base of the hair follicles of the eye lashes. Infection of these is called stye.

Structure of the eye lids: There is a thin layer of skin, then, a thin layer of areolar tissue. The eye lids have two muscles, the orbicularis oculi and levator palpebrae superioris. There is a thin sheet of dense connective tissue, the tarsal plate, and a lining of conjunctiva.

The conjunctiva

It is a thin, transparent mucous membrane which lines the inner surface of the eye lids (Palpebral conjuctiva) and is reflected on to the front of the eye ball (bulbar conjuctiva). The conjunctiva of eye lids is highly vascular. There are less vessels on the corneal conjunctiva. When the eye lids are closed, the conjunctival sac is a closed one. This sac contains lacrimal fluid which protects the cornea and eye ball, and keeps the cornea, always moist. The upper and lower eye lids meet at the medial and lateral angles, called medial canthus and lateral canthus. Numerous sebaceous glands are present at the edge of the eye lids. Some ducts open into the hair follicles of eye lashes and some ducts open at eye lid margin between the hairs. Meibomian glands(tarsal glands) are modified sebaceous glands situated in tarsal plates with ducts open into the margin of the eye lids. They secrete an oily material that spread over the conjunctiva by blinking that delays the evaporation of tears. The eye lids and eye lashes protect the eye from injury and prevent the foreign bodies entering into the eye.

Lacrimal apparatus

1 lacrimal gland and its ducts

2 lacrimal canaliculi

1 lacrimal sac

1 naso lacrimal duct.

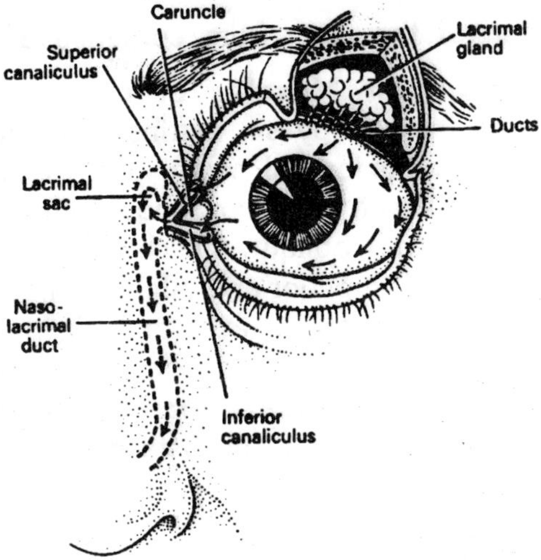

Figure 116. The lacrimal apparatus.

The Lacrimal glands:

These glands are situated in the supra lateral fossa of the orbital cavity. Its size may be of almond and composed of secretory epithelial cells. They secrete tears which is composoed of water, salts and lysozyme, which is a bactericidal enzyme. Each gland has a dozen ducts that convey tears to superior fornix of conjundival sac. By blinking of the eye, the lacrimal fluid moves towards lacrimal puctum situated at the medial ends of lid margins. Each punctum is continuous as two canaliculi and opens into the lacrimal sac, which is an expanded sac situated in the lacrimal fossa. This sac continues downwards as nasolacrimal duct. It is about 2 cms long and opens into the inferior meatus of the lateral wall. When a foreign body or other irritant enters in the front side of eye, the secretion of tears increase and conjunctival blood vessels dilate. Secretion of tears is also increased in emotional states. The tears washes away all irritating materials like dust particles. The lysozyme has bactericidal action, and the oily secretion of the meibomian glands prevents the evaporation of the tears from conjunctival sac.

Extra ocular Muscles of the eye ball: The eye balls are moved by six extrinsic muscles attached to the walls of the orbital cavity and to the eye ball. They are the 4 recti and two oblique muscles, superior oblique and inferior oblique muscles. The recti muscles are medial, lateral, superior and inferior. They are striated muscles. Movement of the eyes to look in a particular direction is under the voluntary control but co-ordination of movement, essential for convergence and accommodation to near or distant vision, is under autonomic control.

Movements: The medial rectus rotates the eye ball inwards. The lateral rectus rotates the eye ball outwards. The superior rectus rotates the eye ball upwards. The inferior rectus rotates the eye ball downwards. The superior oblique rotates the eye ball so that the cornea turns in a downward and outward direction. The inferior oblique rotates the eye ball so that the cornea turns upwards and outwards.

Convergence movement

Light rays from objects enter the two eyes at different angles for clear vision on two retina. Extra ocular muscles, move and rotate the eye balls, so that, they converage on the object viewed. This co-ordinated muscle action is under the autonomic control if the object viewed is nearer to the eyes, the greater the eye rotation is needed to achieve convergence. If the convergence is not complete, there are double (Diplopia) vision.

Nerve Supply

The oculo motor (3rd cranial) nerve supplies the;

Superior rectus

Inferior rectus

Medial rectus

Inferior oblique

The trochlear (4th cranial) nerve supplies the superior oblique.

The abucent (6th cranial) nerve supplies the lateral rectus.

Optic Nerves

The fibres originate in the retina and converge to form the optic nerve about 0.5 cms to the nasal side of the macula lutea, pierces the choroid and sclera to pass out. The convergence of nerve fibres on the retina is called optic disc. The optic nerve passes backward through the optic foramen to meet the opposite optic nerve to form optic chiasma.

Optic chiasma: It is situated in front and above the pituitary gland. In the optic chiasma the nasal side fibres from the retina cross over the opposite side. The temporal side fibres do not cross and continue backwards on the same side as optic tracts.

Optic tracts: It is the pathways of the optic nerves, from posterior to the optic chiasma. Each tract consists of the opposite side of nasal fibres and same side of temporal fibres of the retina. The optic tracts pass backwards and relay in the lateral geniculate bodies, from there, the nerve fibres proceed backwards and medially as the optic radiations to terminate in the visual area of the occipital lobe of cerebral cortex. Other neurons originating in the lateral geniculate bodies convey the sensory impulses to the cerebellum to maintain the balance of the body.

Accommodation of the Eyes to light

Accommodation means alteration of the convexity of the lens of the eye to adjust for vision at various distances.

There are three factors involved in this process, the pupils, lens and movements of the eyeballs.

Size of the Pupils

The diameter of the pupil influences accommodation by controlling the amount of light entering the eye. In a bright light, the pupils are constricted. In a dim light, they are dilated. If the pupils were dilated in a bright light that damages the retina. In dim light, if the pupils are constricted, insufficient light enters the eye, which does not activate the photosensitive pigments in the rods and cones.

The iris consists of one layer of circular and another layer of radiating muscle. Contraction of circular muscle fibres constricts the pupil, and contraction of the radiating muscle fibres dilates the pupil. The pupil is under the autonomic nervous control. Sympathetic stimulation dilates the pupils and parasympathetic stimulation causes their constriction.

Binocular vision

Stereoscopic or Binocular vision has certain advantages. Each eye sees a scene at different angles. There is an overlap in the middle but the left eye see more on the left than can be seen by the right eye and vice versa. So, the images from the two eyes are fused in the cerebrum to form, only one image is perceived. Binocular vision provides more accuracy than monocular vision. Binocular vision has more appreciation of the image and its distance, depth, height and width.

Refraction of the light rays

When light rays pass from a medium of one density to a different density, they are refracted or bent. So, the same principle is used in the eye to focus light rays on the retina. The light rays passes through the cornea, aqueous humour, lens and vitreous body (refractive media). They are all more dense than air and with the exception of the lens, they have a constant refractory power. Lens is a biconvex, elastic transparent body suspended behind the iris. It is the only structure that can change its refractory power. All light rays entering the eye, need to be refracted (bent) to focus them on the retina,. Light from the distant objects, needs least refraction, and the objects near the eye needs more refraction. To increase refractive power, the ciliary muscle contracts. The anterior surface of the lens bulges forward, increasing its convexity. When the ciliary muscle relaxes it slips backwards, then the lens becomes thinner.

Light and colours of the visual spectrum

The light waves travel at a speed of 300,000 kilometers per second. Light rays are reflected into the eyes by objects within the field of vision. White light is a combination of all colours of the visual spectrum i.e., red, orange, yellow, blue, green, indigo and violet. Red light has the longest wave length and violet has the shortest. This range of colour is the spectrum of visible light.

Physiology of vision

The eye may be compared to a camera. The eyelids are the shutters. Cornea is an entrance window for light. The iris acts as a diaphragm which regulate the size of the pupil and in this way regulate the amount of light entering. The lens focuses the image. The choroid forms darkness in the interior of the eyeball. The retina which is sensitive to light receives the image.

A source of light is required to see an object. Darkness exists if there is no source of light and no object can be seen.

Three processes are involved in the formation of images on the retina.

1. Refraction of light rays by the cornea and lens.
2. Accommodation of the lens and

3. Constriction of the pupil.

When objects are seen, light rays from the objects pass through the cornea, acqueous humour, lens and vitreous humour and the image focussed on the retina is inverted (upside down). The nerve endings are stinulated in the retina. The light is coverted into action potentials that are conveyed to the brain through the visual pathway.

Visual pathway

The nerve impulses are conveyed from the rods and cones of the retina to the bipolar cells and then to the ganglion cells whose axons form the optic nerve. The following structures constitute the visual pathway, the optic nerve, optic chiasma, optic tract, lateral geniculate body of the thalamus and the primary visual cortex in the occipital lobe.

Though the images focussed on the retina are inverted the primary visual cortex through experience reverses them so that one sees things the right way up.

Questions

1. Describe the tongue as a sensory organ.
2. Name the three types of taste buds.
3. Draw a neat diagram of the ear and label the parts.
4. Write the mechanism of hearing.
5. Draw a neat diagram of the eye-ball.
6. Name the accessory organs of the eye.
7. Name the muscles of the eye.
8. Write short notes on the following:

8. Write short notes on the following:

a) Cebum

b) Cerumen

c) Auditory Ossicles

d) Refraction of the light rays

e) Physiology of vision

f) Conjunctiva

g) Retina

UNIT 13

The Reproductive Systems

The reproductive systems are essential for the continuation of human generation. In human beings, the off spring or infant is delivered by females. The process is one of sexual reproduction in which the male and female organs differ anatomically and physiologically. Both males and females produce specialised reproductive germ cells called gametes. In the male, they are spermatozoa and in the female, ova. They contain genetic material or chromosomes. Gametes contain only 23 chromosomes. When the two gametes fuse, then it is called zygote which contains 23 pairs of chromosomes. The zygote embeds itself in the wall of the uterus and develops during 40 weeks of gestation period before birth. So the function of female reproductive system is to produce ova, and provide nutrition during development, then delivery of infant. After the delivery of infant, the female feeds the child with breast milk until the child can take the semisolid foods. The function of male reproductive system is to form the spermatozoa and transmit them to the female reproductive system.

FEMALE REPRODUCTIVE SYSTEM

This system consists of external and internal organs. External organs are external genitalia and mammary gland. The external genitalia are known as the vulva (Pudendum) which consists of,

Mons pubis	vestibule
Labia majora	hymen
Labia minora	greater vestibular glands.
Clitoris	

Mons Pubis

It is a slight elevation caused by a pad of fatty tissue over the symphysis pubis. It is covered by skin and course pubic hair.

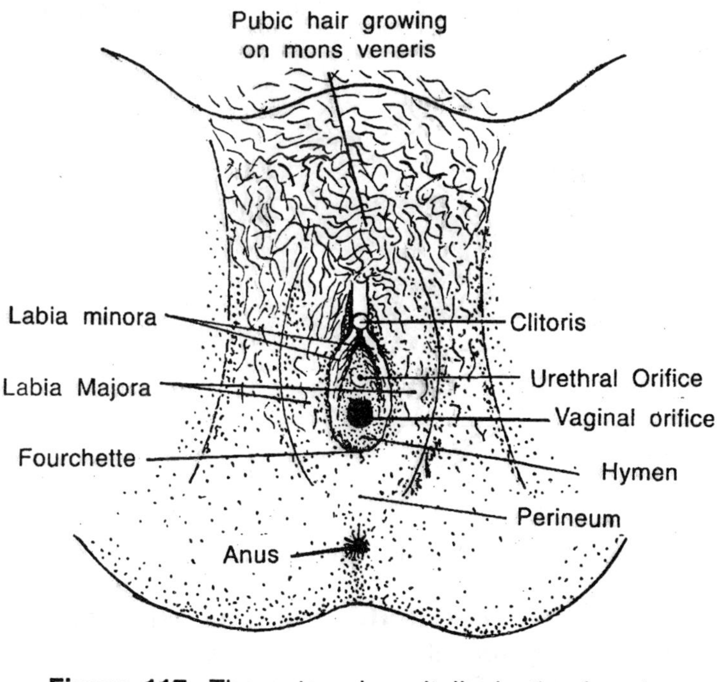

Figure 117. The external genitalia in the female.

Labia majora: It has two large folds which form the boundary of the vulva. It is composed of skin, fibrous tissue and fat. Its medial surfaces contain large number of sebaceous and sweat glands. The lateral surfaces of the labia majora are covered by coarse hair.

Labia minora: These are two smaller folds of skin between the labia majora. They contain numerous sebaceous glands and few sweat glands. The labia minora is devoid of pubic hair and fat. They fuse to form a fold posteriorly called fourchette.

Vestibule: The cleft between the labia minora is the vestibule. The vagina, urethra and ducts of the greater vestibular glands open into the vestibule.

Clitoris: It corresponds to the penis in the male and contains erectile tissue. The exposed portion of the clitoris is the glans. It plays a role in sexual exitement of the female. It is located in the anterior margin of the vestibule.

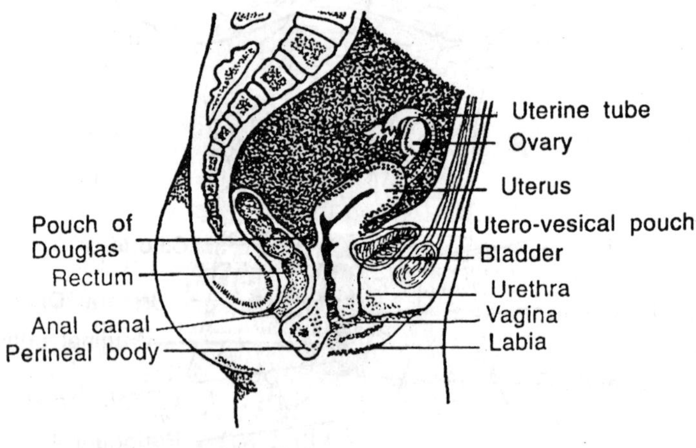

Figure 118. The female reproducing organs in pelvis

Greater vestibular glands (Bartholin's glands): They are situated one on each side near the vaginal opening. They are about the size of a small pea and have ducts opening into the vestibule immediately lateral to the attachment of the hymen. They secrete mucus that keeps the vulva moist.

Blood Supply: The internal and external pudental arteries supply arterial blood.

The venous blood is drained by the veins which form large plexus into internal iliac veins.

Lymph is drained through the superficial inguinal nodes.

Perineum: It is the area extending from the pubic symphysis to the anal canal. It is roughly triangular in shape. It consists of connective tissue, muscle and fat.

Breasts or mammary glands: These are situated on the front side of chest wall. They are the accessory glands of the female reproductive system. The breasts exist in the male but they are in a rudimentary form. The female breasts are quite small until puberty. Thereafter they grow and develop to mature adult size under the influence of oestrogen and progesterone. The alveoli are stimulated by prolactin hormone from the anterior pituitary to produce milk soon after the birth of the infant. Oxytocin from the posterior pituitary gland contracts the alveoli and the ducts propel milk towards nipple.

External surface of the breast: In the centre of the breast there is a projection called Nipple. On the surface of the nipple, there are 15 to 20 small openings of lactiferous ducts. The nipple is surrounded by areola which is a pigmented area of skin. The areola contains numerous sebaceous glands. They produce oily secretion, which lubricates the nipple in pregnancy. The nipples contain smooth muscle. They are very sensitive to tactile stimulation. The nipples become erect when the smooth muscle contracts in response to stimuli such as touch, cold and sexual arousal.

Structure: The mammary glands consist of glandular, fibrous and fatty tissue. Each breast consists of 15 to 20 lobes of glandular tissue. Each lobe is made up of a number of lobules. The lobules consist of numerous alveoli. All the secretion is collected by small ducts which unite to form large lactiferous ducts and they open on the surface at the nipple. The fibrous tissue is situated between among lobes and skin, and also there is deep fascia to the skin. The fat is situated around lobes and underneath the skin. Both fibrous and fatty tissue give shape to the breast. In old age both connective tissue is reduced and the breast becomes pendulous.

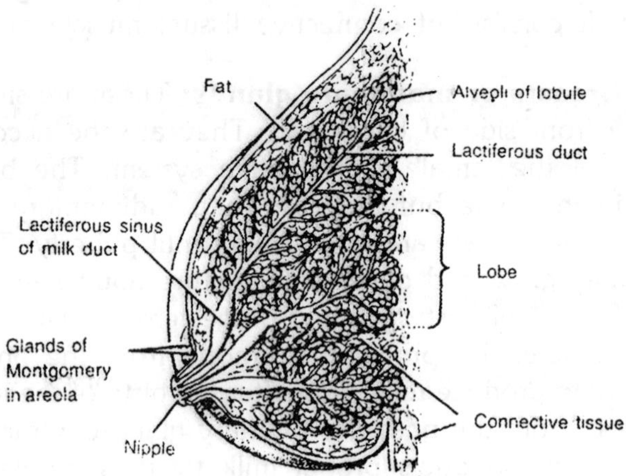

Figure 119. The Breast.

Function: During later months of pregnancy and after child birth the breasts become active to produce milk. The production and release of milk by the mammary glands is called lactation. Prolactin, a hormone of anterior pituitary gland stimulates lactation of milk.

Oxytocin, a hormone secreted by anterior pituitary causes ejection of milk by myometrial contractions. Nervous reflex initiated by suckling or psychological anticipation of suckling releases oxytocin from neurohypophysis. This explains why emotional stress may disturb lactation.

Blood supply: By the thoracic branches of axillary arteries and from the internal mammary artery and intercostal arteries.

Venous drainage: An anastomatic venous circle is situated at the base of the nipple and drains into axillary and internal mammary veins.

Lymphatic drainage: The lymph of the breast is drained into axillary lymph vessels and nodes.

Nerve Supply: The branches of 4th, 5th and 6th intercostal nerves supply the breasts. Plenty of sensory nerve endings are situated in the nipple and areola. When baby sucks the nipple, the touch receptors impulse pass through these nerves to the hypothalamus and flow of the oxytocin hormone enters the blood, then through this, it acts on the glandular tissue to propel the milk towards the nipple.

INTERNAL ORGANS

The internal organs of the female reproductive system lie in the pelvic cavity and consist of the vagina, uterus, two uterine tubes and two ovaries.

Vagina

It is a fibro muscular tube lined with mucous membrane and consists of stratified epithelium. It opens externally at the vestibule of vulva, and another end opens internally with the uterus. It is situated between the urinary bladder in front and behind this is the rectum and anus. It runs obliquely upwards and backwards where it attaches to the uterus. In adult the anterior wall is about 7.5 cms and posterior wall is about 9 cms. The difference is due to the opening of the cervix of uterus through the anterior wall.

Structure: The vagina has an outer areolar tissue, a middle layer of smooth muscle and an inner lining of stratified squamous epithelium. The lining epithelium is thrown into flods called rugae. There is absence of secretory glands but the inner surface is kept moist by cervical secretions. The pH of vagina is between 3.5 and 4.5. The acidity inhibits the growth of most microbes.

Blood supply: An arterial plexus around the vagina formed by the branches of uterine artery and vaginal arteries.

Venous drainage is to the internal iliac veins.

Nerve supply: By autonomic nerve plexus.

This acid pH is due to glycogen which is present in large amounts in the mucosa. Lactobacillus acidophilus acts upon the glycogen and produce lactic acid. The mucosa also contains dentritic cells (antigen presenting cells). It is believed that these cells take part in the transmission of HIV virus (that causes AIDS) to a female during intercouse with an infected male.

The muscular layer contains many elastic fibres so that it can stretch considerably to receive the penis during sexual intercourse. It stretches greatly during child birth.

The vagina allows menstrual flow from puberty till menopause.

Hymen: It is a thin layer of mucous membrane which partially covers the opening of the vagina. It is perforated at monarche. Sometimes it completely covers the vaginal orifice. This condition is called imperforate hymen which may be opened surgically to allow menstrual flow. The hymen may be torn as a result of certain activities or sternous exercise. The condition of the hymen is therefore not a reliable indicator of virginity.

Vaginal examination

The vagina is examined by introducing two fingers, the index and the middle finger which can palpate, not only the vagina itself, but also the cervix, the uterus and the ovaries. The vagina and cervix can also be inspected by using a speculum.

Uterus

It is hollow, muscular, pear shaped organ. It is flattened antero-posteriorly. It is situated in the pelvic cavity in the median plan between urinary bladder in front and rectum behind. It expands upto xiphoid process during pregnancy.

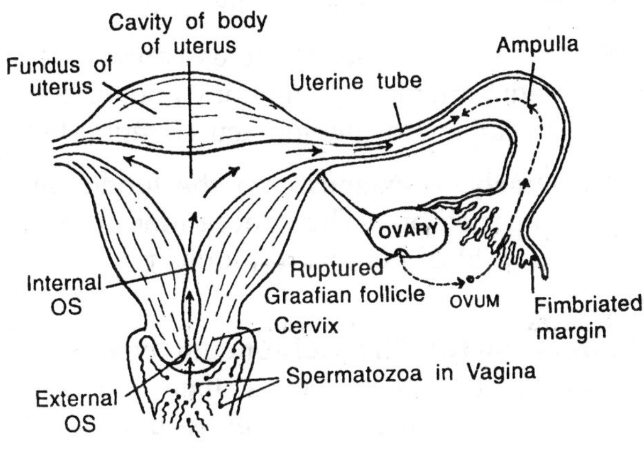

Figure 120. Diagram of a section of the Uterus

Position: It is anteverted, means bends forward and anteflexion means it is bent forward almost at right angles to the vagina with its anterior surface resting on the urinary bladder. Anteflexion is slightly reduced when the bladder is filled, with urine.

The length of uterus is about 7.5 cms, width 5 cms and thickness about 2.5 cms. Its parts are the fundus, body and cervix. The fundus is the dome shaped part above the openings of the uterine tubes. The body is the main part, it is below the openings of the uterine tubes, extends upto the level of internal os. It is narrower below, and continuous with the cervix. The cervix is about 1 cm in length and the thickest part opens into the vagina in the anterior wall. It acts as sphincter. The cervical canal is very small in diameter. It is constricted at each end. It communicates with the uterus as internal os and opens below with vagina as external os.

Between the internal os and external os in the cervical canal is the histological os. The part of the cervix between histological os and the internal os is known as the lower segment of the uterus because in pregnancy it is incorporated into the uterine body.

Structure: The wall of uterus consists of 3 layers of tissue perimetrium, myometrium and endometrium. Perimetrium consists of peritoneum covering the uterus.

Anteriorly, it extends over the fundus and body where it is reflected on to the upper surface of the urinary bladder. This fold of peritoneum forms the utero- vesical pouch.

Posteriorly: The peritoneum covers over the fundus, the body and the cervix, then it is reflected on to the rectum forming recto-uterine pouch (Pouch of Douglas).

Laterally: The peritoneum covers the fundus. The folds on lateral side continue as folds of broad ligament enclosing uterine tubes and attached to the sides of pelvis.

Myometrium: It is the thickest smooth muscular layer of the uterus. It consists of three layers of smooth muscle fibres, the inner layer consists of longitudinal fibres. the middle layer is circular and the outer layer is oblique. The myometrium is thickest in the fundus and thinnest in the cervix.

The wall of the uterus also contains areolar tissue, blood vessels and nerves.

The hormone oxytocin from the posterior pituitary gland causes coordinated contractions of the muscles during childbirth and helps expel the foetus from the body of uterus.

Endometrium: It is the inner layer composed of columnar epithelium. It contains simple tubular glands and this layer gives nutrition to growing foetus. It consists of two layers. 1) The stratum functionalis (functional layer) which is closer to uterine cavity, is shed during menstruation. 2) The stratum basalis (basal layer) is permanent. From this layer new stratum functionalis is developed after each menstruation.

Blood supply: A pair of uterine arteries situated at the sides of the broad ligament to supply the uterus and the uterine tubes. These arteries anastomose with vaginal arteries to supply the vagina.

Venous drainage is by uterine veins to internal iliac veins. The uterus has a rich blood supply This is essential to support regrowth of a new stratum functionalis after menstruation, implantation of a fertilized ovum and development of the placenta.

Lymphatic drainage: Wide distribution of lymphatic vessels are present in the terus. Lymph from the fundus drain with the ovarian vessels into the aortic nodes. Lymph from the lower part of the body and of the cervix drain into the inguinal, external and interval iliac nodes.

Nerve supply is by sympathetic and parasympathetic fibres from the autonomatic nerve plexus.

Supports of the uterus: The uterus enlarges upto xiphoid process during pregnancy and to expel the foetus, it needs strong support. The support is given by the pelvic muscles and ligaments.

1. Two broad ligaments are formed by a double layer of peritoneum on lateral side of the uterus and enclosing uterine tubes. Laterally, the ligaments are attached to the sides of the pelvic wall.
2. The round ligaments: They are composed of fibrous tissue between the two layers of the broad ligament, one on each side of the uterus. They pass to the sides of the pelvis through the inguial canal and fuses with the labia majora.
3. Two utero sacral ligaments originate from the posterior walls of the cervix and vagina and extend backwards, one on each side of the rectum and attached to the sacrum.
4. Two transverse cervical ligaments (cardinal ligaments) extends from the sides of the cervix and vagina to the side walls of the pelvis.
5. The pubocervical fascia extends forward from the transverse cervical ligaments on each side of the bladder and is attached to the posterior surface of the pubic bones.

Functions: After puberty the uterus bleeds regularly once in 28 days. This cycle is called Menstrual cycle. This cycle prepares the endometrium to receive, nourish and protect the fertilized ovum for 40 weeks of gestation period. The cycle usually occurs at regular intervals of 28 days. If the ovum is not fertilised, a new cycle begins with menstruation. At the end of gestation period labour begins and ends when the baby is born and the placenta is expelled. During labour, the muscular layer of the fundus and body of the uterus goes on contracting intermittently and the cervix relaxes and dilates. As labour progresses, the uterine contractions become stronger and more frequent until the foetus is expelled out.

Uterine tubes (Fallopian tubes): They are also called oviducts.

The uterine tubes are about 10 cms long and extend from the sides of the uterus between the body and the fundus. They lie in the upper free border of the broad ligament. Other lateral ends open into peritoneal cavity. Close to the ovaries, the end of each tube is a funnel shaped structure called infundibulum which has finger like processes called fimbriae. The longest fimbriae is in contact with ovary. The ampulla of the uterine tube makes up about two thirds of its length. The isthmus of the uterine tube is joined to the uterus.

Structure: The outer peritoneal layer (broad ligament), middle layer is composed of the smooth muscle layer and the inner layer is composed of ciliated columnar epithelium and secretory cells which have microcilli and may provide nutrition for the ovum.

Function: The movements of the fimbrie produce local currents after ovulation and sweep the secondary oocyte into the uterine tube. The spermatozoa usually fertilizes a secondary oocyte in the ampulla of the uterine tube near the ovary. Few hours after fertilization, the sperm and the haploid ovum unite and become a diploid fertilized ovum which is now called zygote. The zygote undergoes several cell divisions in the uterine tube and reaches the uterus about six days after ovulation. Now it is called a blastocyst which attaches itself to the uterine wall.

Ovaries: The ovaries are the female gonads and are situated in a shallow fossa on the lateral wall of pelvic cavity one on eachside of the uterus. Each ovary measuress abouut 3 cms in length, 2 cms wide and 1 cm thickness. The blood vessels and nerves enter and leave the ovary at hilus. Each ovary is attached to the broad ligament of the uterus by a short fold of peritoneum called mesovarium.

Structure: On cut section of the ovary, it has an outer portion is cortex and inner portion is medulla. The cortex surrounds the medulla. The cortex has a framework of connective tissue or stroma covered by Germinal epithelium. It contains ovarian (GRAAFIAN) follicles. During each menstrual cycle, about 5-6 follicles go for maturation. Among these follicles, only one follicle matures to form the Graafian follicle and others go for atrophy called atreatic follicle. The matured follicle is expelled out on the surface as ovum surrounded by a few granulosa cells - the corona radiata cells. It is liberated into the peritoneal cavity during mid menstrual cycle. The liberated ovum enters into the uterine tube. The maturation of follicle is stimulated by follicle stimulating hormone (F.S.H.) from the anterior pituitary. While maturing the follicle, the theca cells become interstitial cells and produce the hormone oestrogen. After ovulation, the granulosa and thecal cells become corpus luteum, which produces the hormone progesterone under the influence of the luteinizing hormone (LH), from the anterior pituitary. If the ovum is fertilized and implanted in the uterus, the growing embryo produces the human chorionic gonodotrophin which stimulates the corpus luteum to continue to produce progesterone for the first 3 months of pregnancy. If the ovum is not fertilized, then the corpus luteum goes atrophy called corpus.

Six types of oestrogens are present in the plasma of human females. Three of them are present in high quantities, they are beta (b) oestradiol, oestrone and oestriol. Beta (b) oestrodiol is the principal oestogen present in the nonpregnant woman. Ovaries synthesize this hormone from cholesterol.

Functions of oestrogens

1. They promote development and maintenance of female reproductive organs. They influence female sexual behaviour.

2. They play an important part in the control of fluid and electrolyte balance.

3. They increase protein anabolism.

4. They lower blood cholesterol level.

The corpus luteum secretes the hormone progesterone. It also produces two other hormones in small quanitty. They are (1) relaxin and 2) inhibin. Inhibin is also secreted by granulosa cells of growing follicles.

Albicans: Sometime abnormally, two ova are released and multiple pregnancy occurs.

Medulla of ovary contains loose connective tissue containing blood vessels, lymphatics and nerves. They enter and leave the hilum.

Blood supply: Arterial blood supply is by ovarian arteries, a branch of abdominal aorta.

Venous drainage: The right ovarian vein drains blood into interior vena cava, the left ovarian vein drains blood into left renal vein.

Lymph drainage: Lymph drains into para aortic and pre arotic lymph nodes.

Nerve supply: The ovaries are supplied by parasympathetic nerves from the sacral outflow and sympathetic nerves from the lumbar outflow.

The Perineum

It is an area medial to thighs and buttocks of both males and females that ocntains external genitalia and anus. It may be divided into an anterior urogenital triangle that contains the external genitalia and a posterior anal triangle that contains the anus.

FEMALE REPRODUCTIVE HORMONES AND TARGET TISSUES

Hypothalamus

↓

luteinizing hormone releasing hormone (LHRH)

↓

Anterior pituitary

↙ ↘

Follicle stimulating hormone	Luteinizing hormone
↓	↓
Ovarian follicle	Corpus luteum
↓	↓
Oestrogen	Progesterone.

Puberty in the female (Monarche)

Puberty in females is marked by the first episode of menstrual bleeding. The age of puberty varies between 10-14 years. During puberty, the internal reproductive organs reach maturity. The ovaries are stimulated by gonadotrophins from the anterior pituitary, follicle stimuulating hormone and the luteinizing hormone. During this time, a number of physical and psychological changes take place.

1. The uterus, the uterine tubes and the ovaries reach maturity.
2. The menstrual cycle and ovulation begin.
3. The breasts develop and enlarge.
4. Pubic and axillary hair begins to grow.
5. The pelvis increases in all diameter.
6. Amount of fat deposition increases in subcutaneous tissue to give female shape.

MENSTRUAL CYCLE

This is a series of events, occurring regularly in females every 26 to 30 days throughout the reproductive age of women i.e., may be 40 years. The cycle consists of a series of changes in the ovaries and uterine wall which are stimulated by changes in the blood concentration of hormones. The hypothalamus secretes luteinizing hormone releasing hormone (LH-RH) to stimulate the anterior pituitary to secrete LH.

1. Follicle - stimulating hormone (FSH) promotes the maturation of ovarian follicles and the secretion of oestrogen, leading to ovulation.

2. Luteinizing hormone (LH) stimulates the development of corpus luteum and the secretion of progesterone. The hypothalamus responds to changes in the blood levels of oestrogen and progesterone. The average length of the menstrual cycle is about 28 days. The menstrual cycle begins with menstruation, lasts for 4 or 5 days. This is followed by the proliferative phase, which is about 10 days. Then follows the secretory phase which is about 14 days.

Menstruation

When the ovum is not fertilised, the high level of progesterone in the blood inhibits the activity of the pituitary gland and production of luteinizing hormone is reduced. The with drawal of this hormone causes degeneration of the corpus luteum and thus, progesterone is decreased. After ovulation, the lining of the uterus degenerates and breaks down and menstruation begins, the menstrual flow starts. It consists of the secretions of glands, endometrial cells, blood and unfertilised ovum. Then next cycle begins by FSH which stimulates the ovarian follicles and proliferative phase begins in the walls of uterus.

Proliferative phase

Oestrogen stimulates the proliferation of the endometrium in preparation for reception of a fertilized ovum. The endometrium becomes thicker to about 4-6 mm by rapid cell multiplication. Nutritional materials are secreted by tubular glands and there is rich blood supply during proliferation. Ovulation occurs on about day 14 of the 28 day menstrual cycle. It varies from individual to individual and can vary within an individual from one menstrual cycle to next. Ovulation means the rupture of mature follicle and release of the secondary oocyte into the pelvic cavity. This phase ends when ovulation occurs and oestrogen production stops.

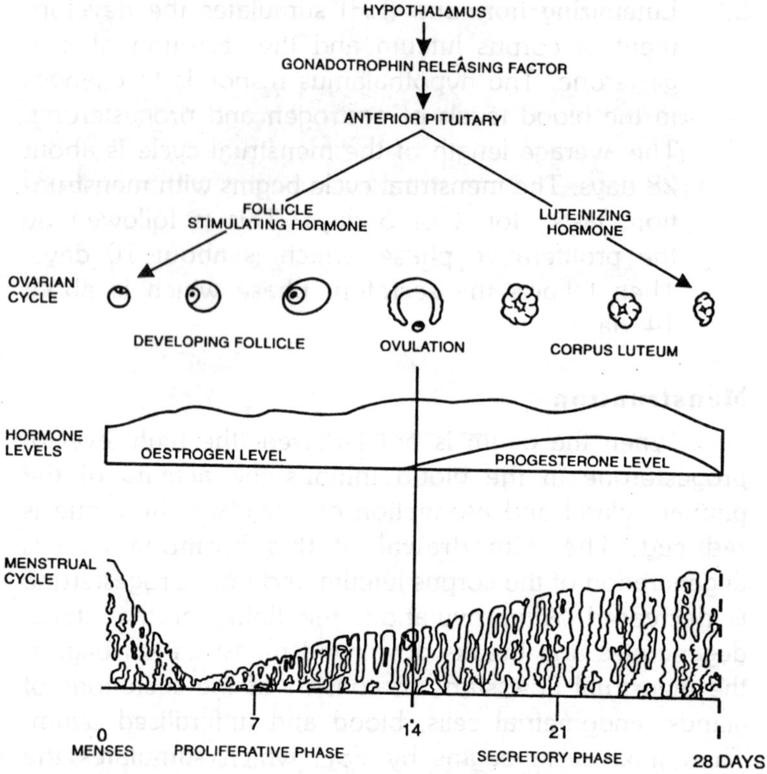

Figure 121. Diagram showing the relationship of ovarian and menstrual cycles

Secretory phase

After ovulation, the follicle cells are stimulated by LH to develop the corpus luteum which produces progesterone. Under the influence of progesterone, the endometrium becomes oedematous and secretory glands secrete more glycogen in the uterine tubes. The glands secrete more watery mucus to assist the passage of ovum and spermatozoa. If the ovum is not fertilised, mestruation occurs and a new cycle begins.

If the ovum (now it is secondary oocyte) is fertilised and implanted, then there will be no menstrual flow. The fertilized ovum is called zygote which travels through uterine tube. During 4.1/2 to 5 days travel the zygote undergoes several cell divisions and it is then called a blastocyst which enters the uterus and implanted in the wall of the uterus 6 days after the fertilization. The placenta formation starts, and produces hormone i.e., human chorionic gonadotrophin (HCG). This hormone keeps development of corpus luteum and produces progesterone for the first 3 months of pregnancy, inhibiting the maturation of ovarian follicles. During this time the placenta produces oestrogen, progesterone and gonadotrophins.

Placenta provides indirect connection to mother and foetus. Through the placenta the foetus obtains nutritional materials, oxygen and antibodies and expels waste products and carbon dioxide.

MENOPAUSE

This stage occurs usually between the ages 40-45 years and ends uo child bearing period. It is due to changes in the sex hormones. The ovaries gradually become less responsive to the FSH and LH. The ovulation and the menstrual cycle becomes irregular, eventually ceasing. Complete cessation of menstrual cycles is called female climacteric. The ovaries undergo atrophy, and certain changes occur in the women.

1. The sex organs atrophy
2. The breasts become pendulous
3. Axillary and pubic hair become sparse.
4. Short term unpredictable vasodilation with flushing, sweating and plapilations, disturbance of normal sleep.
5. Sometimes uncharacteristic behaviour.

MALE REPRODUCTIVE SYSTEM

The male reproductive system consists of the following organs

2	testes	Both are in the scrotum
2	epididymes	
2	ductus-deferens (vas deferens)	
2	spermatic cords	
2	seminal vesicles	
2	ejaculatory ducts	
1	prostate gland	
1	penis.	

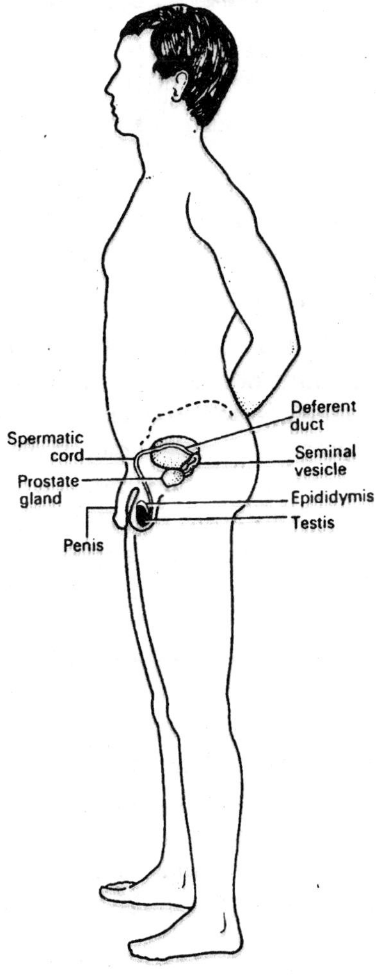

Figure 122. The Male reproductive organs.

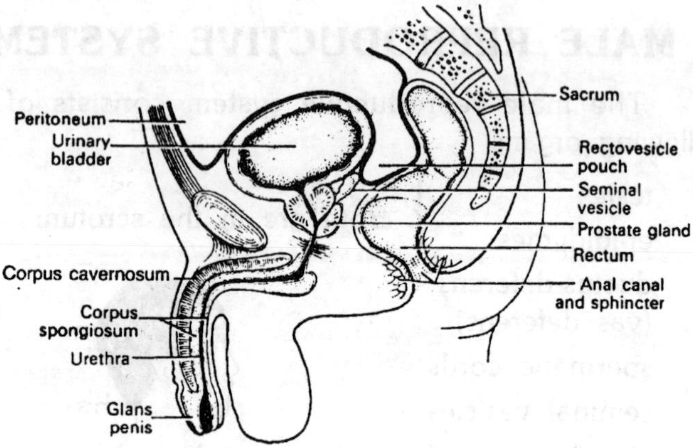

Figure 123. The Male reproductive organs and their associated structures.

Scrotum

It is a pouch in the perineum. The skin is pigmented, contains fibrous and connective tissue and smooth muscle called dartos muscle. The scrotum also contains the cremaster muscle which is an extension of internal oblique muscles. The two muscles help in the regulation of the temperature of the testes lesser than normal body core temperature. As the scrotum is outside the body cavities, it provides an environment about 3° C below body temperature which is required for normal sperm cell development. It is divided into two internal compartments by a connective tissue septum. A ridge called raphe, indicating the division of compartments can be seen on the surface. This raphe is continuous forwards along the under surface of the penis and backward to the penis. Each compartment contains one testis, one epididymis and the testicular end of a spermatic cord. It lies below the symphysis pubis and behind the penis.

Testes

The testes are the reproductive glands (gonads) of the males, situated in the scrotum. They are equivalent of the ovaries in the female. They are about 4.5 cms long, 2.5 cms wide and 3 cms thick, and are covered by three layers of tissue. The tunica vaginalis, a serous membrane, has two layers i.e. outer parietal layer lines the inner surface of the scrotum, and another layer lines the testis and epididymis. In between these two layers, there is a potential space containing a film of fluid. The tunica albuginea is a fibrous covering surrounding the testes situated under the tunica vaginalis. The tunica albuginea extends inward and forms septa and divides each testis into lobules. The tunica vasculosa consists of a net work of capillaries supported by delicate connective tissue.

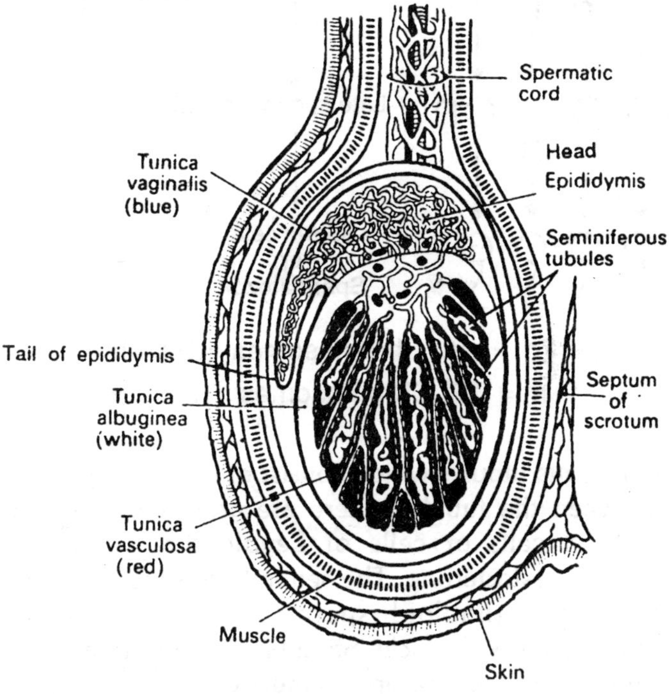

Figure 124. Stucture of Testis and its covering.

Structure

In each testis there are 250 to 300 lobules. Within each lobule, there are 1 to 3 convoluted loops of

Spermatogenesis

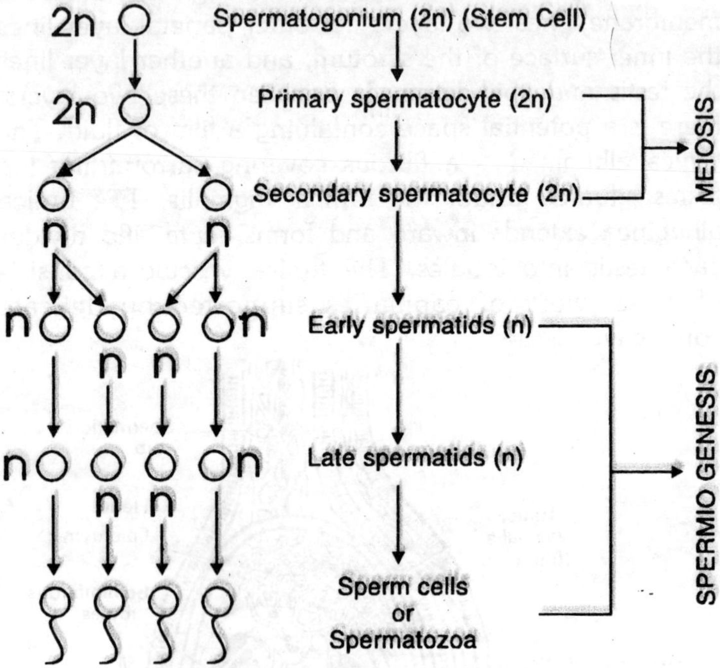

2n = 46 Chromosomes (Deploid)

n = 23 Chromosomes (Haploid)

seminiferous tubules which consist of spermatogenic cells. In between the tubules, there are groups of cells called interstitial cells or cells of Leydig that produce the hormone - testosterone. The seminiferous tubules produce spermatozoa (haploid sperm) by a process called spermatogenesis. Follicle Stimulating Hormone (F.S.H.) together with testosterone stimulates sperm production by the seminiferous tubules. At the time of puberty, the interstitial cells increase in size and number. The seminiferous tubules enlarge and spermatogenesis begins.

The seminiferous tubules contain germ cells and sertoli cells (subtentacular cells). The sertoli-cells extend from the basement membrane to the lumen of the tubule. These cells support, protect and nourish the sperm cells. They mediate the effects of testosterone and follicle-stimulating hormone (F.S.H.). They also control the movements of spermatogenic cells and release the sperm into the lumen, produce fluid for sperm transport and secrete the hormone inhibin.

Inhibin helps to regulate production of sperm by inhibiting secretion of follicle stimulating hormone (F.S.H.) by the anteriory pituitary gland.

In humans, spermatogenesis takes about 65-70 days.

After development, the sperms enter the lumen of the seminifeous tubules and flow towards ducts of the testes.

Sperm

About 300 million sperms mature in 24 hours. After ejaculation they retain their fertilizing capacity in the female reproductive tract for 48 hours only, although most of them degenerate by 24 hours. A sperm cell has the ability in reaching and penetrating a secondary oocyte.

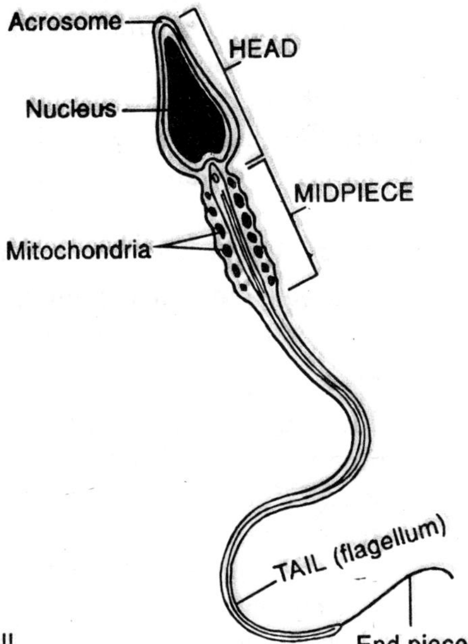

Figure 125. Sperm cell

Structure

Each sperm cell is composed of a head, a midpiece and a tail. The head contains the nucleus. There is a vesicle called acrosome just anterior to the nucleus. It contains enzymes (hyaluronidase and proteinases) that facilitate the penetration of a sperm cell into secondary oocyte. The midpiece contains numerous mitochondria. They carry on metabolic activities that provide Adenosine Triphosphate (ATP) for locomotion. The tail, a typical flagellum propels the sperm cell along its way. The sperm contains very little cytoplasm.

The endocrine function of the testis

At the onset of puberty the secretion of gonadotrophic hormones are increased by the anterior lobe of pituitary gland. They are luteinizing hormone (LH) and follicle stimulating hormone (FSH). Their release is controlled by gonadotrophin releasing hormone (GNRH) secreted by the hypothalamus. LH stimulates the interstitial cells to secrete testosterone, the male sex hormone. This hormone is synthesized from cholesterol in the testes. In the prostate gland and seminal vesicles testosterone is converted into dihydrotestosterone (DHT) which is more potent than testosterone.

Effects of male sex hormones:

1. In foetal life, they stimulate the male pattern of development of reproductive system.
2. At puberty testosterone and DHT stimulate further development and enlargement of the male sex organs. They also produce masculine secondary sexual characteristics such as muscular and skeletal growth, growth of hair on the face, chest axilla and the male distribution of pubic hair, thickening of skin, enlargement of the larynx and "breaking of the voice".

3. Sexual functions: They maintain male sexual behavior and support spermatogenesis and bring about sex drive (libido).
4. They have anabolic action i.e. they stimulate protein synthesis.

Ducts of the testis

From each lobule the seminiferous tubules unite to form a straight tubule. The straight tubules are joined to a network of ducts in the testis called the rete testis, which lead toward the epididymis. The sperms and fluid pass from seminiferous tubules to the epididymis through the structures described above.

The epididymis

It consists of a tightly coiled structure ductus epididymis is about 20 feet long, which is site of sperm maturation and acts as a storage for the sperms for a month or more. The epididymis consists of a head, body and and a tail. The tail joins the vas deferens or seminal duct. It is about 45 cms. (18 inches) long. It ascends and enters the pelvic cavity through the inguinal canal. The vas deferens keeps the sperms upto several months. It joins with the duct of seminal vesicles to form ejaculatory duct.

The spermatic cord

The vas deferens, the testicular artery, autonomic nerves, veins that drain the testes and carry testosterone into circulation, lymphatic vessels and the cremaster muscle constitute the spermatic cord.

There are two spermatic cords and ilioinguinal nerve pass through the inguinal canal. (In female, the round ligament of the uterus and ilioinguinal nerve pass through inguinal canal).

The testicular artery branches from the abdominal aorta. The pampiniform plexus of veins are continuous as testicular veins. The right testicular vein drains into inferior vena cava. The left testicular vein drains into left renal vein. The lymphatic drainage is to the para aortic lymph nodes in the abdominal cavity.

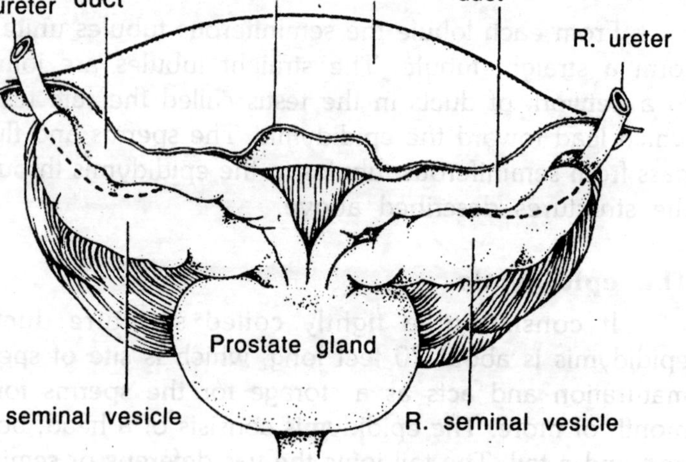

Figure 126. Structures associated with the prostate gland. Posterior view

Ductus deferens

The ductus deferens is the continuation of epididymis. It passes upwards from the testis, through the inguinal canal and ascends medially towards the posterior wall of the urinary bladder, where it is joined by the duct from the seminal vesicle which together form the ejaculatory duct.

Branches from the 10th and 11th thoracic nerves provide the nerve supply.

Seminal vesicles

A pair of seminal vesicles are situated on the

posterior surface of the urinary bladder. They are fibroglandular organs which secrete seminal fluid, which is alkaline in reaction. The duct of each seminal vesicle joins with vas deferens to form the ejaculatory duct.

Ejaculatory ducts: These are two ducts about 2 cms in length and pass through the prostate gland. These ducts open into the prostatic urethra on either side of prostatic utricle. They transmit seminal fluid and spermatozoa to the urethra.

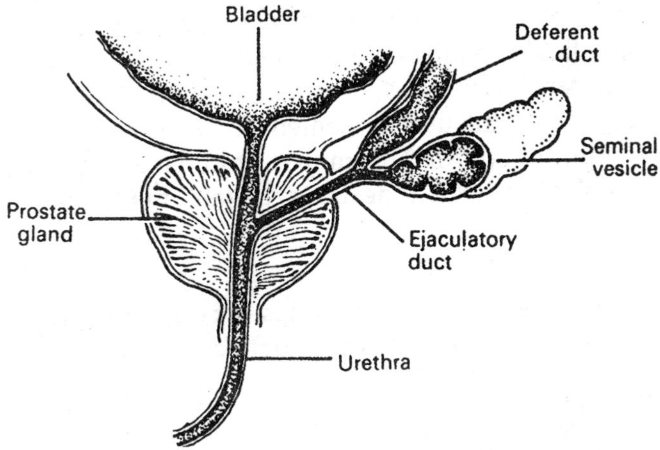

Figure 127. Section of the Prostate gland

Prostate gland: It is a fibro musculo glandular organ situated at the posteroinferior part of the urinary bladder surrounding the 1st part of the urethra. It consists of an outer fibrous layer. Inside, it consists of smooth muscle and glandular substance composed of columnar epithelial cells. It secretes prostatic fluid that enters into the prostatic part of urethra through numerous ducts.

The prostatic fluid is a milky, slightly acidic fluid (pH 6.5) that contains citrate (ionized citric acid), acid phosphatase and several proteolytic enzymes. These secretions make up about 25% of the volume of semen and contribute to sperm motility and viability.

Bulbo urethral glands (Cowper's glands): They are paired glands. Each is about a size of a pea. They lie on either side of the membranous urethra within the urogenital diaphragm below the prostate gland. Their ducts open into the spongy urethra. They secrete an alkaline fluid and mucus. The mucus lubricates the lining of the urethra and end of the penis. In this way sperm injury is decreased during ejaculation.

Semen

It is a milky white viscous fluid alkaline in reaction pH 7.2 to 7.7. It contains sperms and seminal fluid. Seminal fluid is a mixture of secretions of the seminiferous tubules, seminal vesicles, prostate gland and bullourethral glands. One millititre of semen contains about 100 to 300 million sperms. Semen contains an antibiotic seminaplasmin which destroys certain microbes.

Urethra

The male urethra provides a common pathways for urinary system and reproductive system, i.e. urine and semen. It is about 20-25 cms long. It has three parts. The prostatic part starts at urethral orifice at the neck of urinary bladder and pass through the prostate gland. The membranous part is the shortest and narrowest part that extends from the prostate gland, to the bulb of the penis, after passing through the perineal membrane. The spongy part lies within the corpus spongiosum of the penis and terminates at the external urethral orifice in the glans penis. There are two urethral sphincters, one at the neck of urinary bladder above the prostate gland, another at the membranous part of urethra, both the sphincters are made up of smooth muscles.

Voiding

It is otherwise called micturition. When the urinary bladder is filled with urine the person feels the sensation of voiding. This sensation is brought about by the action of sympathetic and parasympathetic nerves. Though the sensation of fullness of the bladder is felt the person can withold or control this sensation for some more time till he reaches a suitable place to void. When the act of voiding is ready, the sphincter muscles relax and allow the free flow of urine to the exterior. The sphincter muscles both external and internal relax and contract during the voiding of urine and remain intact after the act of urination.

Penis

It has a root and a body. The root lies in the perineum and the body surrounds the urethra. It is formed by three erectile tissues of cylindrical masses and smooth muscle. The erectile tissue is supported by fibrous tissue and covered by skin and it has a rich blood supply. The two lateral columns are corpora cavernosa and another column between them is the corpus spongiosum, containing the urethra. The corpus spongiosum at the tip expands into glands penis. Just above the glans the skin is folded upon itself and forms a movable double layer, the foreskin or prepuce. The arterial supply is by deep, dorsal and bulbar arteries of the penis which are the branches of the internal pudendal arteries. The venous drainage is to the internal pudendal veins. The penis is supplied by autonomic and somatic nerves. The parasympathetic stimulation leads to enlargement with blood and erection of the penis.

Circumcision is a surgical procedure in which the part or all of the prepuce is removed.

Function

Both the female and male reproductive organs are stimulated by the gonadotrophic hormones from the anterior lobe of the pituitary gland. In males the follicle stimulating hormone, stimulates the seminiferous tubules of the testes to produce male germ cells, the spermatozoa.

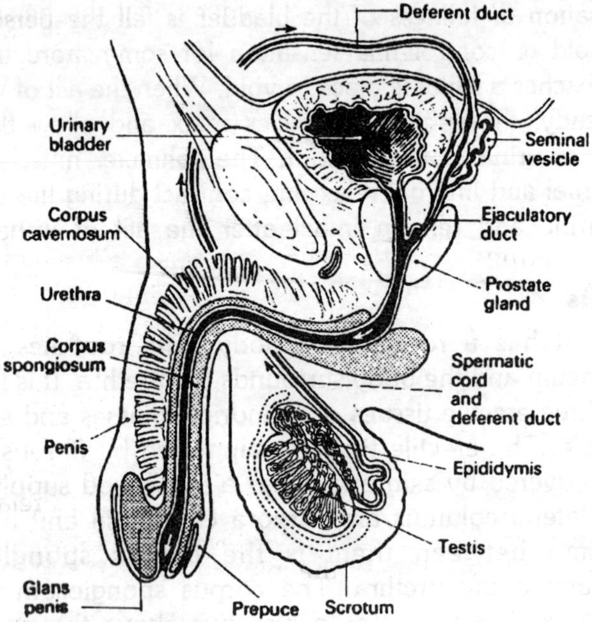

Figure 128. The Penis.

The sprematozoa in semen pass through the ejaculatory ducts and the urethra to the vagina during coitus. An ejaculation, usually, consists of 2 to 5 ml of semen containing 100 to 300 millions of spermatozoa per millilitre.

The successful spermatogenesis takes place at a temperature of about 3°C lower than normal body temperature.

Ejaculation is a reflex action in which the sympathetic nervous system is involved.

As a part of reflex, the smooth muscle sphincter at the base of the urinary bladder closes. Thus urine is not expelled during ejaculation and semen does not enter the urinary bladder. Before ejaculation, emission of a small volume of semen occurs. Emission may also occur during sleep (nocturnal emission).

The human sexual response

Both male and female experience the similar sequence of physiological and emotional changes before, during and after intercourse. This is termed the human sexual response. William Masters and Virginia Johnson described these changes as occuring in four stages.

1) Excitement
2) Plateau
3) Orgasm
4) Resolution

1. Excitement

During excitement various physical and psychological stimuli increase parasympathetic reflexes. This results in vasocongestion, engorgement with blood of genital organs. The first sign of sexual excitement is erection. The enlargement and stiffening of the penis. The bullourethral glands secrete mucus. Female contributes most of the secretion of lubricating fluid. In females erection of clitoris, engorgement of the labia and relaxation of vaginal smooth muscle occurs. The breasts may also swells and erection of the nipples of the breasts may occur.

2. Plateau stage

The changes that begin during excitement are sustained at an intense level in this stage. This stage may last for few seconds to many minutes. Many females and some males display a sex flush - a rashlike redness of the face and chest. In males the diameter of the penis increases and the testes swell up. In females the distal third of the vagina swells the tissue which narrows the opening. The vagina grips the penis more firmly.

3. Stage of orgasm

Generally this is the briefest stage. The penis ejaculates semen into the vagina of the female. Both sexes experience intense pleasurable sensations. As the orgasm begins, rhythmic sympathetic impulses cause peristaltic contraction of smooth muscle in the ducts of each testis, epididymis, the vas deferens as well as the walls of the seminal vesicles and prostate gland. These contractions propel semen and fluid into the urethra.

In females, if effective sexual stimulation continues, orgasm may occur. This is associated with 3-15 rhythmic contractions of vagina, uterus and surrounding skeletal muscles. Females may experience two or more orgasms in rapid succession.

In both sexes, orgasm is a total body response that may produce varied sensations milder to more intensive.

4. Stage of resolution

This stage begins with a sense of profound relaxation. The genital organs, the heart rate, blood pressure, breathing and muscle tone return to unaroused state.

Questions

1. Name the structures of female reproductive system.
2. Give a brief account of mammary glands.
3. Draw a neat diagram of the uterus and label the parts.
4. Write the position and structure of the uterus.
5. Explain the menstrual cycle.
6. Name the organ of male reproductive system.
7. What are the changes that could take place at puberty in a male?
8. Write short notes on the following:
   a) Uterine tubes
   b) Ovaries
   c) Menopause in a female
   d) Testes
   e) Prostate gland